THE
ITALIAN DIABETES
COOKBOOK

DELICIOUS AND HEALTHFUL DISHES
FROM VENICE TO SICILY AND BEYOND

AMY RIOLO

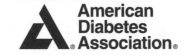

**American
Diabetes
Association.**

Director, Book Publishing, Abe Ogden; *Managing Editor,* Greg Guthrie; *Acquisitions Editor,* Victor Van Beuren; *Project Manager,* Boldface LLC; *Production Manager, Composition,* Melissa Sprott; *Cover Design,* pixiedesign, llc; *Photography,* Renée Comet Photography; *Printer,* Versa Press.

Printed in the United States of America
1 3 5 7 9 10 8 6 4 2

The suggestions and information contained in this publication are generally consistent with the *Standards of Medical Care in Diabetes* and other policies of the American Diabetes Association, but they do not represent the policy or position of the Association or any of its boards or committees. Reasonable steps have been taken to ensure the accuracy of the information presented. However, the American Diabetes Association cannot ensure the safety or efficacy of any product or service described in this publication. Individuals are advised to consult a physician or other appropriate health care professional before undertaking any diet or exercise program or taking any medication referred to in this publication. Professionals must use and apply their own professional judgment, experience, and training and should not rely solely on the information contained in this publication before prescribing any diet, exercise, or medication. The American Diabetes Association—its officers, directors, employees, volunteers, and members—assumes no responsibility or liability for personal or other injury, loss, or damage that may result from the suggestions or information in this publication.

♾ The paper in this publication meets the requirements of the ANSI Standard Z39.48-1992 (permanence of paper).

American Diabetes Association titles may be purchased for business or promotional use or for special sales. To purchase more than 50 copies of this book at a discount, or for custom editions of this book with your logo, contact the American Diabetes Association at the address below or at booksales@diabetes.org.

American Diabetes Association
1701 North Beauregard Street
Alexandria, Virginia 22311

DOI: 10.2337/9781580405652

Library of Congress Cataloging-in-Publication Data
Riolo, Amy.
  The Italian diabetes cookbook : delicious and healthful dishes from venice to sicily and beyond / Amy Riolo.
     pages cm
  Summary: "This book will help the reader see that Italian food is not off limits for people with diabetes. It will help change the way Italian cuisine is viewed abroad, and demonstrate ways in which traditional Italian food can be part of a diabetes-friendly eating plan"-- Provided by publisher.
  Includes bibliographical references and index.
  ISBN 978-1-58040-565-2 (paperback)
  1. Diabetes--Diet therapy--Recipes. 2. Cooking, Italian. I. Title.
  RC662.R514 2015
  641.5'6314--dc23
                    2015018201

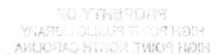

TABLE OF CONTENTS

iv Acknowledgments

vi Introduction

ix Seasonal Menus

1 Appetizers/*Antipasti*

29 First Courses/*Primi*

89 Second Courses/*Secondi*

157 Side Dishes/*Contorni*

181 Salads/*Insalate*

207 Bread/*Pane*

225 Sauces and Condiments/*Salse e Condimenti*

233 Desserts/*Dolci*

279 How to Cook like an Italian

293 The Italian Pantry

295 Italian Culinary Glossary

299 Where to Buy Guide

301 Resources

303 Index

ACKNOWLEDGMENTS

I owe my ability to write this book entirely to destiny. If I had been born into another family or culture and had not had the opportunity to live in Italy and the U.S., it would never have been possible. It was my mother's battle with diabetes that gave this cause such a large place in my heart and mind.

Destiny is also to thank for the opportunity I've had to get to know so many people and places in Italy on such an intimate level. I believe that it truly "takes a village" to make a good chef—and in my case, that village is a global one. I am honored and proud to say that I have learned from amazing cooks in places that I never dreamed I would even visit. For all of you who have shared a kitchen or a meal with me, I thank you.

My *nonna*, Angela Magnone Foti, taught me to cook and bake and gave me valuable lessons that served me outside of the kitchen as well. Because of her and our heritage, my first tastes of "Italian food" were Calabrian dishes. Those edible time capsules formed a culinary link between the two of us and our relatives in southern Italy. Because of her, I am able to prepare many of the same dishes that my Italian relatives do, even though I am a fourth-generation American. Nonna Angela gave me my first cookbook and showed me how cooking was not a mundane chore, but a form of magic that could unite people across distances and time. I owe my career to her and would give anything to be able to share more time in the kitchen with her. Cooking was so important to her that a few weeks before she passed, at 90 years old, she refused to go into the hospital because it was Christmastime. She told the doctors that she needed to be home so that she could "make cookies with Amy." It is an honor for me to be able to pass her knowledge on to my readers. My *yia yia*, Mary Michos Riolo, also shared her beloved Greek traditions with me, and I am happy to say that they have become woven into my culinary fabric as well—which is not surprising, since many Italian regions were Greek colonies in antiquity.

My earliest memories of cooking were with my mother, Faith Riolo, who would sit me on the counter and roll more meatballs and cookies than I could count. She taught me that food was not just something we eat to nourish ourselves, but an edible gift that could be given to express love. I owe my love of food history and anthropology to my father, Rick Riolo. He planted in me the desire to answer the question, "I wonder what they eat." This is a type of culinary curiosity that is never completely satisfied and gives me the motivation to continue my work each day.

I would probably never have published a cookbook if it weren't for my mentor, Sheilah Kaufman, who patiently taught me much more than I ever planned on learning. I am proud to pass her knowledge on to others. My special thanks to my partner, Chef Luigi Diotaiuti, for being a continuous source of inspiration and motivation, for sharing my passions for maintaining culinary traditions that are on the verge of being forgotten, and for promoting all of the splendor that southern Italy and the Mediterranean region have to offer.

In Italy, I thank my cousin Angela Riolo for sharing my passion and continuously supplying me with authentic Calabrian recipes. In Rome, I thank Liana Mari, Mauro Lesti, and Marialuisa DiMatteo for their continued support. I also thank Luigi and Maria Fabbiano for sharing so much with me over the years.

Thank you to Dr. Norton Fishman, Dr. Beth Tedesco, and Dr. Mary Lee Esty for enabling me to overcome my illness and fulfill my dreams. To my dear friends Dr. Amira Mohsen and Susan Simonet, you are the sisters I never had. To Kathleen Ammalee Rogers, my "adopted" sister, trusted healer, and wellness coach—thank you for your love and support, for guiding me to realize my full potential, and for enabling me to achieve my dreams. I have you to thank for the goodness I have created in my life.

At the American Diabetes Association, I would like to thank Abraham Ogden, Director of Book Publishing; Greg Guthrie, Managing Editor; and Lauren Wilson for assisting me with the creation of this book. I truly appreciate the food styling of Lisa Cherkasky and Renée Comet's great food photography. I also appreciate the assistance of Robert Schueller and Melissa's Produce for providing produce for our photo shoot, and Anthony Quinn of Cleveland Park Wine and Spirits for providing Calabrian wine. I would also like to thank every shopkeeper, housewife, taxi driver, chef, fisherman, farmer, and restaurateur who took the time to discuss food with me and provide me with additional insights.

This book is dedicated to my mother, Faith Riolo—I owe everything to you.

It is also dedicated to everyone suffering from this disease—may you always enjoy the sweetness of life.

INTRODUCTION

"La cucina di un popolo è la sola esatta testimonianza della sua civiltà."
"The cuisine of a people is the only true testimony of their civilization."
—Italian proverb

If you think Italian food is off-limits for people with diabetes, think again. My motivation for writing this book was to change the way Italian cuisine is viewed abroad and to demonstrate ways in which traditional Italian food can be part of a diabetes-friendly eating plan. While thoughts of the *bel paese* ("beautiful country") generally conjure up the image of platters of carbohydrate-rich pastas and fat-laden sauces, authentic Italian cuisine is both healthful and delicious.

The inspiration for this book came to me years ago. I was 15 years old when I began preparing many of these recipes for my family after my mother's diabetes diagnosis. Since I didn't want to create two separate meals for our family, I strove to make the recipes that fit into my mother's eating plan delicious enough for the whole family to eat. Who knew that it would turn into a career?

When I visited our ancestral hometown of Crotone, Italy, for the first time, I was struck by how much healthier our Italian family members were than our American ones. While we share the same genes, it is the diet and lifestyle of our southern Italian relatives that make the difference to their health. While living in Rome, I was struck by how fit even the elderly citizens were. Belying the stereotypical figurines, even most Italian chefs are in good shape. Ever since that stay, it has been my goal to demon-strate that fantastic food and good health don't have to be mutually exclusive.

The secret to my success with cookbooks, teaching, and lecturing has been to focus on what people with diabetes can eat, instead of what they can't. Vegetables, fruits, grains, beans and legumes, nuts, dairy, seafood, poultry, lean meats, and wholesome baked goods can all be part of a healthful lifestyle. Fortunately, each of these food groups offers scores of ingredients to choose from—many of which include nutrients that are particularly beneficial to people seeking optimal health. Best of all, preparing these foods in a traditional Italian fashion helps to coax the ultimate flavor, texture, and aroma out of them.

Italian food is currently the most popular cuisine in the world. At its core, true Italian cuisine is all about preparing fresh ingredients using time-honored techniques that preserve both tradition and flavor. This book contains over 150 easy-to-prepare, satisfying, and robust Italian dishes that can be enjoyed by the whole family.

Some of the recipes in this book are well known and 100% authentic. Others have been adapted slightly to meet the American Diabetes Association's nutrition guidelines. For recipes that aren't naturally gluten-free, I have offered gluten-free alternatives. (Those who do not suffer from gluten sensitivities can simply ignore these alternatives.) Since foreigners' perception of Italian food usually consists of regional dishes offered at "Italian" restaurants abroad or foods tasted in popular tourist destinations, I was sure to include authentic recipes from each of Italy's regions. I specifically chose recipes ranging from the very famous to the obscure—coming from both large cities and small villages. By sampling dishes from all of Italy, readers can gain insight into the land and the people as well as the food.

Many researchers maintain that the longevity of the Italian population is due to their diet and lifestyle. Unfortunately, as Italians are beginning to abandon their traditional ways of living and eating, diabetes is on the rise in Italy just as it is in the U.S. *The Italian Diabetes Cookbook* combines a respect for the culinary and cultural traditions of Italy's past with easy-to-recreate recipes and healthy living tips that are perfectly suited for those with diabetes. My mission is to help fine-food lovers everywhere achieve their health goals by utilizing the bountiful array of nutritious eating options that Italy has to offer.

Wine/*Vino*

"*Nessun poema è mai stato scritto da
un bevitore di acqua.*"
"No poem was ever written by a drinker of water."
—Italian proverb

Wine originated in Mesopotamia, the area which is now modern-day Iran and Iraq. It was the Romans who made the most significant contributions to the development and spread of viticulture, the study of grape cultivation, around the Mediterranean. Today, as a result, Italy is the largest producer of wine in the world. In Italy, wine has been enjoyed with meals for millennia. Because viticulture is such an important part of the Italian lifestyle, culture, traditions, economy, and food scene, I have decided to offer a wine-pairing suggestion for several of the recipes in this book. These pairings have been made by award-winning chef, sommelier, and restaurateur Luigi Diotaiuti, who is a Certified Italian Sommelier. Note that in the Italian tradition, recipes with a high citrus content and vinegar are not served with wine.

When the ancient Greeks settled in southern Italy and Sicily, they introduced the wine-making tradition, as they believed that this region was the perfectly suited place for wine production. They referred to Italy as Oenotria, or "land of trained vines." My ancestral homeland of Calabria was settled by two tribes: the Oenotrians (vine cultivators) and the Itali. Calabrian wine was so revered by the Greeks that they used to serve it during Olympic ceremonies in Greece.

The Romans improved upon Etruscan and Greek techniques and began introducing vines to Gaul (modern-day France) and other areas in the empire. Wine demand increased greatly with the beginning of the Christian Era in 300 BCE (before Common Era). Over the years wine making became a practice that farmers, businessmen, and priests alike could partake in. Because of its sacramental significance in the Catholic Church, many wineries and wine-making traditions were tightly guarded in monasteries. In addition to the sensual pleasure of drinking wine, its consumption also became a way to strengthen relations—with the divine, family members, friends, and new acquaintances.

The Mediterranean diet allows for wine in moderation. The American Diabetes Association recommends no more than one alcoholic drink (5 ounces of wine) per day for women and two alcoholic drinks per day for men. Of course, for those with diabetes, the carbohydrate content of alcoholic beverages must be factored into the carbohydrate count for the overall meal.

Recent research demonstrates that the polyphenols and flavonoids (antioxidants that prevent blood clotting, prevent tumors from growing, and reduce arterial plaque) found in the skin of grapes provide cardiovascular protection. Since red wine is fermented with its skin, it contains a more concentrated amount of antioxidants than white wine. However, most doctors do not advise patients who currently abstain from alcohol to begin drinking specifically for this benefit, because antioxidants can also be found in a wide variety of other plant-based foods.

Italian Wine Quality Labels

The wine pairings in this book are types and varietals of wine rather than specific brands. While shopping for the Italian wines mentioned in this book, you may notice the letters "DOC" or "DOCG" on some of the labels. Here's a breakdown of what these acronyms mean when they appear on wine labels:

- DOC *(Denominazione di origine controllata):* Wines with this designation are produced within a limited area, using precise grape varieties, and adhering to strict production controls.
- DOCG *(Denominazione di origine controllata e garantita):* An indicator of the highest-quality wines, this designation is given to wines that are subject to the strictest varietal, processing, and production controls.
- IGT *(Indicazione geografica tipica):* Wines with this designation are produced from approved grape varieties within a defined geographical region.

SEASONAL MENUS

To me, making menus is one of the most pleasurable experiences that life has to offer. I love pairing foods and courses together, and giving careful thought to each dish and its role in the overall effect of the meal. In a well-planned menu, seasonality, nutrition, taste, texture, aroma, and terroir (flavors imparted by the local terrain) work together through a series of courses to create a perfectly balanced eating experience. While it might sound intimidating to some, so many of the principles of food pairing are so embedded in our memories that it seems as though certain foods just naturally go together. If you've never created a menu before, use the following guidelines until you are comfortable with the process. Notice how the elements of the Italian meals you enjoy the most work together, and apply those principles in your own kitchen.

Here are a few tips:

1. Traditional, complete Italian meals consist of an appetizer, a first course, a second course with a side dish, salad, fruit and cheese, and/or a dessert and a cup of espresso—in that order.

2. In today's hurried culture, even in Italy, the full traditional meal is often only served on Sundays (when most Italians still participate in the ritual family meal), when entertaining, in fine-dining situations, or on holidays.

3. Workday lunches may now consist of a *primo* (first course), salad, and espresso (often omitting the second course).

4. Workday dinners may consist of a second course, side dish, salad, fruit and cheese, and espresso (often omitting the appetizer and first course).

5. Pasta, risotto, or gnocchi is typically present in Italian lunches.

6. Fresh, seasonal, local, organic foods are always preferred.

7. Pasta dishes are never preceded by soup. Soup can be enjoyed on its own, or as a first course.

Spring Menu
Tuscan Crudités with Olive Oil Dip (page 5)
Chickpea Soup with Rosemary-Infused Shrimp (page 38)
Sea Bass with Fennel Baked in Parchment (page 114)
Chargrilled Asparagus with Balsamic and Parmesan (page 178)
Val d'Aosta–Style Dandelion Salad (page 193)
Espresso Panna Cotta (page 238)

Summer Menu

Sicilian Sweet-and-Sour Vegetable Medley (page 6)
Spaghetti Squash "Pasta" with Shrimp, Tomatoes, and Basil (page 62)
Swordfish with Olives, Capers, Herbs, and Tomatoes (page 120)
Spinach Sautéed in Garlic and Oil (page 180)
Cauliflower and Herb Salad from Le Marche (page 199)
Fresh Fruit Kabobs (page 237)

Fall Menu

Umbrian Frittata Skewers with Chickpea Dipping Sauce (page 14)
Barley, Chestnut, and White Bean Minestrone (page 54)
Roasted Chicken with Grapes and Chestnuts (page 144)
Mixed Mushroom and Herb Medley (page 172)
Beet, Quinoa, and Arugula Salad (page 185)
Poached Autumn Pears with Vanilla and Ginger Cream (page 243)

Winter Menu

Spinach Fettuccine with Walnut-Ricotta Pesto (page 64)
Cacciatore-Style Chicken (page 140)
Pan-Fried Fennel with Parmesan (page 162)
Arugula Salad with Pears, Parmesan, and Cocoa Nibs (page 192)
Ivrea's Polenta Cake (page 266)

Christmas Eve Feast of the Seven Fishes

Crostini with Chickpea Cream (page 10)
Smoked Fish, Orange, and Radicchio Salad with Olives (page 194)
Seafood Salad (page 200)
Mussels in Saffron-Tomato Broth (page 110)
Pan-Seared Sea Scallops (page 106)
Spaghetti with Fresh Tuna and Fennel (page 72)
Braised, Stuffed Calamari with Tomato Sauce (page 112)
Sea Bass with Fennel Baked in Parchment (page 114)
Make-Ahead Cookie Platter:
Coconut Ball Cookies (page 256),
Pine Nut Cookies (page 258), and
Piemontese "Ugly but Good" Cookies (page 262)

Vegetarian Feast

Vegetable and Parmesan Carpaccio (page 12)
Whole-Wheat Fusilli with Pesto and Cherry Tomatoes (page 66)
Artichoke, Mushroom, and Caramelized Onion Frittata (page 96)
Sautéed Zucchini with Vinegar and Mint (page 173)
Asparagus, Orange, and Fennel Salad (page 188)
Pear, Ricotta, and Pine Nut Cake (page 274)

Calabrian New Year's Celebration

Ricotta, Grilled Eggplant, and Fresh Mint Bruschetta (page 8)
Eggplant Croquettes (page 102)
Holiday Minestrone (page 48)
Classic Meatballs (page 154)
Calabrian-Style Roasted Potatoes (page 176)
Smoked Fish, Orange, and Radicchio Salad with Olives (page 194)
Espresso and Spice–Poached Figs (page 244)

Italian *Sagra* (Festival) Menu

Whole-Wheat Cracker Rings with Black Pepper and Fennel Seeds (page 222)
Southern Italian Fava Bean Purée (page 16)
Trapani-Style Almond Couscous (page 86)
Abruzzese-Style Roasted Baby Goat with Peppers (page 152)
Pepper, Potato, and Eggplant Medley (page 174)
Red Pepper, Yellow Tomato, and Artichoke Salad (page 187)
Crunchy Almond and Pine Nut Cookies (page 260)

Sunday Dinner

Stuffed Eggplant (page 22)
OR
Stuffed Peppers (page 24)

Whole-Wheat Orecchiette Pasta with Broccoli and Garlic (page 68)
OR
Whole-Wheat Ziti with Goat Ragu (page 70)

Vegetable-Stuffed Turkey Breast (page 146)
OR
Herb-Roasted Turkey (page 148)

Haricots Verts with Hazelnuts (page 175)
Tuscan Farro Salad (page 204)
Cinnamon-Infused Apple Cake (page 264)

Southern Italian Picnic

Whole-Wheat Country Loaves (page 220)
Puglian Fava Bean Purée with Sautéed Chicory (page 18)
Cannellini Bean, Tuna, and Red Onion Salad (page 186)
Tomatoes with Balsamic Vinegar (page 190)
Fresh Fruit Kabobs (page 237)

Classic Roman Fare

Roman-Style Rice and Herb–Stuffed Tomatoes (page 20)
Roman-Style Broccoli and Pecorino Soup (page 60)
Roman Chicken, Pepper, and Tomato Stew (page 94)
Artichokes with Garlic and Oil (page 164)
Chocolate and Orange Sponge Cake (page 257)

APPETIZERS
(ANTIPASTI)

5 Tuscan Crudités with Olive Oil Dip/*Pinzimonio*

6 Sicilian Sweet-and-Sour Vegetable Medley/*Caponata*

8 Ricotta, Grilled Eggplant, and Fresh Mint Bruschetta/*Bruschetta Calabrese*

10 Crostini with Chickpea Cream/*Crostini con ceci*

12 Vegetable and Parmesan Carpaccio/*Carpaccio di verdure e parmigiano*

14 Umbrian Frittata Skewers with Chickpea Dipping Sauce/
     Spiedini di frittata con crema di ceci d'Umbria

16 Southern Italian Fava Bean Purée/*Maccu*

18 Puglian Fava Bean Purée with Sautéed Chicory/*Fave e cicoria Pugliese*

20 Roman-Style Rice and Herb–Stuffed Tomatoes/*Pomodori ripieni di riso alla Romana*

22 Stuffed Eggplant/*Melanzane ripiene*

24 Stuffed Peppers/*Peperoni ripieni*

26 Lemon-Scented Shrimp/*Gamberi al limone*

28 Zucchini Carpaccio with Green Peppercorns/*Carpaccio di zucchine al pepe verde*

In the Italian tradition, the word for appetizers *(antipasti)* comes from the Latin term for "before the meal" and the word *pasto,* which means "meal" in Italian. Little tidbits meant to whet your appetite and stimulate digestion before the meal, authentic Italian appetizers can consist of everything from seasonal vegetables sautéed in olive oil to cured meats and aged cheeses, or even a puréed *sformato,* a molded flan-like savory dish often served in restaurants.

Everyday meals in Italian homes don't always begin with appetizers unless someone is entertaining. When entertaining guests, usually one or two appetizers will be served before the first course. Family-style restaurants and *trattorias* often offer a salad bar consisting of already prepared *antipasti* that diners can choose for themselves in more casual establishments, or have selected by a waiter in more formal restaurants.

In order to choose an appetizer for an Italian meal, you must understand a bit about Italian meal planning in general. Italians always plan meals starting with the first course. This is because, in the popular culture, pasta, rice, and soup are the backbones of the diet. In leaner times, these kinds of dishes can be "stretched" into the entire meal, and in times of decadence, they are the ultimate way to showcase even the most expensive products, such as truffles. So once you know which pasta/risotto/soup you are serving first, you can decide which second course will go best and which appetizer is the best way to open the meal.

Let's say, for example, you are serving a first course with tomatoes—then your second course would probably be roasted, grilled, or braised, but without tomatoes, and the appetizers could be a combination of vegetable- , legume- , and cheese-based recipes. If you were serving a first course that was on the lighter side and did not contain tomatoes, and a vegetarian or seafood-based second course, then your appetizer could be something heavier (like stuffed tomatoes, peppers, or eggplant) and might contain other types of seafood.

There are also traditional appetizers that are served for special holidays. On Christmas Eve in Calabria, for example, Crostini with Chickpea Cream (page 10) are usually served, whereas Southern Italian Fava Bean Purée (page 16) is eaten on St. Joseph's Day on March 19. Fresh vegetable-based appetizers, such as Tuscan Crudités with Olive Oil Dip (page 5) and Zucchini Carpaccio with Green Peppercorns (page 28), are only eaten when those particular vegetables are in season.

If you haven't created Italian meals before, this may sound intimidating, but it really isn't. In the U.S., meals are planned according to food groups. Most American dietary plans recommend that we eat a certain combination of carbohydrates, proteins, and vegetables/fruits with our meals. The Italian meal consists of the same components, but they are stretched out in a series of courses, which requires that each dish fits with the others. I like to tell my cooking students that if all of the courses being served in an Italian meal do not look good or seem appetizing when placed on the same table, they do not go together. Use the menus in this book to serve as a guideline for this rule of thumb.

Fine-dining restaurants use *antipasti* to showcase the latest seasonal products and authentic ingredients in new and creative ways—it's a sort of culinary platform to reinforce the restaurant's mission. Appetizers also go hand in hand with the afternoon *apertivo*, or aperitif, which comes from the Latin *aperire*, meaning "to open." The *apertivo* is to many Italians what happy hour is to Americans. You can meet friends in a bar or *enoteca* for an *apertivo*—to have drinks and appetizers. During these occasions, a wide array of appetizers would be served with the drinks after work and prior to dinner.

Among the most popular *apertivo* drinks are the Aperol Spritz and the Bellini. While Milan is known for the most fashionable *apertivi*, Venice is home to some of the most famous. The Venetians even have their own blend of appetizers called *cicchetti*, or small plates similar to Spanish tapas, specifically for the occasion.

If you would like to host your own *apertivo*, I suggest the following menu:

Ricotta, Grilled Eggplant, and Fresh Mint
    Bruschetta (page 8)
Umbrian Frittata Skewers with Chickpea
    Dipping Sauce (page 14)
Stuffed Peppers (page 24)
Lemon-Scented Shrimp (page 26)

TUSCAN CRUDITÉS WITH OLIVE OIL DIP (PINZIMONIO)

Serves: 4 | Serving Size: Approximately 1 cup vegetables
Prep Time: 15 minutes | Cooking Time: 0 minutes

This appetizer is representative of the soul of the Tuscan kitchen, which glorifies the best, ripest, and most beautiful produce by pairing it with fresh, local olive oil. The word pinzimonio *is a combination of two Italian words:* pinze, *meaning "tweezers," and* matrimonio, *meaning "marriage." The terms refer to the romantic act of pinching the fresh, new vegetables between your fingers and "marrying them" in the fruity, local, seasoned oil, which is always first cold-pressed. If possible, use Sicilian sea salt, Tuscan olive oil, and freshly ground Tellichery black pepper in this recipe.*

1 radicchio, rinsed, damaged outer leaves removed, and cut in half lengthwise

1/4 cup fresh cherry tomatoes

1 bulb fennel, rinsed, trimmed, and quartered lengthwise

4 radishes, rinsed

4 slender carrots, peeled, trimmed, and quartered lengthwise

2 red bell peppers, rinsed, trimmed, seeded, and sliced into 1/4-inch strips lengthwise

1/4 cup extra virgin olive oil (preferably first cold-pressed)

1/8 teaspoon unrefined sea salt

1/4 teaspoon freshly ground black pepper

⟡ Italian Living Tradition ⟡

If you're lucky enough to have any vegetables left over after serving this attractive, healthful appetizer, dice them and incorporate them into a salad or minestrone.

1. Arrange all the vegetables attractively on a platter, leaving a hole in the center.

2. Pour the olive oil into a bowl, season with salt and pepper, and place in the center of the platter. Serve.

Choices/Exchanges 1 Starch, 1 Vegetable, 2 1/2 Fat
Calories 210 | Calories from Fat 130
Total Fat 14g | Saturated Fat 2.0g | Trans Fat 0.0g
Cholesterol 0mg
Sodium 220mg

Potassium 660mg
Total Carbohydrate 20g | Dietary Fiber 6g | Sugars 8g
Protein 3g
Phosphorus 85mg

SICILIAN SWEET-AND-SOUR VEGETABLE MEDLEY (CAPONATA)

Serves: 4 | Serving Size: Approximately 1 cup vegetables and 1 slice bread
Prep Time: 15 minutes | Cooking Time: 40 minutes

Caponata is one of my all-time favorite dishes. I used to teach this recipe in a class called "Cooking with Chocolate," and people were always surprised to learn that there is chocolate in the recipe! While the addition of chocolate may seem unorthodox to some, the Sicilian town of Modica— named a World Heritage site by the United Nations Educational, Scientific and Cultural Organization (UNESCO)—is actually famous for its chocolate; it's an ancient Aztec recipe introduced by the Spaniards. Sicily is also known for its sweet-and-sour flavor combinations, which bear testimony to the Arab influence on the Mediterranean's largest island. This agrodolce (sweet-and-sour) eggplant dish is rich and sweetened with caramelized onions and raisins.

1/4 cup extra virgin olive oil

3/4 pound eggplant, cut into 1-inch cubes

1/4 yellow onion, finely chopped

1/3 stalk celery, roughly chopped

1/4 teaspoon freshly ground black pepper

1 tablespoon no-salt tomato paste, thinned with 1/4 cup water

1/3 cup canned crushed tomatoes

2 ounces green olives, drained, rinsed well, pitted, and roughly chopped

1/8 cup white wine vinegar

1/8 cup golden raisins

1 tablespoon finely grated unsweetened chocolate

3 tablespoons finely shredded fresh basil

1/2 teaspoon pine nuts

4 very thin slices Italian bread (or gluten-free bread), rubbed with olive oil and grilled or toasted on one side

---

Choices/Exchanges 1/2 Starch, 2 Vegetable, 3 1/2 Fat
Calories 240 | Calories from Fat 170
Total Fat 19g | Saturated Fat 3.5g | Trans Fat 0.0g
Cholesterol 0mg
Sodium 220mg

Potassium 405mg
Total Carbohydrate 19g | Dietary Fiber 5g | Sugars 7g
Protein 3g
Phosphorus 70mg

1. Heat oil in a 12-inch skillet over medium-high heat. Working in batches if necessary, add eggplant to skillet and fry, tossing occasionally, until browned, about 3–4 minutes. Using a slotted spoon, transfer eggplant to a large bowl.

2. Add onions and celery to skillet, and season with pepper. Cook, stirring often, until vegetables begin to brown, about 10 minutes. Reduce heat to medium, add tomato paste, and cook, stirring, until vegetables are caramelized and paste is almost evaporated, 1–2 minutes.

3. Add crushed tomatoes and continue cooking for 10 minutes. Stir in olives, vinegar, raisins, and chocolate, and cook, stirring occasionally, until thickened, about 15 minutes.

4. Transfer mixture to bowl with eggplant. Add basil and pine nuts, and mix together. Let cool to room temperature. Serve over toasted bread slices.

⤏❧ Italian Living Tradition ❧⤎

Caponata is usually served at room temperature as a side dish, but it also tastes great served cold on top of tender lettuce leaves or tossed into hot pasta for a quick, delicious, and satisfying meal.

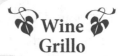

Wine Grillo

RICOTTA, GRILLED EGGPLANT, AND FRESH MINT BRUSCHETTA (*BRUSCHETTA CALABRESE*)

Serves: 4 | Serving Size: 1 slice bread, 2 tablespoons ricotta, and approximately 1/3 cup eggplant
Prep Time: 5 minutes | Cooking Time: 10 minutes

The popular Italian poet Gabriele D'Annunzio once described the view of the sea from Reggio Calabria as "the most beautiful kilometer in Italy." Known as the ancestral homeland to 20% of the Italian-American population, the southern Italian region was once home to powerful Greek and Byzantine colonies like the city of Crotone, where Pythagoras once formed a secret society of intellectuals. This recipe is popular in Calabria because it incorporates eggplant and ricotta—two widely celebrated ingredients—on their beloved country-style bread.

2 baby eggplants (1/2 pound total), ends trimmed and cut lengthwise into 4 × 1/4-inch slices
2 tablespoons good-quality extra virgin olive oil (preferably Calabrian; see Where to Buy Guide), divided
1/8 teaspoon unrefined sea salt, divided
4 (1/2-inch) slices ciabatta or other light, crusty, country bread
1/2 cup ricotta cheese, divided
1/4 teaspoon freshly ground black pepper
1/4 cup finely chopped fresh mint

Choices/Exchanges 1/2 Starch, 1 Vegetable, 1/2 Medium-Fat Protein, 1 Fat
Calories 150 | Calories from Fat 90
Total Fat 10g | Saturated Fat 2.6g | Trans Fat 0.0g
Cholesterol 10mg

Sodium 170mg
Potassium 225mg
Total Carbohydrate 11g | Dietary Fiber 3g | Sugars 2g
Protein 5g
Phosphorus 85mg

1. Preheat broiler to high or grill to medium-high.

2. Lightly brush the eggplant slices with 1 table-spoon olive oil and set on a baking sheet. When the grill is ready, use tongs to place slices directly on the grill and cook each side until grill marks appear and slices are nicely browned, 3–4 minutes per side. Or, if broiling, place baking sheet directly under broiler, and broil each side until golden, 1–2 minutes per side.

3. Remove baking sheet from oven or, if grilling, use tongs to transfer eggplant back to the baking sheet, and sprinkle with about half the salt. When slices are cool enough to handle, cut into 1/4-inch cubes, place in a bowl, and set aside.

4. When ready to serve (do not prepare these ahead of time or the bread will get soggy), grill the bread slices on both sides until grill marks appear, or place under the broiler until golden brown. Slather each piece evenly with 2 table-spoons ricotta. Sprinkle with remaining salt and the pepper. Top with the chopped eggplant. Drizzle with remaining 1 tablespoon olive oil and garnish with mint. Serve immediately.

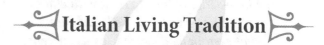

Italian Living Tradition

A great deal of Italy's olive oil is produced in Calabria. There are three main varieties of Calabrian olive oil:

Alto Crotonese
Production of this type of oil can be traced to the Byzantine period, when Basilian monks settled in the region and improved olive cultivation. Made using at least 70% *Carolea* olives, this is a lighter Calabrian oil, suited for drizzling over fish or seasoning greens.

Bruzio
The olives used to make this oil were introduced to the region by the ancient Greeks. Bruzio's Protected Designation of Origin (*Denominazione di origine protetta* in Italian) is limited to the province of Cosenza. This oil has a light green color with hints of yellow.

Lamezia
Olive production in Lamezia is limited for quality, and the harvesting season is heavily regulated. Olive oil from Lamezia is made from at least 90% *Carolea* olives, and the acidity of the oil is restricted to 0.5%, giving it a smooth, full flavor.

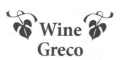

Wine
Greco

CROSTINI WITH CHICKPEA CREAM (CROSTINI CON CECI)

Serves: 6 | Serving Size: 1 1/3 slices bread and 1/3 cup chickpea purée
Prep Time: 5 minutes | Cooking Time: 10 minutes

Chickpeas are an important staple in the Sicilian diet, and are called ciceri *in the local dialect. The knowledge of how to cook with chickpeas (as well as knowing how to pronounce the term) is what has separated the locals from foreigners for centuries. It is important to remember that certain foods were used as currency prior to the invention of coins. According to his contemporaries, the ancient Roman philosopher Cicero (*cicer *means "chickpea" in Latin) was so called because he came from a family that flourished due to the sale of this ancient legume. During times of war, Sicilians would often ask foreigners suspected of espionage to pronounce the word* ciceri *(chee-chee-ree); if they pronounced it incorrectly, they were taken as prisoners of war.*

2 cups cooked chickpeas (cook dried chickpeas without salt)

1/4 cup extra virgin olive oil (preferably Sicilian, first cold-pressed, and unfiltered), plus extra for drizzling

1 clove garlic, minced

Juice of 1 orange

Juice of 1 lemon

1/4 teaspoon freshly ground black pepper

Pinch crushed red chile flakes

8 (1/4-inch) slices sesame-semolina or gluten-free bread

1/4 cup sun-cured black Sicilian olives, pitted

Choices/Exchanges 2 Starch, 1 Lean Protein, 1 1/2 Fat
Calories 250 | Calories from Fat 110
Total Fat 12g | Saturated Fat 1.7g | Trans Fat 0.0g
Cholesterol 0mg
Sodium 210mg

Potassium 230mg
Total Carbohydrate 30g | Dietary Fiber 5g | Sugars 4g
Protein 7g
Phosphorus 125mg

1. Preheat oven to 350°F.

2. Place chickpeas, olive oil, garlic, orange juice, lemon juice, pepper, and crushed red chile flakes in a food processor. Purée until smooth. Add a few tablespoons of water until mixture resembles a light purée. Set aside.

3. Place bread slices on a baking sheet. Toast 2–3 minutes per side in the oven.

4. Remove bread from the oven and spread chickpea purée on top. Garnish each slice with an olive, drizzle extra olive oil on top, and serve.

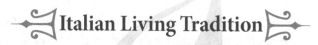

Italian Living Tradition

Today this easy appetizer is served in many parts of southern Italy—including Calabria, where it is usually a part of the Christmas appetizer lineup. Simple, healthful Italian ingredients appeal to palates everywhere. Try serving these crostini with your favorite soup or salad.

I have prepared this appetizer for many professional occasions, including a "Sacred Foods of Italy" presentation with the U.S. Department of State's American Chefs Corps and the Les Dames d'Escoffier's Global Culinary Initiative for a Global Culinary Dialogue at Al Tiramisu restaurant in Washington, D.C.

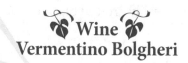

Wine
Vermentino Bolgheri

VEGETABLE AND PARMESAN CARPACCIO (CARPACCIO DI VERDURE E PARMIGIANO)

Serves: 6 | Serving Size: Approximately 3/4 cup
Prep Time: 15 minutes | Cooking Time: 0 minutes

Based on Carne all'Albese, a traditional dish of sliced raw beef from the Piedmont region, carpaccio received its now-popular name when it was served at Harry's Bar in Venice by Giuseppe Cipriani in 1950. One of Cipriani's customers, Countess Amalia Nani Mocenigo, was instructed to eat raw meat by her doctor. Inspired by the red and white hues of Venetian painter Vittore Carpaccio, who was exhibiting at the time, Cipriani served her Carne all'Albese and called it "carpaccio." Today, when raw fish, seafood, and vegetables are dressed in a similar fashion, they are called by this same name.

1 cup large, firm radishes

2 large carrots

2 stalks celery (from the heart)

2 firm leeks, white and tender green only

1 small bulb fennel, halved and cored

1/2 lemon plus 3 tablespoons fresh lemon juice

1 teaspoon good-quality balsamic vinegar

3 tablespoons extra virgin olive oil (preferably first cold-pressed), plus more for drizzling

1 medium, firm artichoke

2 ounces parmigiano-reggiano cheese, for shaving

1/4 teaspoon freshly ground black pepper

Choices/Exchanges 3 Vegetable, 2 Fat
Calories 160 | Calories from Fat 90
Total Fat 10g | Saturated Fat 2.7g | Trans Fat 0.0g
Cholesterol 10mg
Sodium 250mg

Potassium 435mg
Total Carbohydrate 15g | Dietary Fiber 5g | Sugars 5g
Protein 6g
Phosphorus 130mg

1. Using a manual mandoline-type slicer or a food processor with slicing disc attachment, trim and very thinly slice the radishes, carrots, celery, leeks, and fennel bulb. Set aside.

2. In a large bowl, combine the 3 tablespoons lemon juice with the balsamic vinegar and whisk lightly with a fork. Beat in the 3 tablespoons olive oil.

3. Trim the artichoke, rubbing the cut portions with the lemon half as you go to prevent discoloration. Cut off the stem and pull off all the dark outer leaves around the base. Cut the artichoke crosswise about 1 1/2 inches from the base to remove the remaining leaves. Scoop out the hairy choke, and trim around the top and bottom of the heart.

4. Slice the artichoke heart very thin and toss with the dressing. Add the other sliced vegetables and toss gently.

5. Arrange the carpaccio on plates or on a platter. Using a vegetable peeler, shave parmesan on top. Season with pepper, drizzle with olive oil, if desired, and serve.

⊰ Italian Living Tradition ⊱

A popular new trend in Italian homes and restaurants is to serve healthful, extremely light dishes in elegant forms. Feel free to use whichever vegetables you have on hand to create this dish. Note how doling out vegetables with style seems to make them taste better!

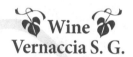

**Wine
Vernaccia S. G.**

UMBRIAN FRITTATA SKEWERS WITH CHICKPEA DIPPING SAUCE (*SPIEDINI DI FRITTATA CON CREMA DI CECI D'UMBRIA*)

Serves: 8 | Serving Size: 1 skewer (or 1/8th frittata)
Prep Time: 10 minutes | Cooking Time: 40 minutes

Umbria is a breathtaking Italian region nestled between Lazio and Tuscany. The region's simple, straightforward flavors are combined in a unique way in this recipe. Both hearty and healthful, this dish is a vegetarian dream. If you prefer not to serve this frittata on skewers, you can simply cut it into individual slices and serve them on top of a "bed" of the Chickpea Dipping Sauce. [Note: You will need eight (6-inch) wooden skewers and a medium-size (10-inch) nonstick ovenproof skillet to complete this dish.]

Frittata

2 tablespoons extra virgin olive oil, divided

1 medium yellow onion, diced

1 cup shiitake, cremini, or portobello mushrooms, cleaned, stems removed, and chopped into bite-size pieces

1/4 teaspoon unrefined sea salt

1/4 teaspoon freshly ground black pepper

6 large eggs, beaten

Chickpea Dipping Sauce

2 cups cooked chickpeas (cook dried chickpeas without salt)

1/4 cup fresh lemon juice

2 cloves garlic, minced

1 teaspoon finely chopped rosemary plus 1 rosemary sprig for decoration

4 tablespoons extra virgin olive oil

Choices/Exchanges 1/2 Starch, 1 Vegetable, 1 Lean Protein, 1 1/2 Fat

Calories 200 | Calories from Fat 100

Total Fat 11g | Saturated Fat 2.2g | Trans Fat 0.0g

Cholesterol 140mg

Sodium 120mg

Potassium 275mg

Total Carbohydrate 16g | Dietary Fiber 4g | Sugars 5g

Protein 9g

Phosphorus 165mg

1. Preheat oven to 400°F.

2. Heat 1 tablespoon olive oil in a medium-size (10-inch) nonstick, ovenproof skillet over medium heat. Add the onion and sauté 3–5 minutes, or until tender and translucent. Add the mushrooms and remaining 1 tablespoon olive oil. Sauté mushrooms approximately 10 minutes with the onions until the water from the mushrooms has evaporated and the mushrooms are browned.

3. Whisk salt and pepper into the eggs. Add eggs to skillet and cook, uncovered, over medium-low heat until the bottom is set, about 5–10 minutes.

4. Transfer frittata to the oven and bake for 10–15 minutes, or until top is dry and eggs are cooked through.

5. Combine all Chickpea Dipping Sauce ingredients in a food processor. Purée until smooth. Add water 1 tablespoon at a time and continue processing until a thin, creamy, sauce-like consistency is reached.

6. When the frittata is cool enough to handle (after about 5 minutes), cut it into 1-inch pieces and slide them onto skewers. Serve on a platter with the dipping sauce in the middle.

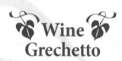

SOUTHERN ITALIAN FAVA BEAN PURÉE (MACCU)

Serves: 6 | Serving Size: Approximately 1/3 cup
Prep Time: 5 minutes (plus 1 hour bean-soaking time) | Cooking Time: 1 hour 5 minutes

Maccu is a popular dish in my ancestral homeland of Calabria, Italy. The word calabria *is derived from a Byzantine term meaning "fertile land." This region lives up to its name with rich agricultural traditions that continue today. The word* maccu *comes from the dialect word for "mashed" and refers to a purée that is made of fava beans, one of the world's oldest agricultural crops. Fresh and dried fava bean dishes are served in Calabria for St. Joseph's Day. Serve this appetizer alone, drizzled with olive oil as a side dish, or with crackers, flatbread, or Whole-Wheat Cracker Rings with Black Pepper and Fennel Seeds (page 222). Use first cold-pressed olive oil and pecorino Crotonese—a high-quality, aged sheep-milk cheese from Calabria, if possible. This dish, like many popular Italian appetizers, can be served hot or at room temperature. Chickpeas and cannellini beans can be substituted for the fava beans.*

2/3 cup peeled, dried fava beans, soaked in boiling water for 1 hour and drained

1 small onion, quartered

1 dried bay leaf

2 tablespoons pecorino Crotonese or Romano cheese

2 tablespoons extra virgin olive oil (preferably first cold-pressed), divided

1 teaspoon fennel seeds, plus extra for garnish

Crushed red chile flakes, to taste

1/8 teaspoon unrefined sea salt

1/4 teaspoon freshly ground black pepper

Choices/Exchanges 1/2 Starch, 1 Fat
Calories 80 | Calories from Fat 50
Total Fat 5g | Saturated Fat 1.0g | Trans Fat 0.0g
Cholesterol 0mg
Sodium 120mg

Potassium 90mg
Total Carbohydrate 6g | Dietary Fiber 2g | Sugars 1g
Protein 2g
Phosphorus 45mg

1. Place beans, onion, and bay leaf in a large saucepan. Cover with water and bring to a boil over high heat. Reduce heat to medium-low, cover, and cook until tender, approximately 1 hour.

2. Drain beans and place in a food processor with cheese, 1 tablespoon olive oil, and fennel seeds. Purée until smooth. Taste and season with crushed red chile flakes, salt, and pepper.

3. Spoon onto a serving platter and smooth out the top with a spatula. Drizzle with remaining 1 tablespoon olive oil, and sprinkle crushed red chile flakes and fennel seed on top, if desired.

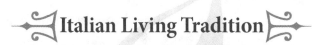

Italian Living Tradition

Many of Italy's most beloved dishes were created to honor and commemorate the lives of saints. In the Catholic faith, St. Joseph is known as the patron saint of the family, children, the Universal Church, and pastry chefs!

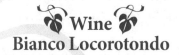

Wine
Bianco Locorotondo

PUGLIAN FAVA BEAN PURÉE WITH SAUTÉED CHICORY (FAVE E CICORIA PUGLIESE)

Serves: 6 | Serving Size: 1/3 cup
Prep Time: 5 minutes (plus bean-soaking time) | Cooking Time: 1 hour 10 minutes

Fava beans served with chicory is one of the most beloved traditional dishes of Italy's beautiful Puglia region, which is the most popular vacation destination in Italy for Italians. This version of the dish was shared with me by Puglian native chef Rocco Cartia, whose culinary skills have taken him to Australia and the U.S., and who is proud to prepare traditional, healthful foods from his homeland.

Puntarelle is an Italian word that means "little tips"; in the kitchen, the term is used to refer to a variety of Catalonian chicory that southern Italians enjoy in the winter months. When possible, use puntarelle in this recipe. If they are not available, regular chicory is a perfect substitute. If using puntarelle, be sure to remove the outer leaves in order to use the shoots. Note that the beans in this recipe need to be soaked prior to cooking. Serve with Whole-Wheat Country Loaves (page 220).

1/2 cup peeled, dried fava beans, soaked in cold water for a minimum of 2 hours or overnight

2 cups Catalonian chicory* or regular chicory, washed, trimmed, and cut in half

1 cup fresh fava beans, shelled

1/4 cup extra virgin olive oil (preferably first cold-pressed and Puglian), divided

1/8 teaspoon unrefined sea salt

*If using Catalonian chicory, be sure to remove the outer leaves in order to use the shoots. Reserve leaves for garnish, if desired.

Choices/Exchanges 1/2 Starch, 1 Vegetable, 2 1/2 Fat
Calories 140 | Calories from Fat 80
Total Fat 9g | Saturated Fat 1.3g | Trans Fat 0.0g
Cholesterol 0mg
Sodium 65mg

Potassium 220mg
Total Carbohydrate 10g | Dietary Fiber 4g | Sugars 1g
Protein 4g
Phosphorus 75mg

1. Drain and rinse the dried fava beans and place them in a pot. Cover with double the amount of water and add a pinch salt. Bring to boil over high heat, then reduce heat to low. Simmer uncovered, stirring occasionally, until tender, approximately 45 minutes. Remove from heat, drain, and allow to cool slightly.

2. In the meantime, place chicory in a saucepan and cover with water. Bring to a boil over high heat. Reduce the heat to low and simmer, uncovered, for 15 minutes.

3. Add the fresh fava beans to the saucepan and continue to simmer another 5 minutes. Remove from heat and drain. Pat dry, and let cool slightly.

4. Add the cooked dried fava beans, 2 tablespoons olive oil, and the salt to a food processor. Purée until smooth.

5. To serve, spoon fava bean purée onto the bottom of a plate. Top the purée with the cooked chicory and scatter the cooked fresh fava beans around the dish. Garnish with chicory leaves, if using Catalonian chicory, and drizzle with remaining 2 tablespoons olive oil.

Italian Living Tradition

Beans and greens are a classic combination that pleases both the palate and the figure. While this dish may have roots in the *cucina povera* (or "poor kitchen"), the fiber, iron, protein, and other nutrients in the dish make it fit for a king.

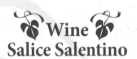

Wine
Salice Salentino

ROMAN-STYLE RICE AND HERB–STUFFED TOMATOES (POMODORI RIPIENI DI RISO ALLA ROMANA)

Serves: 4 | Serving Size: 1 tomato
Prep Time: 5 minutes | Cooking Time: 45 minutes

Stuffed tomatoes are one of the ultimate delicacies of the Roman diet and the pride of many home cooks—some of whom bake tiny, matchstick-size pieces of potato along with the tomatoes. Simple and delicious, they are a great accompaniment for grilled seafood and meat. Save this recipe for summer, when tomatoes are at their peak.

1/2 cup arborio rice or calrose rice

1 cup Homemade Chicken Stock (page 289), low-sodium chicken stock, or water

4 beefsteak tomatoes, approximately 6–8 ounces each

4 tablespoons extra virgin olive oil, divided

1/4 cup minced basil

1/4 cup minced mint

1/8 teaspoon unrefined sea salt

1/4 teaspoon freshly ground black pepper

Choices/Exchanges 1 1/2 Starch, 1 Vegetable, 2 1/2 Fat
Calories 250 | Calories from Fat 130
Total Fat 14g | Saturated Fat 2.0g | Trans Fat 0.0g
Cholesterol 0mg
Sodium 100mg

Potassium 505mg
Total Carbohydrate 28g | Dietary Fiber 3g | Sugars 5g
Protein 4g
Phosphorus 85mg

1. Preheat oven to 350°F.

2. Place rice and chicken stock in a saucepan. Bring to boil over a high heat. Cook, stirring constantly, for 20 minutes, or until rice is tender but firm (al dente). Add more water, 1/4 cup at a time, if rice begins to stick to the bottom of the pan. When rice is finished cooking, set aside.

3. Meanwhile, wipe off the tomatoes, discard the stem without damaging the skin, and lay the tomatoes stem side down. Cut a round slice from the side opposite to the stem; you will be using it as a lid. With a melon scoop, scrape out the flesh of the tomato, being careful not to break the skin. Reserve the pulp and the juice.

4. Chop the pulp and mix it with the juice (you can use a food processor). In a bowl, combine the pulp and juice with the rice, 3 tablespoons olive oil, basil, mint, salt, and pepper.

5. Stuff hollow tomatoes with the rice mixture. Cover with the tomato lids and arrange in a greased baking dish, standing the stuffed tomatoes with the lid side up. Drizzle with the remaining 1 tablespoon olive oil and bake for 20–30 minutes, or until the tomatoes are cooked through. Serve hot or at room temperature.

⊰ Italian Living Tradition ⊱

Roman and Italian cooks love using a variety of mint called *mentuccia* instead of *menta,* which is the word for regular mint. The English name for *mentuccia* is lesser calamint. I highly recommend growing some on your own. The beautiful shrub produces leaves with the aroma of both mint and oregano combined, and they are known to attract butterflies. *Mentuccia* is a wonderful addition to tomato- , vegetable- , and egg-based dishes. Regular mint, oregano, or a combination of the two are all perfect substitutions.

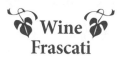

**Wine
Frascati**

STUFFED EGGPLANT
(MELANZANE RIPIENE)

Serves: 12 | Serving Size: 1 eggplant half
Prep Time: 10 minutes | Cooking Time: 50 minutes

I adapted this recipe from noted Puglian chef Rocco Cartia, who has the pleasure of cooking in beautiful masseria (farmhouses) and trulli (white stone huts with conical roofs) when he is in his homeland. His recipe calls for both eggplant and zucchini, but because I have a hard time finding zucchini that work well for this purpose in the U.S., I have decided to use only eggplant. Eggplants were introduced to Sicily by the Arabs in the 9th century. Although it took a while for them to grow in popularity, they are now one of the most popular vegetables in Italy. This is a great dish to make in advance, since resting allows the flavors of the sauce, olives, cheese, and seasonings to slowly seep into the dish.

6 small Italian eggplants (about 1 1/2 pounds total)

1/4 cup extra virgin olive oil, divided

2 medium yellow onions, diced, divided

4 cloves garlic, finely chopped

1 cup Fresh Tomato Sauce (page 228)

Crushed red chile flakes, to taste

1/4 cup black olives (such as gaeta or kalamata), pitted

1/4 cup grated parmigiano-reggiano cheese, divided

1 cup Fresh Bread Crumbs (page 291) or almond flour

Choices/Exchanges 1/2 Starch, 1 1/2 Vegetable, 2 Fat
Calories 160 | Calories from Fat 100
Total Fat 11g | Saturated Fat 1.9g | Trans Fat 0.0g
Cholesterol 0mg
Sodium 130mg

Potassium 220mg
Total Carbohydrate 14g | Dietary Fiber 3g | Sugars 4g
Protein 3g
Phosphorus 55mg

1. Preheat oven to 400°F.

2. Halve the eggplants lengthwise. Scoop out any seeds, then scoop out the flesh, leaving a 1/2-inch shell. Cut the eggplant flesh into small cubes. In a large nonstick skillet, over medium-high heat, heat 2 tablespoons olive oil. Brown the inside of the eggplant shells, cut side down, in the oil, about 2 minutes. Remove from skillet and place in an oiled baking dish, cut side up.

3. In the same skillet, heat the remaining 2 tablespoons olive oil. Add the eggplant flesh, onions, and garlic. Once the eggplant has begun to wilt, add the tomato sauce, crushed red chile flakes, and olives. Cook until the eggplant is tender but the tomatoes still retain their shape, about 5 minutes.

4. Scrape the eggplant/tomato mixture into a bowl, stir in 1/8 cup parmigiano-reggiano and the bread crumbs. Stuff the filling into the eggplant shells and top with the remaining 1/8 cup parmigiano-reggiano. Cover with foil and bake for 30 minutes. Uncover, and bake until the eggplant shells are tender and the top is browned, about 10–15 minutes more. Serve hot or at room temperature.

Italian Living Tradition

In southern Italy, being considered a good chef and/or a good wife depends on your creativity with eggplants. Since eggplants yield particularly large crops, are low in calories and have a low glycemic index, and are high in fiber, vitamins, and minerals, they are a great vegetable to experiment with.

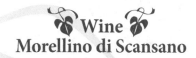

Wine
Morellino di Scansano

STUFFED PEPPERS
(PEPERONI RIPIENI)

Serves: 4 | Serving Size: 1 pepper
Prep Time: 15 minutes | Cooking Time: 30 minutes

This is one of those classic recipes that takes many Italians back to their childhood. While different versions abound, including peppers stuffed with rice and meat, this recipe uses a simple bread-crumb mixture as a filling. This filling also works well when stuffing tomatoes, artichokes, baby calamari, and zucchini blossoms.

1/2 cup Fresh Bread Crumbs (page 291)

2 tablespoons extra virgin olive oil, divided

1/4 cup finely chopped fresh parsley

2 tablespoons finely chopped fresh basil

4 anchovy fillets, drained, rinsed, and finely chopped

2 tablespoons freshly grated pecorino Romano cheese, divided

2 tablespoons pickled capers

2 cloves garlic, finely chopped

1/4 teaspoon freshly ground black pepper

4 red, green, or yellow bell peppers, tops cut off and reserved, seeds and pith removed

---

Choices/Exchanges 1/2 Starch, 1 Vegetable, 1/2 Lean Protein, 1 1/2 Fat

Calories 150 | Calories from Fat 80

Total Fat 9g | Saturated Fat 1.5g | Trans Fat 0.0g

Cholesterol 5mg

Sodium 220mg

Potassium 410mg

Total Carbohydrate 14g | Dietary Fiber 4g | Sugars 7g

Protein 5g

Phosphorus 80mg

1. Preheat oven to 350°F.

2. Place bread crumbs and 1 tablespoon olive oil in a medium bowl. Add the parsley, basil, anchovies, 1 tablespoon cheese, capers, and garlic, and mix well to combine. Season with pepper. Mix in the remaining 1 tablespoon olive oil to form a fairly soft paste.

3. Divide the mixture evenly among the 4 hollowed peppers (do not pack the mixture in too tightly) and top with the remaining 1 tablespoon cheese. Replace the top of each pepper, and place peppers in a baking dish that has been brushed with extra virgin olive oil.

4. Bake in the oven until peppers are tender, approximately 30 minutes. Serve hot or cold.

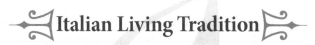

Italian Living Tradition

The use of anchovies in recipes as a condiment dates back to Roman times. In those days, salt was heavily taxed. One way people could avoid paying the tax on salt was to import salt-cured fish, such as anchovies, instead of salt. People began to flavor their foods with the salt-preserved fish. Over time, the complexity of flavors that the anchovies imparted to food was preferred to that of plain salt.

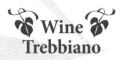

**Wine
Trebbiano**

LEMON-SCENTED SHRIMP
(GAMBERI AL LIMONE)

Serves: 4 | Serving Size: Approximately 4 ounces shrimp
Prep Time: 5 minutes | Cooking Time: 5 minutes

All of the bodies of water that border Italy—from the Adriatic to the Ionian, Mediterranean, and Tyrrhenian seas—contain multiple varieties of shrimp, making shrimp popular everywhere. If you've never prepared shrimp before, you'll be amazed at how easy it is. In my seafood cooking classes, I often tell students that, if they've had bad luck making shrimp in the past, it's because they're doing too much, not too little. The key to preparing good shrimp is choosing the freshest shrimp possible and cooking them just until done—not a second longer. Baby, regular, and jumbo shrimp all work in this recipe, so feel free to use whatever is freshest.

1 tablespoon extra virgin olive oil
1 pound shrimp, peeled and deveined
1/2 teaspoon kosher salt
1/4 teaspoon freshly ground black pepper
Crushed red chile flakes, to taste
Juice and zest from 1 lemon

Choices/Exchanges 2 1/2 Lean Protein, 1/2 Fat
Calories 130 | Calories from Fat 25
Total Fat 3g | Saturated Fat 0.0g | Trans Fat 0.0g
Cholesterol 140mg
Sodium 110mg

Potassium 245mg
Total Carbohydrate 1g | Dietary Fiber 0g | Sugars 0g
Protein 18g
Phosphorus 190mg

1. Heat olive oil in a large skillet over medium-high heat.

2. When olive oil begins to release its aroma, add shrimp, salt, black pepper, and crushed red chile flakes. Cook shrimp on one side just until the tail of the shrimp is bright pink, approximately 1–2 minutes.

3. Turn shrimp over and squeeze lemon juice over top. Cook shrimp until all gray color is gone and they are pink and cooked through, approximately 1–2 more minutes. At this point, shrimp should be coiled slightly tighter than when they were raw. Shrimp will continue to sizzle in the pan.

4. When they are cooked completely through, transfer shrimp to a serving platter, garnish with lemon zest, and serve immediately.

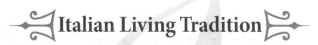

Italian Living Tradition

In addition to serving this as an appetizer, you can toss these shrimp into pasta with fresh parsley or add into a finished soup or salad. They also taste great on top of the Crostini with Chickpea Cream (page 10).

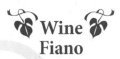

Wine
Fiano

ZUCCHINI CARPACCIO WITH GREEN PEPPERCORNS (CARPACCIO DI ZUCCHINE AL PEPE VERDE)

Serves: 8 | Serving Size: 1 cup
Prep Time: 15 minutes | Cooking Time: 0 minutes

This recipe borrows from the same tradition as the Vegetable and Parmesan Carpaccio (page 12). I suggest serving this dish as an appetizer along with a hearty soup or stew as a second course for an easy weeknight meal, or as one of several appetizers for an elegant dinner party. It tastes best in the summer when zucchini are in season. Black pepper can be substituted for green, if necessary.

2 medium zucchini (about 3/4 pound total)

1/8 teaspoon unrefined sea salt

1/4 teaspoon freshly cracked green pepper

2 tablespoons extra virgin olive oil
   (preferably first cold-pressed)

2 tablespoons finely chopped fresh chives

1 tablespoon good-quality balsamic vinegar

1 1/2 tablespoons grated parmigiano-reggiano
   cheese

1. Using a mandoline or very sharp knife, slice zucchini into very thin (1/32-inch rounds).

2. Overlap zucchini disks to form a single layer on a plate. Season with salt and pepper. Drizzle olive oil over the top and scatter with chives. Drizzle balsamic vinegar over the top, sprinkle with cheese, and serve immediately.

⊷ Italian Living Tradition ⊶

Green peppercorns, which are drupes of the pepper plant, are treated so they retain their green color. They are commonly used in a sauce for beef fillets and in this recipe to enhance the green color of the zucchini.

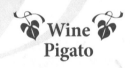

**Wine
Pigato**

Choices/Exchanges 1 Vegetable, 1 Fat
Calories 60 | Calories from Fat 50
Total Fat 5g | Saturated Fat 1.4g | Trans Fat 0.0g
Cholesterol 5mg
Sodium 115mg

Potassium 140mg
Total Carbohydrate 2g | Dietary Fiber 1g | Sugars 1g
Protein 3g
Phosphorus 55mg

FIRST COURSES
(PRIMI)

34   Tuscan Seafood Stew/*Cacciucco Livornese*

36   Pumpkin Soup/*Crema di zucca*

38   Chickpea Soup with Rosemary-Infused Shrimp/*Crema di ceci con gamberi*

40   Cannellini Bean Soup with Seafood/*Zuppa di fagioli con frutti di mare*

42   Cream of Chestnut Soup/*Crema di castagna*

44   Zucchini Soup with Crostini/*Zuppa di zucchini con crostini*

46   Rustic Lentil Soup/*Zuppa di lenticchie*

48   Holiday Minestrone/*Millecosedde*

50   Calabrian Wedding Soup/*Minestra maritata*

52   Sardinian Fava Bean Soup/*Zuppa di fave Sarda*

54   Barley, Chestnut, and White Bean Minestrone/*Minestra d'orzo, castagne, e cannellini*

56   Cannellini Bean, Tomato, and Orzo Soup/*Zuppa di cannellini e pomodoro con pasta di riso*

58   Farmhouse Vegetable and Farro Soup/*Zuppa di verdure e farro*

60   Roman-Style Broccoli and Pecorino Soup/*Zuppa di broccoletti*

62   Spaghetti Squash "Pasta" with Shrimp, Tomatoes, and Basil/*"Pasta" di zucca con gamberi, pomodori, e basilico*

64   Spinach Fettuccine with Walnut-Ricotta Pesto/*Fettuccine di spinaci con pesto di noci e ricotta*

66   Whole-Wheat Fusilli with Pesto and Cherry Tomatoes/*Fusilli con pesto e pomodori*

68   Whole-Wheat Orecchiette Pasta with Broccoli and Garlic/*Orecchiette integrale con broccoli*

70   Whole-Wheat Ziti with Goat Ragu/*Ziti integrale con ragù di capra*

72   Spaghetti with Fresh Tuna and Fennel/*Pasta con tonno e finocchio*

74   Pumpkin Risotto/*Risotto di zucca*

76   Venetian-Style Whole-Wheat Spaghetti with Sauce/*Bigoli in salsa*

78   Potato Gnocchi/*Gnocchi di patate*

80   Tuscan Buckwheat Pasta with Cheese, Potatoes, and Greens/*Pizzoccheri della Valtellina*

82   Red Pepper and Sweet Potato Gnocchi/*Gnocchi di peperoni rossi e patate dolce*

84   Turnip Gnocchi with Herb Sauce/*Gnocchi di rapa con salsa d'erbe*

86   Trapani-Style Almond Couscous/*Cuscus alla mandorla Trapanese*

"Chi mangia da solo si strozza in solitudine."
"Who eats alone strangles himself in loneliness."
—Italian proverb

The first course is the most integral part of the Italian meal. Italian cooks always decide on which pasta, risotto, or soup they are serving before they plan the other courses of their meal. This has a lot to do with the Italian meal structure and the importance placed on local, seasonal ingredients in Italy. Thanks to agricultural festivals called *sagre* (see page 159 in Side Dishes/*Contorni* for more information), Italians learn multitudes of ways to use seasonal vegetables.

Italian lunches are the main daily meal. Breakfast in Italy is simply something to end the fast from the night before and provide sustenance until lunch, which is usually eaten at 1:00 P.M. Dinner, which traditionally takes place at 8:00 P.M. or later, requires less food since it is closer to bedtime. Fortunately, this is also a healthy way of eating that translates well into diabetes-friendly lifestyles. The most popular first course for lunchtime is pasta, followed by risotto. Pasta courses weren't traditionally served for dinner, except during the Sunday meal or on holidays. Today, restaurant dining is changing these norms, especially in the U.S. Because most pasta dishes are substantial enough to stand alone, they (usually accompanied by a salad) make up the busy weekday lunches of modern Italians on the go. It is traditional to begin a home or restaurant dinner with a first course of soup, although soups may be enjoyed at other times as well.

Pasta

Whether they're quick, on-the-go lunches or the stars of a holiday meal, healthful Italian pasta recipes are a wonderful addition to anyone's cooking repertoire. Pasta is by far the crowning glory of the Italian kitchen. Throughout history, each province, region, town, and village (and sometimes even individual homes) has had its own fresh pasta recipes that were passed down from generation to generation. Fresh pasta made from quality grains and paired with fresh, seasonal produce, beans, legumes, and seafood can be part of a healthful lifestyle when eaten in moderation. Note that each recipe in this book is either gluten-free or includes a gluten-free ingredient substitution for those who are sensitive to gluten.

In Italy today, many types of pasta and cheese are on the verge of being forgotten. These important pieces of culinary patrimony must be carried forward by new generations in order to maintain Italian cultural identities and protect the traditional way of life, which has centered around the connection between humans and nature for millennia. The first written accounts of pasta date to the Shang Dynasty in China from 1700 to 1100 BCE (before Common Era). In approximately 1000 BCE, accounts of *laganon*, strips of pasta used as mortuary offerings, surfaced as did something called "pasta," which was actually a barley porridge.

In the 7th and 8th centuries BCE, the regions of Basilicata and Calabria were actually unified under

Magna Grecia or "Greater Greece"—colonies which were established by the Greeks in southern Italy. By the 8th century BCE, pasta was enjoyed in Magna Grecia. Due to its Greek heritage, it was called *lagane*, from the Greek name Laganon. *Lagane* pasta, which is flat, thin, and irregularly shaped, is traditionally served for important holidays and occasions, just as it was in ancient Greece. In modern-day Calabria and Basilicata, it is often paired with beans and eaten at harvest times and on St. Joseph's Day.

Often dismissed as *cucina povera* (which literally means "poor kitchen"), pasta and beans are much more dignified than one might think. It's important to remember that both wheat and legumes were forms of currency in antiquity, as opposed to the inexpensive, go-to pantry items that they are today. Not everyone could afford to eat them on a daily basis. One of the reasons that the ingredients were so expensive is the heavy taxes that were imposed on them. Wheat itself was taxed heavily in many areas of Italy in antiquity; milling wheat was even taxed all the way up until the 20th century in some areas. What this meant was that average people, mostly farmers and fishermen in southern Italy, could not afford the finely milled flour that is used to make today's pasta, nor could they always afford the wheat to make flour. As a result, pasta and wheat products were highly prized ingredients in the traditional Italian diet.

Gnocchi

Potatoes were introduced to Italy from the Americas along with peppers, corn, and tomatoes. In addition to serving them roasted and pan-fried, many Italians love to transform potatoes into the tender, puffy little dumplings known as gnocchi. Gnocchi recipes are especially popular in the cooler months due to their rib-sticking, starchy consistency. In addition to potatoes, many other ingredients, such as spinach, ricotta, pumpkins, turnips, and sweet potatoes, can be transformed into gnocchi. The variations on gnocchi offered in this chapter are delicious and perfect for the health-conscious reader, which means that "indulgence" doesn't need to be synonymous with "off-limits."

Risotto

"La storia del risotto e lungo quanto e il mondo."

"The history of risotto is as long as that of the world itself."
—Italian proverb

Italy is now the largest producer of rice in Europe. Rice is grown predominately in the regions of Lombardy, Piedmont, and Veneto. While arborio is the most widely known variety of Italian rice in the U.S., *carnaroli* and *vialone nano* are also very popular rice varieties in Italy. The short, stubby grains of Italian rice varieties are ideal for slowly absorbing liquid and maintaining a firm-to-the-bite texture. In order to master making risotto, one must learn how to make it *all'onda* or "by the wave," meaning that it will have a creamy, firm, yet fluid consistency that resembles the strong waves of the ocean.

Although I personally prefer pasta as my first course, when I test out an Italian restaurant or chef, I often order risotto because of the skill involved in preparing it and the fact that it is difficult to serve properly in a restaurant. Risotto should be served and enjoyed the minute it is finished cooking. Homemade stock must be added one ladleful at a time, at just the right moment, and slowly stirred into the rice until just the right texture is achieved. But don't be intimidated; while it may seem difficult, once a few simple steps are learned, risotto can be a delight to prepare and eat.

Risotto was once enjoyed only in the northern regions of Italy where rice grew. But thanks to the unification of Italy in the 19th century, the increased modes of transportation, as well as the expat community that introduced it to the rest of the world, risotto is now considered a mainstream "Italian" food.

Soups

Italians love soups! They are a hallmark of the *cucina casalinga,* or housewife's kitchen, which is the backbone of the modern Italian table. This book offers a variety of soup styles and flavors from all over Italy. In terms of healthy dishes, it's hard to beat a soup made with quality ingredients and homemade stock.

While I understand the time constraints that a modern cook has to face, I advise taking a few minutes to boil good-quality ingredients into a homemade stock and reserving it until you need it. This is probably the most important health and flavor tip in this book. Making homemade stock saves calories and money while lending nutrients and far more delicious flavor to your food. Italian cooks always keep stock on hand—not only for soups, but also to ladle into risottos, or to use to stew or braise meat in order to give it more flavor. Refer to How to Cook Like an Italian (page 279) to learn how to make your own stock.

In Italy, soups can be a light, elegant way to open an evening meal or large banquet. Some soup recipes in this book are thick and chock full of hearty beans, legumes, chestnuts, and pasta, while others are creamy, smooth purées that can take even leftover ingredients to new heights. Italian soups fall into three main categories—*minestre*, *zuppe*, and *creme*—and, in the Italian language, the correct terms are used to refer to each type of soup. For example, while *Crema di Castagna,* or Cream of Chestnut, would be called a soup in English, it would only be called a *crema* in Italian. Note that these three terms can end with either an "a" or an "e" depending on whether the term is singular or plural; ending in an "e" denotes the plural form of a feminine word in the Italian language.

Minestre

In Italy, a *minestra* is a thick soup made from a multitude of ingredients. The suffix "*-one*" on the end means that it is a "large or big" *minestra*, which explains why there are so many ingredients in *minestrone*.

Zuppe

A soup, in Italy, is something made from a clear stock–base with ingredients added to it. It's a rather "loose" soup, where the ingredients are perceivable and separate from the stock. A vegetable soup or consommé-type soup would fall into this category.

Creme

A *crema* was traditionally a thicker, cream-based soup. It always has a creamy, puréed texture. Nowadays, a *crema* may omit the actual cream for health reasons, but it should still have a luxurious, velvety mouth feel.

TUSCAN SEAFOOD STEW (CACCIUCCO LIVORNESE)

Serves: 8 | Serving Size: Approximately 1 cup
Prep Time: 15 minutes | Cooking Time: 1 hour

This recipe is said to be the ancestor of San Francisco's famous Cioppino stew. This version comes from the western Tuscan town of Livorno, located on the sparkling Ligurian Sea. When making fish soup, local fishermen would traditionally use the fish left behind after more valuable fish have sold. Use your favorite seafood combination to come up with the version of this dish you like best.

1/4 cup extra virgin olive oil
1 tablespoon minced parsley
1 tablespoon minced fresh sage leaves
1/2 teaspoon crushed red chile flakes
5 cloves garlic, minced
12 ounces calamari, cleaned and cut into 1-inch pieces
12 ounces baby octopus, cleaned, and cut into 1-inch pieces, if desired
1 tablespoon unsalted tomato paste
1 cup dry white wine
2 cups chopped fresh tomatoes, juice reserved
1/4 teaspoon freshly ground black pepper
1 cup Homemade Seafood Stock (page 288) or water
1 (1-pound) monkfish fillet, cut into 2-inch pieces
1 (1-pound) mullet or other white fish fillet, cut into 2-inch pieces
12 ounces large shell-on shrimp
12 ounces mussels, scrubbed and debearded

Choices/Exchanges 1/2 Starch, 6 1/2 Lean Protein
Calories 350 | Calories from Fat 110
Total Fat 12g | Saturated Fat 2.3g | Trans Fat 0.0g
Cholesterol 240mg
Sodium 340mg

Potassium 1110mg
Total Carbohydrate 8g | Dietary Fiber 1g | Sugars 2g
Protein 47g
Phosphorus 610mg

1. Heat oil in a 6-quart saucepan over medium heat. Add parsley, sage, chile flakes, and minced garlic, and cook until fragrant, about 1 minute. Add calamari and octopus and cook, stirring occasionally, until seafood is opaque, about 4 minutes. Add tomato paste, stir well, and cook until paste has darkened slightly, about 1 minute. Add wine and cook, stirring often, until the liquid has evaporated, about 20 minutes.

2. Add tomatoes along with their juice, season with pepper, and cook, stirring occasionally, until seafood is tender, about 10 minutes. Stir in stock, cover, and simmer for 10 minutes.

3. Add monkfish and cook, covered, until fish is just firm, about 5 minutes. Add mullet and shrimp to the pot, and scatter mussels over top. Cook, covered, without stirring (so as not to break up the seafood), until the mullet is just cooked through and the mussels have just opened, about 10 minutes.

4. Ladle stew into bowls and serve.

❖ Italian Living Tradition ❖

While variations of this soup abound, the common denominators to an authentic *cacciucco* are octopus, squid, tomatoes, wine, garlic, sage, and dried red chilies. Other types of fish can be added. In Italy, the soup must be served over toasted or grilled garlic-rubbed bread.

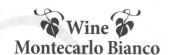

Wine
Montecarlo Bianco

PUMPKIN SOUP
(CREMA DI ZUCCA)

Serves: 6 | Serving Size: 1 cup
Prep Time: 5 minutes | Cooking Time: About 1 hour

In the Italian language, pumpkins, squash, and zucchini are all called a variation of the word zucca. *Pumpkin is most appreciated in the Friuli-Venezia Giulia region, where an annual festival is held in its honor. Throughout Italy, pumpkin is used to stuff ravioli and make soups, risottos, and many other sweet and savory recipes. Available in a wide range of green, orange, yellow, red, white, and gray hues, pumpkins are rich in vitamin A, fiber, and antioxidants. Consuming this nutritional powerhouse is believed to promote better vision and weight loss while reducing the risk of cancer and boosting immunity. Vegetable stock or water can be used instead of chicken stock in this recipe, if desired.*

6 cups Homemade Chicken Stock (page 289) or reduced-sodium chicken stock
1 teaspoon unrefined sea salt
4 cups pumpkin purée
1 medium yellow onion, diced
1 teaspoon finely chopped fresh thyme
1 clove garlic, minced
1/4 teaspoon freshly ground black pepper
1/2 cup low-fat plain yogurt
3 tablespoons freshly chopped parsley

Choices/Exchanges 1 1/2 Starch
Calories 130 | Calories from Fat 20
Total Fat 2g | Saturated Fat 1.0g | Trans Fat 0.0g
Cholesterol 0mg
Sodium 430mg

Potassium 685mg
Total Carbohydrate 21g | Dietary Fiber 5g | Sugars 10g
Protein 9g
Phosphorus 200mg

1. Combine stock, salt, pumpkin, onion, thyme, garlic, and pepper in a large pot. Bring to a boil over high heat. Reduce heat to low and simmer, uncovered, for 30 minutes.

2. Using a food processor (or blender with the center spout removed and the hole covered with a clean kitchen towel), purée the soup in 2 or 3 batches.

3. Return purée to pot and bring to a boil again over high heat. Reduce heat to low and simmer for another 30 minutes, covered. Stir in yogurt.

4. Ladle purée into soup bowls and garnish with fresh parsley.

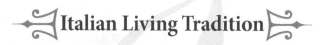

Italian Living Tradition

In Italy, creamy soups like this one are often enhanced by adding handfuls of cooked small pasta, leftover grilled vegetables, or freshly sautéed shrimp.

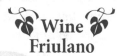

Wine
Friulano

CHICKPEA SOUP WITH ROSEMARY-INFUSED SHRIMP (*CREMA DI CECI CON GAMBERI*)

Serves: 4 | Serving Size: 1 cup
Prep Time: 5 minutes plus bean-soaking time
Cooking Time: 1 hour 5 minutes (dried beans) or 10 minutes (canned beans)

Chickpeas, shrimp, and rosemary might not seem like a natural flavor pairing to Americans, but in Italy it's a classic. Variations of this recipe can be found in almost every region, from Calabria to the Mediterranean island of Corsica, which is now under French control but has a long history of Italian influence. This recipe has been adapted from my Ultimate Mediterranean Diet Cookbook. *The combination of homemade stock, chickpeas, and shrimp with herbs make this soup sing!*

Chickpeas are a good source of protein, calcium, phosphorous, potassium, and magnesium. Consider adding them to salads, soups, pastas, rice, and couscous dishes—the way people in the Mediterranean region do—to take advantage of their health benefits.

1 cup dried chickpeas, soaked overnight, rinsed, and drained well OR
  1 (15-ounce) can chickpeas, drained and rinsed well
6 cups Homemade Seafood Stock (page 288)
1 medium yellow onion, thinly sliced
1 tablespoon extra virgin olive oil
1/2 pound shrimp, deveined
1/2 teaspoon chopped fresh rosemary
1 lemon, juiced (about 1/2 cup)
1/4 teaspoon freshly ground black pepper

Choices/Exchanges 1 1/2 Starch, 1 1/2 Lean Protein, 1 Fat
Calories 220 | Calories from Fat 50
Total Fat 6g | Saturated Fat 0.9g | Trans Fat 0.0g
Cholesterol 70mg

Sodium 440mg
Potassium 475mg
Total Carbohydrate 28g | Dietary Fiber 7g | Sugars 8g
Protein 15g
Phosphorus 260mg

1. Place chickpeas in a large saucepan or stock pot and add seafood stock and onion. Simmer, covered, on medium-low heat until chickpeas are tender (1 hour for dried chickpeas or approximately 5 minutes for canned).

2. Meanwhile, heat olive oil in a large skillet over medium-high heat. When olive oil begins to release its aroma, add shrimp and rosemary. Cook for 1–2 minutes per side, just until shrimp lose their gray color, begin to turn bright pink, and are cooked through. Remove from heat and set aside.

3. When chickpeas are tender, take them off the heat, drain (reserving cooking liquid), and place chickpeas and onions in blender. Add lemon juice and pepper. Blend well until a purée is formed.

4. Return mixture to pot. If soup is too thick, stir in a few tablespoons of the cooking liquid. Stir and simmer over low heat until ready to serve. Garnish soup with shrimp on top before serving.

❧Italian Living Tradition❧

I highly recommend making your own stock for this recipe; it gives the dish a light, clean taste. Homemade stock is delicious and easy to make, and it is a much more healthful alternative to sodium-laden, store-bought stocks.

If you don't have time to make homemade shrimp stock, you can substitute water or seafood stock in this recipe. You can also freeze the shrimp shells to make stock at a later time. If you choose to make homemade stock, it can be made ahead of time and frozen in a plastic container for up to a month. To defrost, place in a bowl in the refrigerator for 24 hours.

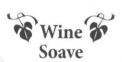

**Wine
Soave**

CANNELLINI BEAN SOUP WITH SEAFOOD (ZUPPA DI FAGIOLI CON FRUTTI DI MARE)

Serves: 10 | Serving Size: 1 cup
Prep Time: 10 minutes | Cooking Time: About 80 minutes

This recipe is based on a lighter, brodetto-style zuppa di pesce, a traditional fish soup, but I've added cannellini beans. This type of soup can be found all over Italy and is typically served with crusty bread. Each area has its own version, determined by the available fresh catches of the day. For maximum flavor, I highly recommend making your own stock and beans. However, canned varieties can be substituted, if necessary.

Stock

3 1/2 pounds fresh plum tomatoes, peeled, seeded, and diced (or passed through a food mill)

1 1/2 cups dry white wine

2 large leeks (white parts only), trimmed, cleaned, and cut into 3-inch pieces (about 2 cups)

2 medium carrots, trimmed and cut into thick slices

1 large onion, cut into thick slices

10 sprigs fresh thyme

Zest of 1/2 lemon, removed in wide strips with a vegetable peeler

1/2 teaspoon loosely packed saffron threads

1/4 cup extra virgin olive oil

Soup

1/4 cup extra virgin olive oil

1 large onion, thinly sliced

2 small leeks (white parts only), trimmed, cleaned, and cut into 1/2-inch slices (about 2 cups)

8 cloves garlic

2 medium calamari, cleaned, with tentacles left whole and bodies cut crosswise into 1/2-inch rings

9 medium dry scallops (about 1/4 pound)

1 pound fresh, firm-textured fish fillets (such as salmon, snapper, or swordfish), skin removed and cut into 1-inch pieces

2 cups cooked cannellini beans (dried beans cooked without salt; see Dried Beans recipe on page 283)

24 mussels (preferably cultivated), cleaned

12 large shrimp, peeled and deveined (about 1/2 pound)

1/4 teaspoon freshly ground black pepper

1/4 cup chopped fresh italian or flat-leaf parsley (for garnish)

Choices/Exchanges 1/2 Starch, 4 Vegetable, 3 1/2 Lean Protein, 1 Fat
Calories 340 | Calories from Fat 70
Total Fat 8g | Saturated Fat 1.3g | Trans Fat 0.0g
Cholesterol 140mg

Sodium 430mg
Potassium 1240mg
Total Carbohydrate 33g | Dietary Fiber 8g | Sugars 11g
Protein 30g
Phosphorus 440mg

1. To make the stock for the soup: In large saucepan over medium heat, combine 2 quarts water, plum tomatoes, wine, leeks, carrots, onion, thyme, lemon, and saffron, and bring to a boil. Reduce heat to low and simmer until reduced by about one-third, about 45 minutes. Stir 1/4 cup olive oil into the stock and continue to simmer until the liquid portion of the base is reduced to about 8 cups, about 20 minutes. Strain the stock into a 3-quart saucepan and keep it warm over low heat. Discard the solids. (The stock may be prepared up to 3 days in advance and refrigerated. If using refrigerated stock to make the soup, return the stock to a saucepan, bring it to a simmer over medium heat, then reduce heat to low and keep warm.)

2. To make soup: In a large (about 8-quart), heavy saucepot, add the olive oil and heat over medium heat about 1 minute. Add the thinly sliced onion, small leeks, and garlic. Sauté and stir until the onion is soft and golden, about 4 minutes. Add the calamari rings and cook, stirring, until they turn opaque, about 2 minutes. Pour in the hot soup base minus 1 cup, and bring to a boil.

3. Stir in the scallops, fish fillets, and beans. Reduce heat to low and simmer until the seafood is barely opaque at the center, about 5 minutes.

4. Meanwhile, add the mussels to the 1 cup soup base remaining in the saucepan. Increase the heat to high, cover the saucepan, and steam mussels over medium heat, shaking the pan occasionally, until the mussels open, about 3 minutes. Resist the urge to remove lid from the saucepan until cooking time is over. Discard any mussels that do not open on their own.

5. Stir the shrimp and steamed mussels into the large pot of soup. Simmer until the shrimp is cooked through, about 1 minute. Check the seasoning and add pepper.

6. Garnish with chopped parsley. Ladle soup into soup bowls and serve.

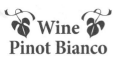

**Wine
Pinot Bianco**

CREAM OF CHESTNUT SOUP
(CREMA DI CASTAGNA)

Serves: 5 | Serving Size: 1 cup
Prep Time: 10 minutes | Cooking Time: 40 minutes

The scent of roasted chestnuts instantly transports me to Rome's Piazza Navona where, during the month of December, the La Befana festival takes place. Freshly roasted chestnuts are traditionally used in this soup, but since that is not an option for many, the jarred variety can be substituted. Despite the health virtues of this soup, it's the luxurious flavors and creamy texture that make it perfect for a family winter holiday. This recipe is easy enough to prepare anytime. You can make it up to 2 days ahead and store it covered in the refrigerator. Serve with Whole-Wheat Rolls (page 218), if desired.

2 tablespoons extra virgin olive oil

1 pound roasted or steamed jarred chestnuts

1 small carrot, peeled and coarsely chopped

1 stalk celery, coarsely chopped

1 small yellow onion, coarsely chopped

2 cloves garlic, sliced

4 cups Homemade Vegetable or Chicken Stock (pages 287, 289) or low-sodium chicken or vegetable stock

1 dried bay leaf

1 teaspoon fresh rosemary, minced OR 1/2 teaspoon dried thyme

1/8 teaspoon kosher salt

1/4 teaspoon freshly ground black pepper

Pinch cayenne (for garnish)

Choices/Exchanges 2 Starch, 1 1/2 Fat
Calories 220 | Calories from Fat 70
Total Fat 8g | Saturated Fat 1.4g | Trans Fat 0.0g
Cholesterol 10mg
Sodium 140mg

Potassium 910mg
Total Carbohydrate 32g | Dietary Fiber 1g | Sugars 2g
Protein 6g
Phosphorus 160mg

1. Heat oil in a large saucepan over medium heat. Add chestnuts, carrot, celery, and onion, stirring to mix well. Sauté until tender, about 7 minutes. Stir in garlic.

2. Add the stock to the vegetables, increase heat to high, and bring to a boil. Reduce heat to medium-low and add bay leaf, rosemary or thyme, salt, and pepper. Simmer, covered, for 20–30 minutes, or until vegetables are tender.

3. Ladle 1/3 of the mixture into 5 serving bowls. Purée the remainder of the soup in a food processor fitted with a metal blade (carefully remove the core of the lid, and cover it with a kitchen towel, so that mixture will not burst out). Process for 20 seconds.

4. Pour the purée over the soup mixture already in the bowls. Sprinkle with cayenne pepper and serve hot.

Italian Living Tradition

La Befana, or the "Italian Witch," as she is sometimes called, originated in pre-Christian Rome. This good witch was thought to sweep away all of the problems from the old year with her broom. When Christmas began to be celebrated in Italy, the lore of this witch was fused with the celebration of Epiphany. Each year, on January 6, she is said to visit the homes of all children (like Santa Claus) and leave them candy and sweets if they're good or coal if they're bad. Today the La Befana festival is celebrated yearly in many Italian cities from December through the Epiphany. It's like a winter version of a state fair with roasted chestnuts, candies, mimes, children's games, inexpensive gifts, and more.

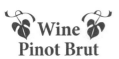

**Wine
Pinot Brut**

ZUCCHINI SOUP WITH CROSTINI (ZUPPA DI ZUCCHINI CON CROSTINI)

Serves: 6 | Serving Size: Approximately 1 1/4 cups
Prep Time: 5 minutes | Cooking Time: 30 minutes

I prepare this soup all summer long—as soon as fresh zucchini are available in the market. I enjoy it because it's a light, broth-based soup, but the cheese, yogurt, basil, and crostini give it texture and rich flavor. You can also serve this soup puréed and/or at room temperature.

1/4 cup extra virgin olive oil

6 medium zucchini, washed and finely diced

6 cups Homemade Chicken Stock (page 289)
   OR 3 cups reduced-sodium chicken stock mixed with 3 cups water

1/8 teaspoon unrefined sea salt

1/4 teaspoon freshly ground black pepper

1 tablespoon freshly chopped mint

1 tablespoon freshly chopped basil

1/2 cup freshly grated pecorino or parmigiano-reggiano cheese, divided

2 tablespoons plain yogurt

6 very thin slices italian baguette, toasted on both sides until golden

---

Choices/Exchanges 1/2 Starch, 2 Vegetable,
1/2 Medium-Fat Protein, 2 Fat
Calories 210 | Calories from Fat 120
Total Fat 13g | Saturated Fat 3.0g | Trans Fat 0.0g
Cholesterol 10mg

Sodium 300mg
Potassium 675mg
Total Carbohydrate 17g | Dietary Fiber 3g | Sugars 5g
Protein 10g
Phosphorus 205mg

1. Heat the olive oil in a large saucepan over medium heat. Add the zucchini, stir, and cook until golden, approximately 3–5 minutes. Add the stock, and season with salt and pepper.

2. Cover the saucepan, reduce heat to medium-low, and cook until zucchini is tender, approximately 20–30 minutes. Remove from heat.

3. In a small bowl, combine the mint, basil, 2 tablespoons cheese, and yogurt. Whisk well to combine. Slowly pour the yogurt mixture into the hot soup, whisking constantly.

4. Place a slice of bread in the bottom of each individual soup bowl. Ladle the soup over the bread. Sprinkle with remaining cheese and serve.

⊷❖ Italian Living Tradition ❖⊷

This is a very versatile recipe because many seasonal ingredients, such as carrots, potatoes, and mushrooms, can be used in place of the zucchini. The soup can be served as is, puréed into a creamy version, or prepared by puréeing half of the ingredients and leaving the other half whole for a unique texture.

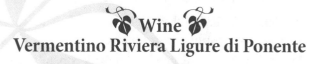

🍃 Wine 🍃
Vermentino Riviera Ligure di Ponente

RUSTIC LENTIL SOUP
(ZUPPA DI LENTICCHIE)

Serves: 6 | Serving Size: 1 cup
Prep Time: 5 minutes | Cooking Time: Approximately 1 hour 15 minutes

During ancient times, Egyptians were the chief exporters of lentils in the world. Since lentils were traded as currency and their shape is reminiscent of small coins, they are often associated with wealth. Italians like to serve lentils during New Year's celebrations to wish guests and themselves a prosperous, healthy new year. I like to serve this soup with Ricotta, Grilled Eggplant, and Fresh Mint Bruschetta (page 8), but any combination of toasted bread and melted cheese would be delicious with this soup.

1 teaspoon extra virgin olive oil

2 carrots, diced

1 onion, diced

2 stalks celery, diced

1 cup brown lentils, rinsed and sorted

1/8 teaspoon unrefined sea salt

1/4 teaspoon freshly ground black pepper

4 cups Homemade Chicken or Vegetable Stock (pages 289, 287) or reduced-sodium vegetable or chicken stock

2 cups Fresh Tomato Sauce (page 228)

1/4 cup plus 2 tablespoons freshly chopped flat-leaf parsley

2 tablespoons parmigiano-reggiano or pecorino Romano cheese

Choices/Exchanges 2 Starch, 2 Lean Protein
Calories 240 | Calories from Fat 45
Total Fat 5g | Saturated Fat 1.3 g | Trans Fat 0.0g
Cholesterol 5mg
Sodium 170mg

Potassium 850mg
Total Carbohydrate 37g | Dietary Fiber 13g | Sugars 10g
Protein 14g
Phosphorus 250mg

1. Heat olive oil in a large saucepan over medium heat. Add carrots, onion, and celery. Sauté until vegetables are translucent, about 3–5 minutes. Stir and add lentils. Cook for 1 minute, and season with salt and pepper.

2. Add stock, tomato sauce, and 1/4 cup parsley. Stir and increase the heat to high. When the stock begins to boil, reduce heat to medium-low and stir. Cover and allow to simmer 45 minutes to 1 hour, or until lentils are tender.

3. Place half of the lentil mixture into a blender or food processor (be sure to remove the cap from the center spout and cover it with a clean kitchen towel to prevent mixture from bursting out). Purée for a few minutes until smooth. Or use an immersion blender to blend half of the mixture until smooth.

4. Return the purée to the pot with the rest of the lentils. Cook over medium heat for an additional 10 minutes. Garnish with remaining parsley and the cheese, and serve.

Italian Living Tradition

Make large batches of Rustic Lentil Soup and freeze single servings in individual containers. That way you'll have a nutritious alternative to canned soup on hand whenever you need it.

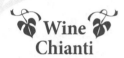

**Wine
Chianti**

HOLIDAY MINESTRONE (MILLECOSEDDE)

Serves: 6 | Serving Size: 1 cup
Prep Time: 10–15 minutes (plus mushroom-soaking time)
Cooking Time: About 2 hours 10 minutes

Many cultures have a New Year's Eve recipe that incorporates leftover pantry items into one fabulous dish, such as Korean Bibimbap. In my ancestral homeland of Calabria, that dish is this soup, called millecosedde *or* millecuselle, *meaning "a thousand little things." I once prepared this soup for an event called "Sacred Foods of Italy" with the Washington, D.C., chapter of Les Dames d'Escoffier and the U.S. Department of State's American Chef Corps at Al Tiramisu restaurant in Washington, D.C.*

1/4 cup dried cannellini beans

1/4 cup dried chickpeas

1/4 cup dried borlotti (cranberry) beans

2 tablespoons extra virgin olive oil

1 stalk celery, diced

1 carrot, diced

1 large yellow onion, diced

2 cloves garlic, finely diced

1/4 cup dried porcini mushrooms, soaked in water for 20 minutes, drained, and rinsed

1/2 pound boxed chopped tomatoes or reduced-sodium diced tomatoes

2 cups chopped savoy cabbage

1/4 cup brown lentils, rinsed and sorted

1/2 teaspoon unrefined sea salt

1/4 teaspoon freshly ground black pepper

3 cups Homemade Chicken or Vegetable Stock (pages 289, 287), reduced-sodium stock, or water

1/2 teaspoon crushed red chile flakes

8 ounces ditalini or gluten-free pasta

Choices/Exchanges 2 Starch, 1 Vegetable, 2 Lean Protein, 1 Fat
Calories 240 | Calories from Fat 50
Total Fat 6g | Saturated Fat 1.0g | Trans Fat 0.0g
Cholesterol 0mg

Sodium 260mg
Potassium 80mg
Total Carbohydrate 37g | Dietary Fiber 10g | Sugars 5g
Protein 13g
Phosphorus 210mg

1. Combine cannellini beans, chickpeas, and borlotti beans in a large pot. Top with enough water to cover plus 2 inches. Bring to a boil, uncovered, over high heat and boil rapidly for 5 minutes. Remove from the heat, cover, and let stand for 1 hour.

2. Add olive oil to a large, heavy-bottomed saucepan or dutch oven over medium heat. Add celery, carrot, onion, and garlic. Sauté until golden, approximately 5 minutes. Stir in mushrooms and sauté for another 2–3 minutes. Add tomatoes, cabbage, lentils, salt, and pepper. Stir and simmer for 5 minutes.

3. Drain the beans, rinse with cold water, and add to the vegetable mixture along with stock or water and the crushed red chile flakes. Bring to a boil over high heat, then reduce heat to medium-low and simmer, covered, for 40 minutes.

4. Add pasta and cook until pasta is done and beans are tender, approximately 10 more minutes. Serve hot.

❧‖Italian Living Tradition‖❧

Stocking your pantry with dried beans and lentils, porcini mushrooms, good-quality tuna, preserved vegetables, olives, and healthful grains makes putting together a nutritious meal easy; it's faster and more delicious than ordering delivery.

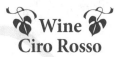

**Wine
Ciro Rosso**

CALABRIAN WEDDING SOUP
(MINESTRA MARITATA)

Serves: 8 | Serving Size: 1 1/2 cups
Prep Time: 15 minutes | Cooking Time: 35 minutes

This soup is called "married soup" in Italy. Hailing from Calabria and neighboring regions, the soup gets its name from the marriage of vegetables, grains, and meat products. Over the years, it actually became a popular wedding dish known as Minestra di sposalizio. *Even the ancient Roman Epicurian Apicius offered versions of it in his cookbook.*

The original versions of this soup combine kale with tiny round pasta (known as pastina), *which is one of the first foods Italian children eat. For a gluten-free version of this dish, substitute quinoa for the pastina. If you cannot find escarole, kale, spinach, or cabbage may be used. Other meats, such as veal, lamb, or even goat, can be used instead of the beef in the meatballs. Many modern cooks incorporate leftover roasted chicken meat along with the other ingredients into this recipe. I highly recommend using homemade chicken stock for best results.*

Soup

9 cups Homemade Chicken Stock (page 289)

1 pound escarole, kale, or cabbage, coarsely chopped

2 stalks celery, trimmed and diced

2 carrots, diced

1 large fresh or canned tomato, chopped

1 medium onion, diced

1/2 teaspoon unrefined sea salt

8 ounces pastina, cooked until al dente
OR 1 cup cooked quinoa

1/4 cup freshly grated pecorino Crotonese (see Where to Buy Guide) or pecorino Romano cheese

Meatballs

1/2 cup dry bread cubes, drizzled with 1/4 cup skim milk, drained, and squeezed of excess liquid

3/4 pound very lean ground beef (85% lean)

1 egg, lightly beaten

2 tablespoons fresh parsley or basil, finely chopped

1/2 teaspoon unrefined sea salt

1/4 teaspoon freshly ground black pepper

Pinch crushed red chile flakes (preferably Calabrian; see Where to Buy Guide)

Choices/Exchanges 1/2 Starch, 2 Vegetable, 2 Lean Protein, 1 Fat
Calories 240 | Calories from Fat 100
Total Fat 11g | Saturated Fat 3.8g | Trans Fat 0.0g
Cholesterol 55mg

Sodium 450mg
Potassium 860mg
Total Carbohydrate 19g | Dietary Fiber 4g | Sugars 4g
Protein 20g
Phosphorus 305mg

1. In a large stock pot, bring stock to a boil, uncovered, over high heat. Reduce heat to medium-low. Add escarole, celery, carrots, tomato, and onion to the pot. Season with salt. Cover and simmer for 15 minutes.

2. Meanwhile, make the meatballs by combining all of the meatball ingredients in a large bowl. Mix well with hands to thoroughly combine. Shape mixture into uniform 1/2-inch meatballs and set on a clean baking sheet or cutting board.

3. Add meatballs to the stock pot, stir, cover, and cook for approximately 15 minutes, or until meatballs are cooked through. Add the cooked pasta, and stir. Cook for an additional 5 minutes.

4. Sprinkle with pecorino cheese and serve.

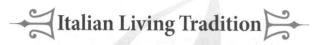

Italian Living Tradition

When I was growing up, knowing how to prepare this soup was synonymous with being an expert in the kitchen. Preparation of this soup is an almost sacred tradition in Calabria. At one time, this soup was prepared every Holy Monday and was made in a traditional clay pot called a *pignata*. It is impossible to reproduce the exact taste of the *pignata*-prepared soup today, partly because the clay pots were placed in coal-burning ovens, covered with ashes, and allowed to cook very slowly in order to produce maximum flavor.

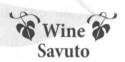

Wine
Savuto

SARDINIAN FAVA BEAN SOUP
(ZUPPA DI FAVE SARDA)

Serves: 6 | Serving Size: 1 cup
Prep Time: 10 minutes (plus bean-soaking time) | Cooking Time: 1 hour

This vegan-friendly, Mediterranean soup comes from the Italian island of Sardinia, known for its unique cuisine. Sardinia is considered to be a "blue zone," boasting a high number of people who live to be over 100 years old, and the diet of Sardinia is one of the healthiest, and most delicious, around.

The fava beans used in this soup are one of the world's oldest agricultural crops. If you are buying them for the first time, specifically for this recipe, keep in mind that they can also be used for the Puglian Fava Bean Purée with Sautéed Chicory recipe (page 18) or to make traditional Egyptian falafel. Regular yogurt is used in this recipe, but in Sardinia this soup would be made with sheep or goat's milk, or a combination of the two. Note that the beans need to be soaked overnight.

1/4 cup extra virgin olive oil, plus extra for drizzling

1 large yellow onion, diced

4 cloves garlic, minced

1 teaspoon fennel seeds, crushed

1/2 cup raw almonds, toasted and finely chopped, divided

1 sun-dried tomato

2 cups dried, shelled fava beans (see Where to Buy Guide), sorted, rinsed, soaked overnight covered with 4 inches hot water, and drained

1/8 teaspoon unrefined sea salt

1/4 teaspoon freshly ground black pepper

1/2 cup nonfat plain yogurt

1/4 cup finely chopped fresh mint or parsley

Choices/Exchanges 1 Starch, 1 Lean Protein, 2 Fat
Calories 200 | Calories from Fat 140
Total Fat 15g | Saturated Fat 1.8g | Trans Fat 0.0g
Cholesterol 0mg
Sodium 90mg

Potassium 300mg
Total Carbohydrate 12g | Dietary Fiber 4g | Sugars 3g
Protein 6g
Phosphorus 135mg

1. Heat oil in a large stock pot over medium heat. Add the onion, cover, and cook until soft, about 5 minutes. Add the garlic, fennel seeds, half the almonds, and the sun-dried tomato. Cook 1 minute.

2. Add the beans and 6 cups water, and stir to combine. Bring to a boil over high heat. Reduce the heat to low, cover partially, and simmer until the beans are falling apart, about 45 minutes to 1 hour. Taste, and season with salt and pepper.

3. Remove the sun-dried tomato from the pot, let it cool slightly, and then cut into thin strips.

4. Using an immersion blender (or regular blender with center spout removed and the hole covered with a clean kitchen towel), purée the bean mixture, working in batches if necessary, until smooth. If the soup seems too thin, return to the stove and continue simmering, uncovered, until it reduces. If it is too thick, add water 1/4 cup at a time, stirring, until you achieve the desired consistency.

5. Serve soup warm. Top each bowl with a spoonful of yogurt and a splash of olive oil. Garnish with the remaining chopped almonds, sun-dried tomato strips, and herbs.

Italian Living Tradition

Beans are an important staple ingredient throughout Italy. Packed with protein and fiber, they are integral to the Mediterranean diet. See How to Cook like an Italian (page 279) to learn how to properly cook a variety of beans Italian style.

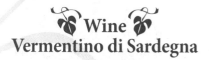

Wine
Vermentino di Sardegna

BARLEY, CHESTNUT, AND WHITE BEAN MINESTRONE (*MINESTRA D'ORZO, CASTAGNE, E CANNELLINI*)

Serves: 6 | Serving Size: 1 cup
Prep Time: 10 minutes | Cooking Time: 30 minutes

When Americans hear the word minestrone, *a tomato broth–based soup chock-full of meat, vegetables, and pasta usually comes to mind. In Italy, however, the word* minestra *refers to a thick soup of almost porridge-like consistency that includes various grains, beans, and vegetables. The addition of the suffix* -one *to the word* minestra *means a "bigger* minestra," *and this type of soup usually contains meat or other ingredients to make it extra hearty.*

Many Italian regions, such as Valle d'Aosta, Basilicata, and Calabria, hold annual chestnut festivals where scores of these delectable treats are prepared in too many ways to count. I love the homey combination of warm barley, chestnuts, and beans in this recipe. You can use canned cannellini beans in this recipe if you'd like, but be sure to rinse and drain them first. Serve this soup in the winter and let the hearty flavors warm you.

2 tablespoons extra virgin olive oil

1/2 cup finely chopped peeled chestnuts

1 cup diced savoy cabbage

1/2 cup medium diced yellow onion

1/2 cup sliced carrot (1/4-inch-thick slices)

1/4 cup medium diced celery

2 cloves garlic, minced

1 quart Homemade Chicken or Vegetable Stock (pages 289, 287) or low-sodium stock

8 ounces reduced-sodium canned or boxed diced tomatoes, juices reserved

1/4 cup pearl barley, rinsed

1 large sprig fresh rosemary

1 (2-inch) square parmigiano-reggiano cheese rind (optional)

1/8 teaspoon unrefined sea salt

1/2 cup cooked cannellini beans (see Dried Beans recipe on page 283)

1/4 teaspoon freshly ground black pepper

1/4 cup freshly grated parmigiano-reggiano cheese (for garnish)

Choices/Exchanges 1 1/2 Starch, 2 Vegetable, 1 1/2 Fat
Calories 230 | Calories from Fat 70
Total Fat 8g | Saturated Fat 1.8g | Trans Fat 0.0g
Cholesterol 5mg
Sodium 220mg

Potassium 590mg
Total Carbohydrate 33g | Dietary Fiber 4g | Sugars 3g
Protein 9g
Phosphorus 170mg

1. Heat the oil in a heavy, 6-quart (or larger) pot over medium heat. Add the chestnuts, cabbage, onion, carrot, celery, and garlic. Cook, stirring frequently, until the vegetables begin to soften, about 6 minutes.

2. Add the broth, tomatoes with their juices, barley, rosemary, parmigiano rind (if using), salt, cannellini beans, and 1 cup water. Bring to a boil over high heat. Then reduce the heat to a simmer and cook until the barley and vegetables are tender, about 20 minutes. Discard the rosemary sprigs and parmigiano rind. Season soup with pepper.

3. Serve the soup sprinkled with the grated parmigiano-reggiano.

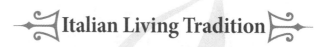

Italian Living Tradition

Leftover remnants of rind from cheese are popular additions to soups and sauces in Italy. Slowly simmering the rind in liquid adds rich flavor and saltiness to recipes.

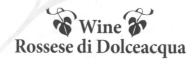

Wine
Rossese di Dolceacqua

CANNELLINI BEAN, TOMATO, AND ORZO SOUP (ZUPPA DI CANNELLINI E POMODORO CON PASTA DI RISO)

Serves: 6 | Serving Size: 2/3 cup
Prep Time: 5 minutes | Cooking Time: 20 minutes

This hearty and succulent soup is my father's favorite. It offers the flavor of a recipe that spent the entire day simmering on the stove, but without the effort! My favorite way to make tomato soup is to start with a traditional Italian tomato sauce as a base (see the recipe for Fresh Tomato Sauce on page 228). In a pinch, you can use a good-quality, low-sodium jarred tomato sauce to make this recipe; however, this soup is so easy to make, there's really no need for jarred sauce. For a real treat, serve with Homemade Bread with Mother Yeast from Molise (page 216).

1 tablespoon extra virgin olive oil
3 cloves garlic, minced
1 cup Fresh Tomato Sauce (page 228)
1/8 teaspoon kosher salt
1/4 teaspoon freshly ground black pepper
1/4 cup freshly chopped flat-leaf parsley or basil
3 cups Homemade Vegetable or Chicken Stock (pages 287, 289)
   or reduced-sodium vegetable or chicken stock
1 (15.5-ounce) can reduced-sodium cannellini beans, drained and rinsed
1/2 cup orzo or other small gluten-free pasta or rice
1/4 cup grated pecorino Romano cheese

Choices/Exchanges 1 Starch, 3 Vegetable, 1 Lean Protein, 1 Fat
Calories 240 | Calories from Fat 50
Total Fat 6g | Saturated Fat 1.6g | Trans Fat 0.0g
Cholesterol 5mg

Sodium 150mg
Potassium 590mg
Total Carbohydrate 37g | Dietary Fiber 5g | Sugars 4g
Protein 11g
Phosphorus 165mg

1. Heat oil in a large saucepan over medium heat. Add garlic and sauté until it releases its aroma. Add tomato sauce, salt, pepper, and parsley or basil. Increase heat to high and bring to a boil.

2. Reduce heat to low and stir in stock and cannellini beans. Bring to a boil, uncovered, over high heat.

3. Reduce heat to low, stir in orzo, and cook 10–15 minutes until pasta is al dente.

4. Garnish with cheese and serve hot.

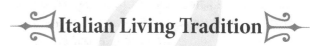

Italian Living Tradition

In Italy, the rinds of hard cheeses like Parmesan and Romano are added to soups and stews while cooking to give them extra flavor. People buy blocks of cheese, grate it themselves, and reserve the rinds for this reason. If you have rinds at home, you could substitute them for the grated cheese in this recipe. If you prefer not to grate your own cheese, many specialty food stores now sell rinds alone. If you don't see them, ask the person at the cheese counter. A little bit of aged, flavorful cheese rind goes a long way! Just be sure to remove the rind before serving.

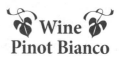

**Wine
Pinot Bianco**

FARMHOUSE VEGETABLE AND FARRO SOUP
(ZUPPA DI VERDURE E FARRO)

Serves: 6 | Serving Size: 1 cup
Prep Time: 15 minutes | Cooking Time: 45 minutes

The now-fashionable grain farro has been enjoyed for millennia in Italy. Farro is a generic Italian term for hulled wheat, but it usually refers to hulled emmer wheat or spelt. For a gluten-free version of this soup, use barley instead of farro. You can use canned cannellini beans in this recipe if you'd like, but be sure to rinse and drain the beans first.

2 teaspoons extra virgin olive oil

1 cup chopped onion

1 cup chopped leek

1/2 cup chopped carrot

3 cloves garlic, minced

3/4 cup uncooked farro, rinsed and drained

1/2 teaspoon salt

1/2 teaspoon freshly ground black pepper

2 cups Homemade Chicken or Vegetable Stock (pages 289, 287)
   OR 1 (14.5-ounce) can reduced-sodium chicken stock

2 bay leaves

1 sprig thyme

2 cups chopped baby spinach

2 cups cooked cannellini beans (see Dried Beans recipe on page 283)

1 (14.5-ounce) can reduced-sodium diced tomatoes, undrained

1/4 cup (1 ounce) grated parmigiano-reggiano cheese

Choices/Exchanges 1 1/2 Starch, 4 Vegetable, 1/2 Fat
Calories 230 | Calories from Fat 25
Total Fat 3g | Saturated Fat 0.8g | Trans Fat 0.0g
Cholesterol 0mg
Sodium 180mg

Potassium 815mg
Total Carbohydrate 42g | Dietary Fiber 8g | Sugars 6g
Protein 13g
Phosphorus 230mg

1. Heat oil in dutch oven over medium-high heat. Add onion, leek, carrot, and garlic. Sauté for 5 minutes, stirring frequently.

2. Stir in 2 cups water, farro, salt, pepper, stock, bay leaves, and thyme, and bring to a boil. Cover, reduce heat, and simmer for 30 minutes.

3. Add spinach, beans, and tomatoes, and bring to a boil. Reduce heat and simmer for 5 minutes. Discard bay leaves and serve. Garnish each serving with cheese.

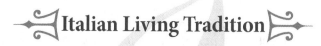

Italian Living Tradition

In addition to being used in soups, cooked farro can be cooled and tossed into salads or mixed with cooked vegetables for a side dish. One of my favorite ways to serve it is tossed with pesto sauce, slightly blanched string beans, and cherry tomatoes.

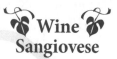

Wine
Sangiovese

ROMAN-STYLE BROCCOLI AND PECORINO SOUP (*ZUPPA DI BROCCOLETTI*)

Serves: 6 | Serving Size: 1 cup
Prep Time: 10 minutes | Cooking Time: 25 minutes

Italians first introduced broccoli to Americans in the early part of the 20th century; it wasn't widely used in America before then. In Italy, however, it was a popular ancient Roman ingredient. Nowadays, many varieties are available, the most common being Calabrese broccoli, which originally came from Calabria. In Rome, this soup might be made with broccoletti, smaller broccoli, which we call "broccolini" in the U.S. I enjoy this recipe with all varieties of broccoli.

4 tablespoons extra virgin olive oil
1 1/2 pounds fresh broccoli or broccolini
1 large onion, chopped
1 carrot, peeled, trimmed, and chopped
1/2 teaspoon unrefined sea salt
1/4 teaspoon freshly ground black pepper
3 tablespoons all-purpose flour
4 cups Homemade Chicken Stock or Vegetable Stock (pages 289, 287)
  or low-sodium chicken or vegetable stock
1/4 cup nonfat plain yogurt
1 cup Homemade Croutons (page 292)

Choices/Exchanges 1/2 Starch, 2 Vegetable, 2 1/2 Fat
Calories 210 | Calories from Fat 120
Total Fat 13g | Saturated Fat 2.0g | Trans Fat 0.0g
Cholesterol 0mg
Sodium 280mg

Potassium 600mg
Total Carbohydrate 18g | Dietary Fiber 4g | Sugars 5g
Protein 8g
Phosphorus 160mg

1. Heat olive oil in a heavy-bottomed Dutch oven or saucepan over medium-high heat. Add broccoli, onion, carrot, salt, and pepper. Sauté, stirring occasionally, until onion is translucent, approximately 5 minutes.

2. Add the flour, stir, and cook for another minute, until the flour takes on a golden hue. Add stock, increase heat to high, and bring to a boil. Reduce heat to medium-low and simmer, uncovered, until broccoli is tender, approximately 15 minutes.

3. With an immersion blender (or in a blender with the center spout removed and the hole covered with a clean kitchen towel), purée the soup. Return to saucepan and stir in yogurt.

4. Serve hot and garnish with croutons.

Italian Living Tradition

While the quality and freshness of broccoli probably seem unimportant to most, freshly picked, organic broccoli has a much more intense flavor than the broccoli that is available at the supermarket. Look for fresh, organic broccoli when it is in season in your area and try purchasing it from a local farmers' market or farm. Rich in vitamins A and C, calcium, folate, and iron, sautéed broccoli is a great addition to your favorite pasta and frittata recipes.

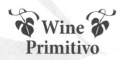

**Wine
Primitivo**

SPAGHETTI SQUASH "PASTA" WITH SHRIMP, TOMATOES, AND BASIL ("PASTA" DI ZUCCA CON GAMBERI, POMODORI, E BASILICO)

Serves: 4 | Serving Size: 1 cup
Prep Time: 15 minutes | Cooking Time: 1 hour 15 minutes

While spaghetti squash is hardly a grain, its tender strands do resemble golden noodles. Doling it out like pasta allows its naturally sweet taste to shine through. An added bonus: it's gluten-free!

1 (approximately 3 1/2-pound) spaghetti squash, halved and seeded

1/4 cup extra virgin olive oil, divided

1 pound shrimp, any size, peeled and deveined

2 tablespoons freshly squeezed lemon juice

1 1/2 pints cherry or grape tomatoes, halved

4 cloves garlic, minced

1/8 teaspoon unrefined sea salt

1/4 teaspoon freshly ground black pepper

6 fresh basil leaves, finely chopped

4 tablespoons finely chopped fresh flat-leaf parsley

Choices/Exchanges 1 Starch, 4 Vegetable, 3 Lean Protein, 2 Fat

Calories 380 | Calories from Fat 150

Total Fat 17g | Saturated Fat 2.5g | Trans Fat 0.0g

Cholesterol 180mg

Sodium 290mg

Potassium 1240mg

Total Carbohydrate 37g | Dietary Fiber 9g | Sugars 16g

Protein 27g

Phosphorus 345mg

1. Preheat oven to 425°F.

2. Line a 15 × 10 × 1/2-inch baking pan with aluminum foil. Brush the cut surface of squash with 1 tablespoon oil; place squash flesh side down on the foil-lined pan. Roast on bottom rack 40 minutes, or until you can easily pierce the squash shell. Remove from oven and cool (do not turn off oven). When cool enough to handle, use a fork to scrape strands of spaghetti squash into a large bowl.

3. Heat 1 tablespoon oil in a large skillet over medium heat. Add shrimp and cook, uncovered, without turning, until the tails begin to turn coral, approximately 1–2 minutes. Turn shrimp and cook just until opaque, about 1 minute. Squeeze lemon juice over shrimp and set aside.

4. Place tomatoes, garlic, and the remaining 2 tablespoons oil in a 13 × 9-inch baking dish. Roast on top rack for 30 minutes, or until tender.

5. Toss shrimp with roasted tomatoes and garlic. Season with salt and pepper, and stir in basil. Spoon over spaghetti squash. Sprinkle with parsley and serve.

Italian Living Tradition

Use this simple method of sautéing shrimp whenever you need a quick dinner. They can be served over beans, polenta, pasta, salad, or soup for a meal in minutes.

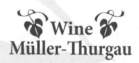
**Wine
Müller-Thurgau**

SPINACH FETTUCCINE WITH WALNUT-RICOTTA PESTO (FETTUCCINE DI SPINACI CON PESTO DI NOCI E RICOTTA)

Serves: 8 | Serving Size: Approximately 1 cup
Prep Time: 5 minutes | Cooking Time: 10–15 minutes

Pesto made with ricotta and walnuts is a creamy alternative to the traditional basil and pine nut version. It pairs beautifully with spinach pasta—but feel free to use any type of pasta, including gluten-free pasta, that you prefer. Fusilli, spaghetti, fettuccine, and linguine are the best shapes to compliment the velvety "sauce" in this recipe. Sometimes called "Sicilian pesto" in Italy, this pesto can be blended together in a bowl while the pasta water is heating up. You can have a distinctive pasta appetizer or main course in minutes! In order to retain its vibrant, fresh flavors, it is important not to cook the pesto, just toss it with the pasta and serve.

1 cup walnut halves or pieces, toasted

1 clove garlic, peeled

1/2 cup fresh basil

6 tablespoons extra virgin olive oil, divided

3/4 cup skim ricotta (preferably fresh)

3 tablespoons grated pecorino Romano cheese

1/4 teaspoon freshly ground black pepper

16 ounces spinach fettuccine or other pasta

Choices/Exchanges 2 1/2 Starch, 1 Lean Protein, 3 Fat
Calories 390 | Calories from Fat 180
Total Fat 20g | Saturated Fat 2.6g | Trans Fat 0.0g
Cholesterol 0mg
Sodium 50mg

Potassium 280mg
Total Carbohydrate 45g | Dietary Fiber 7g | Sugars 2g
Protein 10g
Phosphorus 250mg

1. Start boiling the water for the pasta (using the amount of water suggested on the pasta package).

2. Put the walnuts and garlic in a food processor and pulse until the nuts are chopped into very tiny bits (but don't grind them to a powder). Add in basil and pulse until a paste forms. Add in 4 tablespoons olive oil and pulse until smooth. Scrape the ground nut/garlic mixture into a large bowl. Stir in the ricotta, grated cheese, and pepper until thoroughly blended.

3. When the pesto is ready and the water is boiling, drop all the pasta into the pot at once, and stir to loosen and separate the strands. Cook the pasta until it is perfectly al dente. Drain pasta, reserving pasta water, and place in a large bowl.

4. Drizzle the remaining 2 tablespoons olive oil over the hot pasta, and toss with tongs until all the strands are nicely coated. Add the pesto and toss to combine. If the sauce is too thick, loosen it with a bit of the hot water reserved from the pasta pot as you toss—I normally use 1/4 cup.

5. Toss and serve quickly; the sauce thickens as it cools.

Italian Living Tradition

Sicilian ricotta is often made from goat or sheep's milk, or a combination of the two. If you can get your hands on this variety, I highly recommend it for its flavor and nutritional value. A typical rustic Sicilian breakfast consists of a large dollop of ricotta smeared on a slice of artisan bread and drizzled with local honey. Delicious!

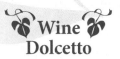

Wine
Dolcetto

WHOLE-WHEAT FUSILLI WITH PESTO AND CHERRY TOMATOES (FUSILLI CON PESTO E POMODORI)

Serves: 8 | Serving Size: 3/4 cup
Prep Time: 5 minutes | Cooking Time: 15 minutes

This is one of my favorite dishes to make during the summer when I am short on time. If you keep basil in your garden, this satisfying, flavorful, and nutritious dish can be whipped up quickly with a few Italian kitchen staples. I like the extra texture and nutritional properties that whole-wheat pasta provides. Farfalle (bow-tie) and penne pasta shapes also work well in this recipe.

Pesto

1/2 cup extra virgin olive oil (preferably first cold-pressed and unfiltered)

3 cups fresh basil leaves

2 cloves garlic

1/4 cup pine nuts

1/4 cup grated parmigiano-reggiano cheese

1/4 cup pecorino Romano cheese

Pasta

1/8 teaspoon unrefined sea salt

16 ounces whole-wheat fusilli OR 3 cups cooked pearl barley

1 pint cherry tomatoes, halved

2 tablespoons parmigiano-reggiano or pecorino Romano cheese (for garnish)

Choices/Exchanges 2 1/2 Starch, 1 Vegetable, 1/2 High-Fat Protein, 2 1/2 Fat
Calories 390 | Calories from Fat 180
Total Fat 20g | Saturated Fat 3.5g | Trans Fat 0.0g
Cholesterol 5mg

Sodium 125mg
Potassium 340mg
Total Carbohydrate 45g | Dietary Fiber 1g | Sugars 2g
Protein 13g
Phosphorus 245mg

1. Mix all pesto ingredients except cheeses in a food processor. Add parmigiano-reggiano and pecorino Romano and stir. You may add less oil to the pesto if you would like a thicker consistency. Or, to thin out the pesto without adding more oil, simply add some of the water used to boil the pasta once it is done cooking. If you do not have a food processor, a pestle can be used to grind the pesto ingredients together.

2. Bring a large pot of water to a boil over high heat. Add salt and fusilli. Reduce heat to medium, and stir. Cook pasta, stirring occasionally, until al dente, approximately 10 minutes. Drain pasta (or barley, if using) and stir in pesto sauce.

3. Spoon pasta onto a serving platter or individual plates and garnish with cherry tomatoes. Sprinkle cheese over the top. Serve hot or at room temperature.

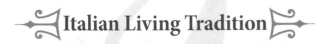

Italian Living Tradition

In addition to being served with pasta, pesto sauce can be used to dress up a side dish of potatoes and green beans, to top potato or ricotta gnocchi, or to slather onto bread for tomato and mozzarella sandwiches. In Italy, it is never reheated or stirred into soup, the way it is in southern France.

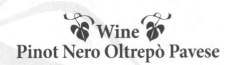

Wine
Pinot Nero Oltrepò Pavese

WHOLE-WHEAT ORECCHIETTE PASTA WITH BROCCOLI AND GARLIC (ORECCHIETTE INTEGRALE CON BROCCOLI)

Serves: 10 | Serving Size: Approximately 3/4 cup
Prep Time: 5 minutes | Cooking Time: 30 minutes

Orecchiette, or "little ears," are popular artisanal pasta shapes in the southern Italian regions of Basilicata, Puglia, and Calabria. This dish is one of the most classic ways to prepare orecchiette. I've replaced the dried white pasta with the whole-wheat version in this recipe for enhanced nutritional benefits.

In its native regions in Italy, the wheat used to make pasta is called grano duro; *it offers a higher amount of protein (16%), vitamin B, folic acid, and phosphorous than other varieties of wheat, and contains no cholesterol. It also contains six of nine essential amino acids, making it an excellent choice for vegetarians. So if you find imported pasta made from* grano duro *wheat while shopping, give it a try!*

1/3 cup good-quality extra virgin olive oil (preferably first cold-pressed and Puglian)

3 cloves garlic, finely chopped

1/2 chile pepper, minced OR 1/2 teaspoon crushed red chile flakes

1/4 cup pine nuts

12 small cherry tomatoes, quartered

1/2 teaspoon salt

1/4 teaspoon freshly ground black pepper

1/2 pound broccoli florets (see Italian Living Tradition)

2 tablespoons freshly chopped basil or flat-leaf parsley

16 ounces whole-wheat orecchiette, or any short rice pasta

1/4 cup pecorino Romano cheese

Choices/Exchanges 2 Starch, 1 Vegetable, 2 Fat
Calories 270 | Calories from Fat 100
Total Fat 11g | Saturated Fat 1.7g | Trans Fat 0.0g
Cholesterol 5mg
Sodium 170mg

Potassium 255mg
Total Carbohydrate 37g | Dietary Fiber 5g | Sugars 1g
Protein 9g
Phosphorus 175mg

1. Heat the olive oil in a large, wide skillet over medium heat. Add the garlic and chile pepper, and sauté approximately 1 minute, just until they release their aroma. Add the pine nuts and sauté until lightly golden. Add the cherry tomatoes, salt, and pepper. Stir, and cook for 2 minutes.

2. Add broccoli florets, basil or parsley, and 1/2 cup water. Stir and cover. Cook until the broccoli is fork tender, 10–15 minutes.

3. Meanwhile, cook the pasta in a large pot of slightly salted boiling water for approximately 12 minutes, or until al dente.

4. Drain pasta, and add it to the cooked vegetables. Toss to combine. Top with cheese and serve.

❖ Italian Living Tradition ❖

Save the unused broccoli stems from this recipe to use as a healthy addition to a soup recipe. Or try boiling and puréeing the stems. Then mix with a little bit of pecorino cheese and olive oil for a delicious and nutritious side dish.

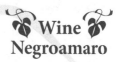

**Wine
Negroamaro**

WHOLE-WHEAT ZITI WITH GOAT RAGU
(ZITI INTEGRALE CON RAGÙ DI CAPRA)

Serves: 10 | Serving Size: Approximately 1/2 cup
Prep Time: 15 minutes (plus marinating time) | Cooking Time: About 1 hour 45 minutes

Goat is the leanest meat eaten in the Mediterranean region. In southern Italy, it was traditionally served for weddings and holidays. While goat is the most commonly eaten meat in the world, it is relatively new to Americans. In March 2014, award-winning chef Luigi Diotaiuti and I gave a presentation at the International Association of Culinary Professionals' annual conference in Chicago on goat, calling it "the meat of the future." The event was so well received that the organization asked us to repeat it in a webinar for the members who couldn't attend.

See the Where to Buy Guide (page 299) for help finding goat meat if it is not readily available in your area. You can substitute lamb, veal, or beef for the goat meat, if necessary. Note that the meat must be marinated a day in advance.

Marinade (to be made one day in advance)

1/2 pound boneless goat leg or shoulder meat, cut into 1-inch cubes

3 sprigs fresh rosemary

3 sprigs fresh thyme

3 cloves garlic

5 fresh bay leaves OR 1 dried bay leaf

2 1/2 cups red wine, divided

Ragu and Pasta

2 tablespoons flour or rice flour

4 tablespoons extra virgin olive oil, divided

3 tablespoons diced onion

3 tablespoons diced carrot

3 tablespoons diced celery

1 tablespoon porcini mushrooms, soaked in cold water for 10 minutes, drained, and chopped

1/3 cup Fresh Tomato Sauce (page 228)

4 cups Homemade Meat Stock (page 290)

1/8 teaspoon unrefined sea salt

16 ounces whole-wheat ziti, penne rigate, or gluten-free pasta

1/4 cup grated parmigiano-reggiano cheese

Choices/Exchanges 2 Starch, 1 Vegetable, 1 1/2 Lean Protein, 1/2 Fat

Calories 280 | Calories from Fat 25

Total Fat 3g | Saturated Fat 1.0g | Trans Fat 0.0g

Cholesterol 15mg

Sodium 125mg

Potassium 390mg

Total Carbohydrate 40g | Dietary Fiber 0g | Sugars 1g

Protein 15g

Phosphorus 225mg

1. To make goat marinade (which should done one day in advance), place goat meat in a bowl with the rosemary, thyme, garlic, and bay leaf. Add wine to reach just below the covering point. Stir, cover, and refrigerate overnight.

2. The next day, drain and reserve the marinade. Place the meat on a plate and sprinkle with flour. Turn to coat well and set aside.

3. To make the sauce, heat 2 tablespoons olive oil in a large saucepan over medium heat. Add the onion, carrot, and celery, and stir. Sauté until vegetables are tender and slightly golden. Add the floured goat cubes, pressing down lightly so that they brown evenly on all sides. Once the goat begins to attach to the bottom of the pan, add the reserved marinade and cook until it evaporates.

4. Add the porcini mushrooms and tomato sauce, and stir well. Cover the goat with beef stock and stir. Cover the pan and reduce the heat to medium-low. Cook for 1 1/2 hours, stirring about every 15 minutes. Add more stock, if necessary, as the sauce cooks down. (You should always have about 1/2 inch stock covering the goat.) The sauce is ready when it is highly aromatic and thickened, yet still quite fluid. Add the salt.

5. Bring a large pot of water to boil over high heat. Add the pasta and cook until al dente, about 10–12 minutes.

6. Drain pasta and add to the goat sauce. Combine gently. Add the remaining 2 tablespoons olive oil and serve with grated parmigiano-reggiano.

Italian Living Tradition

Making *ragù* (or *sugo* or meat sauce) is an important Italian ritual. Too labor-intensive and rich to enjoy daily, *ragù* is one of the recipes enjoyed during the Sunday family meal. Even though the Italian lifestyle is becoming increasingly fast-paced, it is reassuring to note recent studies that have indicated 70% of Italian families still congregate for a family meal on the day of rest. This age-old tradition is viewed not only as a way of socializing, but as a means of promoting cultural identity as well.

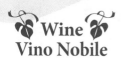

Wine
Vino Nobile

SPAGHETTI WITH FRESH TUNA AND FENNEL (PASTA CON TONNO E FINOCCHIO)

Serves: 8 | Serving Size: 6 ounces
Prep Time: 5 minutes | Cooking Time: About 40 minutes

The southern Italian regions of Calabria and Sicily are known for fresh tuna—fishing tuna has been one of the main economic industries in these regions since ancient times. Leftover grilled tuna or canned tuna can be used instead of fresh tuna in this dish. Many Italians enjoy recipes like this on Christmas Eve, when meat is avoided. If you are used to the Italian-American version of this dish, which uses tomatoes and preserved tuna (also delicious), I recommend you give this version a try as well. The simple, sweet, pure flavors in this recipe are a delight for the senses and are easy on the waistline.

1/4 cup plus 3 tablespoons extra virgin olive oil, divided

3/4 pound fresh tuna fillets

16 ounces whole-wheat or gluten-free spaghetti

2 medium (8-ounce) bulbs fennel

1/2 cup white wine

Juice and zest from 1 lemon

2 tablespoons capers, rinsed and drained

1/4 teaspoon unrefined sea salt

1/4 teaspoon freshly ground black pepper

Choices/Exchanges 3 Starch, 1 1/2 Lean Protein, 1 1/2 Fat

Calories 370 | Calories from Fat 120

Total Fat 13g | Saturated Fat 1.9g | Trans Fat 0.0g

Cholesterol 20mg

Sodium 170mg

Potassium 450mg

Total Carbohydrate 45g | Dietary Fiber 1g | Sugars 2g

Protein 19g

Phosphorus 245mg

1. Preheat oven to 400°F.

2. Heat 1/4 cup olive oil in a large, wide skillet over medium-high heat. Add tuna fillets and sauté until golden on each side, approximately 3 minutes per side. Transfer to oven and cook to desired doneness—approximately 10 minutes for medium-well.

3. Cook spaghetti according to package instructions, omitting salt. Drain, reserving 1 cup pasta water, and return to pot.

4. Trim fennel bulbs, reserving 1/4 cup chopped fronds. Quarter, core, and thinly slice bulbs crosswise. Sauté with 1 tablespoon olive oil in a skillet over medium-high heat. Add in wine, and reduce heat to low. Cover and cook until tender, stirring occasionally, 10–20 minutes.

5. Add fennel to pasta along with fennel fronds, lemon juice, capers, remaining 2 tablespoons olive oil, and reserved pasta water. Season with salt and pepper. Flake in the tuna.

6. Gently toss and garnish with lemon zest. Serve hot.

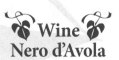

PUMPKIN RISOTTO
(RISOTTO DI ZUCCA)

Serves: 10 | Serving Size: Approximately 1/3 cup
Prep Time: 5 minutes | Cooking Time: Approximately 25 minutes

Documented evidence of "modern-style" risotto recipes can be traced back to the 16th century in Italy thanks to cook and author Bartolomeo Scappi (personal chef to Pope Pio V). The forefathers of Italian rice brought the grain from Egypt to Muslim Spain, and Jewish and Muslim merchants eventually brought the rice to Italy, where it flourished in the Po Valley of the Lombardy region.

The traditional butter and cream in this recipe have been replaced with olive oil and yogurt, in keeping with the dietary guidelines for those with diabetes. Thanks to the addition of the pumpkin, however, the risotto achieves a creamy consistency without the extra fat content. Because of the high amount of nutrients it contains, pumpkin is a good choice for anyone interested in improving their health.

3 tablespoons extra virgin olive oil

1 small yellow onion, minced

2 cups arborio or carnaroli rice

1 1/4 pounds fresh pumpkin, finely chopped

1 cup white wine

6 cups Vegetable Stock (page 287)

4 ounces grated parmigiano-reggiano cheese

2 tablespoons low-fat yogurt

Choices/Exchanges 2 1/2 Starch, 1/2 High-Fat Protein, 1 Fat
Calories 300 | Calories from Fat 80
Total Fat 9g | Saturated Fat 3.0g | Trans Fat 0.0g
Cholesterol 10mg

Sodium 230mg
Potassium 420mg
Total Carbohydrate 41g | Dietary Fiber 2g | Sugars 3g
Protein 11g
Phosphorus 200mg

1. In a heavy-bottomed saucepan, warm the oil over medium heat. When the oil is hot, add the onion and sauté until tender, about 3–5 minutes, but do not let the onion brown.

2. Add the rice and the pumpkin, and stir. Add the wine. Stir and cook until the wine evaporates.

3. Add just enough stock to cover the rice. Mix slowly, making sure the rice does not stick to the bottom of the pan. Once the stock is nearly absorbed, add more stock to cover. Repeat this process until the rice has absorbed all the broth, about 18–19 minutes. The rice should be cooked through with a slightly chewy texture.

4. Remove risotto from heat. Add the parmigiano-reggiano and yogurt. Mix vigorously until the risotto is well blended and has a creamy texture.

5. Serve immediately.

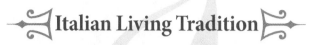

Italian Living Tradition

In the northern Italian regions of Veneto, Lombardy, and Piedmont, there are as many variations on risotto as there are days of the year. Once you have the technique down, you can add different ingredients to create your own version.
Any seasonal vegetable, or even fresh seafood, could be substituted for the pumpkin in this recipe.

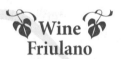

Wine
Friulano

VENETIAN-STYLE WHOLE-WHEAT SPAGHETTI WITH SAUCE
(BIGOLI IN SALSA)

Serves: 8 | Serving Size: Approximately 1/3 cup
Prep Time: 5 minutes (plus 2 hours anchovy-soaking time)
Cooking Time: Approximately 15 minutes

*While this dish is prepared with anchovies, it used to be made with sardines and other salted fish.
Salted fish are extremely popular in Italy because in Roman times heavy taxes were imposed on salt.
In order to avoid the taxes, people imported and used salt-cured fish, such as anchovies, instead of salt.
As a result, the deeply flavored, salted fish became an important culinary ingredient
in many regions, and are now indispensable in Italian cuisine.*

1/3 cup extra virgin olive oil

8 anchovy fillets, soaked in 1/2 cup milk for 2 hours and drained

1/4 teaspoon freshly ground black pepper

2 yellow onions, diced

1 cup dry white wine

16 ounces fresh bigoli pasta (see Where to Buy Guide) or another whole-wheat or gluten-free pasta, cooked until al dente

1/8 teaspoon unrefined sea salt

1/4 cup finely chopped flat-leaf parsley

2 ounces freshly grated parmigiano-reggiano cheese

Choices/Exchanges 3 Starch, 1 Lean Protein, 2 Fat
Calories 340 | Calories from Fat 110
Total Fat 12g | Saturated Fat 2.7g | Trans Fat 0.0g
Cholesterol 10mg
Sodium 290mg

Potassium 185mg
Total Carbohydrate 44g | Dietary Fiber 0g | Sugars 0g
Protein 12g
Phosphorus 215mg

1. Heat olive oil in a large skillet over medium heat.

2. Finely chop anchovies and mash with the side of a chef's knife to form a paste. Add anchovy paste to the olive oil. Season with pepper, and stir to combine. Add onions and sauté until golden and tender, stirring occasionally, approximately 5 minutes.

3. Add the wine, increase heat to high, and allow alcohol to cook down to 1/4 of its original volume. Add the pasta and toss to coat. Taste and season with salt.

4. Place pasta on a large platter or in individual dishes. Sprinkle parsley and cheese over the top. Serve hot.

⊰ Italian Living Tradition ⊱

Homemade *bigoli* was originally made with duck eggs in the Veneto region. The dish was traditionally served on October 7 for the feast of Our Lady of the Rosary. The feast is still celebrated in many towns in northern Italy.

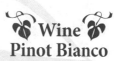

Wine
Pinot Bianco

POTATO GNOCCHI
(GNOCCHI DI PATATE)

Serves: 12 | Serving Size: Approximately 1/2 cup
Prep Time: 15 minutes (plus 1 hour potato-baking time) | Cooking Time: 10 minutes

While they may seem ubiquitous in Italian fare today, gnocchi, when properly prepared, are tender triumphs of bite-sized potato puffs. These culinary masterpieces were, after all, adored by Giacomo Puccini, the great opera legend. In Italy today, most people buy prepared gnocchi from neighborhood pasta shops. But the homemade gnocchi tradition stays alive with the recipes of grandmothers and in trattorias.

Although gnocchi are not difficult to make, it is very hard to find good gnocchi in Italian restaurants in America. The main reason for this is that the amount of flour needed for gnocchi always varies. The type of potato you use, its freshness, how it is cooked, and whether or not you use eggs will determine the taste of the gnocchi. When they are overworked, prepared with too much flour, or left out to sit too long, they will become gummy. Potato gnocchi can be topped with simple tomato sauce, bolognese sauce, pesto sauce, or a variety of vegetable and cheese sauces.

4 medium russet potatoes (about 2 pounds)

1 1/2 teaspoons unrefined sea salt

1 1/2–2 cups unbleached all-purpose flour or a combination of corn and rice flour, plus extra for dusting work surface

2 cups Fresh Tomato Sauce (page 228)

1/4 cup pecorino Romano, pecorino Sardo, pecorino Crotonese, or grana padano cheese

1. Preheat oven to 375°F.

2. Wash and dry potatoes. Make a long incision in the potatoes lengthwise about 1/2 inch deep. Bake the potatoes 45 minutes–1 hour until tender. When cool enough to handle, peel the potatoes and pass them through a ricer into a large bowl.

Choices/Exchanges 2 Starch, 1 Fat
Calories 190 | Calories from Fat 25
Total Fat 3g | Saturated Fat 0.8g | Trans Fat 0.0g
Cholesterol 0mg
Sodium 300mg

Potassium 640mg
Total Carbohydrate 35g | Dietary Fiber 3g | Sugars 4g
Protein 6g
Phosphorus 110mg

3. Add the salt to the potatoes. Add the flour, little by little. You may not need all of the flour. Mix with your hands until the dough begins to stick together. Transfer the mixture to a wooden board. If the dough sticks to the board, add a little flour to the board. When the dough is soft, pliable, and a little sticky, it is ready.

4. Cut the dough into plum-size pieces. Flour your hands and gently roll out each piece of dough with quick back-and-forth motions until you have created a long, thin rope (it should be about the width of your thumb). Cut each rope into 1-inch pieces.

5. Holding a fork so that the curved underside is parallel to the work surface, roll each piece of dough from the curved part of the fork along the length of the tines to make indentations. Let the gnocchi fall onto the board. Place shaped gnocchi onto a lightly floured baking sheet. Repeat with remaining dough until all of it has been shaped.

6. Bring a large pot with 6 quarts water to a boil. Reduce heat to medium. Gently add 1/2 of the gnocchi. Remove gnocchi with a slotted spoon when they float to the top (3–4 minutes). Carefully shake off excess water. Place gnocchi on serving platter and dress with a little of the sauce.

7. Bring water back to a boil. Repeat the cooking process with the remaining gnocchi. Serve immediately with sauce and cheese.

Italian Living Tradition

Here are a few tips to keep in mind when you make gnocchi:

1. Use old russet potatoes because they have the driest consistency.
2. Bake the potatoes instead of boiling them.
3. Always use a ricer instead of a masher when making the dough.
4. Add the flour, little by little, until the potatoes form a dough.
5. Gourmands prefer eggless gnocchi because they are lighter.
6. Gnocchi are meant to be eaten freshly made.

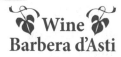

Wine
Barbera d'Asti

TUSCAN BUCKWHEAT PASTA WITH CHEESE, POTATOES, AND GREENS
(PIZZOCCHERI DELLA VALTELLINA)

Serves: 8 | Serving Size: Approximately 2/3 cup
Prep Time: 5 minutes | Cooking Time: 20 minutes

Buckwheat, known as grano saraceno *in Italian, has been around since the 9th century in Siberia. In Italy it was quickly incorporated into pasta recipes. Prized for its high protein content (19%) and generous amounts of iron, selenium, zinc, mineral salts, and antioxidants, buckwheat is believed to help regulate blood glucose as well. Pizzoccheri* are a type of traditional Tuscan pasta that is normally made by hand. Any buckwheat pasta may be substituted in this recipe.*

1/4 cup extra virgin olive oil

2 cloves garlic, peeled

5 large leaves fresh sage

1/8 teaspoon unrefined sea salt

2 medium yukon gold potatoes, peeled and cut into 1/2-inch cubes

12 ounces pizzoccheri (dried buckwheat pasta) or any buckwheat or gluten-free pasta

4 cups baby chard (or regular chard or savoy cabbage, cut into 1-inch pieces), washed

1/4 cup freshly grated parmigano-reggiano cheese

1/4 cup freshly grated fontina cheese

1/4 teaspoon freshly ground black pepper

Pinch freshly ground nutmeg

Choices/Exchanges 2 Starch, 1 Vegetable,
1/2 Medium-Fat Protein, 1 Fat
Calories 250 | Calories from Fat 80
Total Fat 9g | Saturated Fat 2.2g | Trans Fat 0.0g
Cholesterol 5mg

Sodium 410mg
Potassium 355mg
Total Carbohydrate 37g | Dietary Fiber 1g | Sugars 1g
Protein 9g
Phosphorus 165mg

1. In a small saucepan over low heat, heat the olive oil, garlic cloves, and the sage leaves. Keep the mixture over low heat while continuing with the next steps.

2. Bring a large pot of water to a boil over high heat. Add salt and potatoes. Cook potatoes for approximately 10 minutes, or until they are tender. Take the potatoes out with a slotted spoon and set aside.

3. Add pasta to the same water and cook for 5 minutes. Add chard or cabbage in with the pasta and cook until pasta is al dente and vegetables are tender, approximately 5 more minutes.

4. Drain the cooked vegetables and pasta, and layer them, along with the potatoes and both grated cheeses, in a huge serving bowl, ending with a layer of sprinkled cheese.

5. Discard the garlic and sage from the olive oil, and pour the oil over the layers. Add the freshly ground black pepper. Garnish with nutmeg and serve.

Italian Living Tradition

Tuscan cooks use buckwheat to make pizzoccheri pasta and crespelle (crepes). In Calabria, a buckwheat pasta similar to linguine, called struncatura, has also been enjoyed for centuries. Many northern Italian regions even have buckwheat festivals in the springtime. Incorporating buckwheat flour into your diet is a great way to increase your nutrient intake.

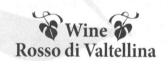

Wine
Rosso di Valtellina

RED PEPPER AND SWEET POTATO GNOCCHI (*GNOCCHI DI PEPERONI ROSSI E PATATE DOLCE*)

Serves: 6 | Serving Size: 1/3 cup
Prep Time: 5 minutes | Cooking Time: 1 hour 20 minutes

While this dish would be served as a first course in Italy, it makes a nice side for roasted poultry and meat in the wintertime. Old, starchy baking (white) potatoes are traditionally used for gnocchi. However, as sweet potatoes continue to gain popularity, gnocchi variations like this one are becoming more common. Sweet potatoes are nutritious and high in fiber, which makes them a good starchy vegetable choice for people with diabetes. If you can't find the peperoni di Senise (crushed, sun-dried peppers from Senise) called for in this recipe, you can crush red chile flakes in a spice blender until they are very fine or substitute good-quality smoked paprika.

1 (8-ounce) sweet potato

1/4 teaspoon unrefined sea salt

1/2 cup skim milk ricotta, divided

1 egg

1 1/2 cups all-purpose flour or a combination of half corn flour and half rice flour, plus extra for dusting work surface

1/4 cup extra virgin olive oil

2 roasted red peppers, finely diced

1 teaspoon peperoni di Senise

1/4 cup grated pecorino Romano, pecorino Sardo, or pecorino Crotonese cheese

---

Choices/Exchanges 2 Starch, 1/2 High-Fat Protein, 2 Fat
Calories 300 | Calories from Fat 120
Total Fat 13g | Saturated Fat 3.0g | Trans Fat 0.0g
Cholesterol 40mg
Sodium 290mg

Potassium 290mg
Total Carbohydrate 35g | Dietary Fiber 3g | Sugars 3g
Protein 9g
Phosphorus 145mg

1. Preheat oven to 425°F.

2. Bake sweet potato for 1 hour, or until very mushy. Remove from the oven, and set aside to cool. Once the potato is cool enough to work with, remove the peel, and mash it or press it through a ricer into a large bowl. Blend in the salt, 1/4 cup ricotta, and egg. Mix in the flour a little at a time until you have soft dough. Use more or less flour as needed.

3. Bring a large pot of water to a boil. While you wait for the water to boil, make the gnocchi: On a floured surface, divide the dough into 10 equally sized small balls. Roll each ball out into a long, 10-inch rope, and cut each rope into 1/2-inch pieces. Holding a fork so that the curved underside is parallel to the work surface, roll each piece of dough from the curved part of the fork along the length of the tines to make indentations. Allow the shaped pieces to fall onto a large baking sheet dusted with flour.

4. Drop the gnocchi into the boiling water, and allow them to cook until they float to the surface. Remove the floating pieces with a slotted spoon, and keep warm in a serving dish.

5. Heat the olive oil in a large, wide skillet over medium heat. Add roasted red peppers and peperoni di Senise. Stir and sauté for 3 minutes, or until golden. Toss gnocchi in oil/pepper mixture and turn to coat.

6. Place on a serving platter and top with the remaining 1/4 cup ricotta in the middle. Sprinkle the grated cheese on top and serve immediately.

◆⊨ Italian Living Tradition ⊨◆

The olive oil and pepper mixture used in this recipe is popular in many regions of southern Italy. In these regions, special varieties of chili peppers are sun-dried and then ground to make a condiment. The *peperoni di Senise* have a slightly sweet taste and are found in both the regions of Basilicata and Calabria. Calabria also sun-dries the "little devil" variety of these chilies, which is the hottest variety. This condiment tastes delicious with pasta and as a condiment for grilled chicken and meats.

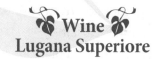

Wine
Lugana Superiore

TURNIP GNOCCHI WITH HERB SAUCE (GNOCCHI DI RAPA CON SALSA D'ERBE)

Serves: 4 | Serving Size: Approximately 1/2 cup
Prep Time: 10 minutes | Cooking Time: 30 minutes

Gnocchi—those puffy little pillows of potato bliss—can be prepared with a variety of root vegetables. Italian chefs often experiment with whatever is on hand to create appealing new recipes. Keep in mind that flour is traditionally added to potatoes to make gnocchi; for a gluten-free alternative, I've incorporated a combination of almond and oat flour into this recipe, but you can substitute all-purpose flour for both if you don't have a gluten sensitivity. You will need a potato ricer to make this recipe.

3 large turnips, peeled and cut into chunks
1/2 cup almond flour
1/4 cup oat flour, plus extra for dusting work surface
2 eggs
1/4 cup extra virgin olive oil
1 tablespoon finely chopped fresh sage
1 tablespoon finely chopped fresh flat-leaf parsley
1 teaspoon finely chopped fresh rosemary
1 teaspoon unrefined sea salt
1/2 teaspoon freshly ground black pepper
1 tablespoon finely grated parmigiano-reggiano cheese

Choices/Exchanges 1 1/2 Starch, 1 Lean Protein, 3 Fat
Calories 290 | Calories from Fat 150
Total Fat 17g | Saturated Fat 2.9g | Trans Fat 0.0g
Cholesterol 95mg
Sodium 400mg

Potassium 185mg
Total Carbohydrate 23g | Dietary Fiber 2g | Sugars 0g
Protein 14g
Phosphorus 165mg

1. Place turnips in a medium saucepan and cover with water. Bring to a boil over high heat. Reduce heat to medium and cook until just fork tender, approximately 10 minutes.

2. Combine almond and oat flours. Pour flour in a mound on table. Pass turnips through a potato ricer; let what extrudes fall in the flour. Make a hole in the flour turnip mixture (it should look like a nest); crack your eggs in the middle of the nest. Mix them in a circular motion slowly, using your fingertips.

3. Mix flour/turnip mixture and eggs well. Knead the dough until it looks like a little loaf. Keep adding the flour mixture until it reaches a dough-like consistency. Divide dough into 6 pieces. On a lightly floured surface, roll pieces into equal-size ropes. Using a sharp knife, cut ropes into 1/2-inch pieces and set pieces on a lightly floured platter.

4. Bring a large pot of water to boil over high heat. Add gnocchi to water, stir gently, reduce heat to medium, and cook until the gnocchi float to the surface, 3–5 minutes. Drain gnocchi.

5. Heat olive oil in a large skillet over medium-low heat. Add sage, parsley, and rosemary, and cook for 3–5 minutes, stirring with a wooden spoon, until herbs begin to release their aroma. Add gnocchi and toss to coat.

6. Taste and season with salt, pepper, and pargmi-giano-reggiano. Serve.

⤖ Italian Living Tradition ⤖

In Italy, turnips are served either thinly shaved and raw, in soups, layered with meats in gratins, stuffed and baked, or puréed (in many regions in northern Italy). Throughout the regions of Piedmont, Trentino-Alto Adige, Tuscany, and Liguria, turnips have been enjoyed for millennia.

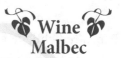

**Wine
Malbec**

TRAPANI-STYLE ALMOND COUSCOUS (CUSCUS ALLA MANDORLA TRAPANESE)

Serves: 4 | Serving Size: 6 ounces
Prep Time: 10 minutes | Cooking Time: 25 minutes

Trapani has been an important fishing port in the Egadi Islands since antiquity. The Arab influence in this Sicilian town has made couscous one of its local specialties. Called the "food of peace," couscous is the star of a yearly international Sicilian festival that hosts cooks from four continents to celebrate this ingredient. The pesto in this recipe is a traditional Trapani-style pesto, made with almonds and tomatoes instead of pine nuts and basil like its Ligurian counterpart.

1/4 cup plus 2 tablespoons blanched almonds, lightly toasted, divided

1 pint small cherry tomatoes, 12 reserved whole and the rest quartered, divided

1/4 cup grated parmigiano-reggiano cheese

2 cloves garlic, peeled

1 cup basil leaves, roughly chopped, plus more for garnish

1/2 teaspoon crushed red chile flakes

1/8 cup plus 2 tablespoons good-quality extra virgin olive oil (preferably first cold-pressed)

1 cup couscous

1 1/4 cups Homemade Vegetable Stock (page 287)

Choices/Exchanges 2 Starch, 2 Vegetable,
1/2 Lean Protein, 3 1/2 Fat
Calories 400 | Calories from Fat 190
Total Fat 21g | Saturated Fat 3.5g | Trans Fat 0.0g
Cholesterol 5mg

Sodium 130mg
Potassium 560mg
Total Carbohydrate 42g | Dietary Fiber 5g | Sugars 4g
Protein 13g
Phosphorus 225mg

1. Put 1/4 cup almonds in a food processor fitted with the blade attachment; pulse them 15–20 times until roughly chopped. Add the quartered tomatoes, cheese, garlic, basil, and red chile flakes. Pulse the machine 8–10 times. Then, with the machine running, use the feed tube to slowly add up to 1/8 cup olive oil in a slow, steady stream. The resulting pesto should be quite grainy but not too chunky and not too wet. You may not need all the oil. Set pesto aside.

2. Heat the remaining 2 tablespoons olive oil in a saucepan over high heat. Add the couscous and cook, stirring often, until toasted, about 5 minutes.

3. Add the stock, cover the pan, and reduce heat to low. Simmer 15–20 minutes until all the liquid has been absorbed. Fluff with a fork and toss in 1/4 cup tomato pesto.

4. Garnish with remaining whole tomatoes, 2 tablespoons chopped almonds, and a few basil leaves. Serve.

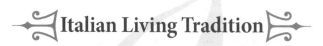

Italian Living Tradition

Try this delicious pesto variation on spaghetti or freshly grilled or broiled tuna for a vibrant dish that's as healthy as it is delicious.

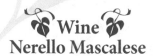

Wine
Nerello Mascalese

SECOND COURSES
(SECONDI)

94 Roman Chicken, Pepper, and Tomato Stew/*Pollo in umido alla Romana*

96 Artichoke, Mushroom, and Caramelized Onion Frittata/
   Frittata di carciofi, funghi, e cipolle caramellate

98 Campania-Style Rustic Vegetable Stew/*Cianfotta*

100 Spiced Chickpea Stew/*Stufato di ceci alle spezie*

102 Eggplant Croquettes/*Polpette di melanzane*

104 Zucchini and Herb Croquettes/*Polpette di zucchine*

106 Pan-Seared Sea Scallops/*Capesante in padella*

108 Fishermen Kabobs/*Spiedini alla marinara*

110 Mussels in Saffron-Tomato Broth/*Cozze in brodo di zafferano*

112 Braised, Stuffed Calamari with Tomato Sauce/*Calamari ripieni in salsa di pomodoro*

114 Sea Bass with Fennel Baked in Parchment/*Branzino con finocchio al cartoccio*

116 Fresh Tuna Steaks with Sautéed Artichokes/*Tonno con carciofi*

118 Trout Fillets with Sun-Dried Tomato and Cured-Olive Crust/
    Filetti di trota impanati con pomodori secchi ed olive curate

120 Swordfish with Olives, Capers, Herbs, and Tomatoes/*Pesce spade alla ghiotta*

122 Sicilian-Style Fish with Vegetables/*Dentice alla Siciliana con verdure al forno*

124 Sea Bream with Duchess-Style Sweet Potatoes/*Orata con patate dolce alla ducchessa*

126 Venetian-Style Sole in a Sweet-and-Sour Sauce/*Sfogi in saor*

128 Fish Stew over Polenta/*Pesce in umido con la polenta*

130 Citrus and Herb–Infused Scallop Stew/*Capesante in umido con erbe ed agrumi*

132 Herb-Marinated Chicken Breasts/*Petti di pollo marinate con erbe*

134 Chicken Stew with Mushrooms and Onions/*Stufato di pollo con funghi e cipolle*

136 Chicken Breasts with Citrus, Capers, and Pine Nuts/*Petti di pollo al limone, caperi, e pinoli*

138 Marinated Chicken with Rosemary and Balsamic Vinegar/
    Pollo marinato con rosmarino ed aceto balsamico

140 Cacciatore-Style Chicken/*Pollo alla cacciatora*

142 Classic Roasted Chicken/*Pollo al forno*

144 Roasted Chicken with Grapes and Chestnuts/*Pollo con le uve e castagne*

146   Vegetable-Stuffed Turkey Breast/*Petto di tacchino ripieno di verdure*

148   Herb-Roasted Turkey/*Tacchino al forno*

150   Veal, Potato, and Pepper Stew/*Spezzatino di vitello*

152   Abruzzese-Style Roasted Baby Goat with Peppers/*Capretto alla Neretese*

154   Classic Meatballs/*Polpette*

"Pisci cottu e carni cruda. (Il pesce deve essere ben cotto, mentre la carne è più saporita se cotta poco.)"
"Fish should be well cooked and meat has more flavor when it's cooked less."
—Calabrian proverb

Both gourmands and the health-conscious home cooks can take pleasure in the wide variety of Italian main dishes that offer great flavor and abundant nutritional value and are relatively low in calories and fat. Authentic, traditional second courses in Italy consist mainly of beans and legumes, eggs and cheese, seafood, poultry, and lean cuts of goat, veal, and lamb. The most popular cooking methods for these ingredients are pan-frying, grilling, roasting, baking, braising, and stewing.

For meal-planning purposes, it is important to remember that heavier second courses pair best with a lighter first course. For dinner, a second course can be served with a side dish/*contorno* and salad. Italian home cooks usually save slow-cooking dishes for Sunday dinners and opt for easy frittatas and grilled or pan-fried seafood, poultry, or meat dishes on weekdays. An advantage to making the stew recipes, which take a little longer, is that you can make them in large quantities and freeze individual portions for lunches or busy weeknight dinners.

Vegetarians and meat lovers alike will love the options in this section, including the Artichoke, Mushroom, and Caramelized Onion Frittata (page 96), Campania-Style Rustic Vegetable Stew (page 98), Spiced Chickpea Stew (page 100), Eggplant Croquettes (page 102), and Zucchini and Herb Croquettes (page 104).

The Italian peninsula is bordered by the Adriatic, Tyrrhenian, Ionian, and Mediterranean seas, and is dotted with numerous lakes, streams, and rivers. So it's no surprise that seafood has been appreciated in Italy since antiquity. The Christmas Eve Feast of the Seven Fishes is a traditional Italian banquet-style meal usually comprised of several different seafood courses. The number of courses or types of fish served at the meal is open to interpretation. Some people maintain that the number seven in this feast stands for the seven sacraments, and others say it refers to the number of days it took God to create the universe. Other variations on the feast call for nine types of fish to be served, signifying the Holy Trinity times three. And still others say the correct number is thirteen, for the twelve apostles and Jesus. Whether or not you celebrate the Feast of the Seven Fishes, this chapter contains many perennial Italian seafood favorites for you to enjoy.

In traditional Italian life, meat and poultry were reserved for Sundays and holidays. Because animals served many purposes, such as providing eggs or dairy, eating their meat was of secondary importance. It was costly to eat meats and poultry because it meant losing a part of a flock, so these proteins weren't eaten daily. Luckily, this created a culinary culture that was predominately centered around plant-based foods, which are more healthful. This chapter contains poultry- and meat-based dishes such as Herb-Marinated Chicken Breasts (page 132), Chicken Breasts with Citrus, Capers, and Pine Nuts (page 136), and Marinated Chicken with Rosemary and Balsamic Vinegar (page 138), all of which can be made in a flash on a weeknight. You'll also find more elaborate dishes such as Vegetable-Stuffed Turkey Breast (page 146), Veal, Potato, and Pepper Stew (page 150), Abruzzese-Style Roasted Baby Goat with Peppers (page 152), and Classic Meatballs (page 154).

I selected the recipes for this chapter because they represent a full range of healthful Italian second courses that often get overlooked abroad, and because they are made with relatively easy-to-find ingredients. In many of the recipes I note possible ingredient substitutions and variations on my version. That is because true Italian cooking is about making the best use of what you have on hand.

Purchasing the freshest, best-quality, organic eggs, seafood, poultry, and meat will make a huge difference in the finished product of your dishes. Many of the recipes in this book are simple enough to let the freshness of the ingredients shine through. Resist the urge to buy less-than-premium ingredients. Italians don't decide what they are going to buy from the market until they see its products. They buy what is freshest and look for the best value. Then, they go home and decide what to make. For those who are not comfortable "winging it" at the grocery store, I recommend looking for an e-book version of whatever cookbook you are using and bringing a mobile device with that e-book to the supermarket. That way, you can determine which foods look best in the store and check the index of the cookbook to see what you can make from them. It is better to make a substitution to a recipe than to prepare ingredients that aren't at their peak.

ROMAN CHICKEN, PEPPER, AND TOMATO STEW (POLLO IN UMIDO ALLA ROMANA)

Serves: 8 | Serving Size: Approximately 1 cup
Prep Time: 5 minutes | Cooking Time: Approximately 1 hour

This is my version of a classic Italian dish that is considered to be a Roman specialty. Chicken has been eaten in Rome since antiquity, as documented by the philosopher/ gourmand Apicius. When I was living in Rome, I prepared this stew on a weekly basis. Its simple, straightforward style, along with its sweet and piquant flavors, makes it a favorite in my family. For an authentic Roman experience, serve Roman-Style Broccoli and Pecorino Soup (page 60) or Spinach Fettuccine with Walnut-Ricotta Pesto (page 64) as a first course.

2 tablespoons extra virgin olive oil

3 pounds chicken thighs

4 green bell peppers, cut into 1-inch strips

4 cloves garlic, minced

1 cup dry white wine

1 cup Homemade Chicken or Homemade Vegetable Stock (pages 289, 287) or reduced-sodium vegetable stock

3 cups canned no-sodium-added crushed tomatoes

1/2 teaspoon unrefined sea salt

1/2 teaspoon freshly ground black pepper

Pinch crushed red chile flakes

1 dried bay leaf

4 tablespoons freshly chopped flat-leaf parsley

Choices/Exchanges 2 Vegetable, 5 Lean Protein, 1/2 Fat
Calories 300 | Calories from Fat 100
Total Fat 11g | Saturated Fat 2.5g | Trans Fat 0.0g
Cholesterol 160mg
Sodium 330mg

Potassium 80mg
Total Carbohydrate 9g | Dietary Fiber 3g | Sugars 5g
Protein 36g
Phosphorus 365mg

1. Heat olive oil in a large skillet over medium heat. Add chicken thighs and brown for approximately 5 minutes on each side, turning once.

2. Add green peppers and cook for about 5 minutes, or until golden. Stir in garlic and cook for 1 minute. Increase heat to high and pour wine over the mixture. Allow to boil until wine has evaporated.

3. Add stock and tomatoes, and stir. Add in salt, pepper, chile flakes, and bay leaf. When mixture comes to a boil, reduce heat to low and cover. Simmer for 45 minutes, or until peppers are tender and chicken is cooked through.

4. Discard bay leaf. Transfer to a serving plate and garnish with parsley. Serve hot.

⇥ Italian Living Tradition ⇤

The "sauce" of this stew also tastes delicious when served on pasta, rice, pizza, or polenta. When making this dish, double the tomato and pepper quantities and reserve the extra sauce to use with another dish during the week.

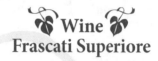

🍃 Wine 🍃
Frascati Superiore

ARTICHOKE, MUSHROOM, AND CARAMELIZED ONION FRITTATA (FRITTATA DI CARCIOFI, FUNGHI, E CIPOLLE CARAMELLATE)

Serves: 6 | Serving Size: 1 (2-inch) slice
Prep Time: 10 minutes | Cooking Time: About 1 hour

The difference between a frittata and an omelet is that frittate *(the plural in Italian) are cooked on only one side, while omelets are cooked on both.* Frittate *can be downsized into mini portions for the perfect appetizer, or served in large slices for a hearty breakfast, lunch, or dinner. You can make frittatas more or less "formal" by playing with their size and shape. In 2011, when CNN.com asked me to prepare my ultimate menu for Prince William's wedding, I included bite-size frittatas as part of the hors d'oeuvres course. The sautéed onions in this recipe are so delicious that I recommend doubling or tripling the quantity and saving the extras to use for sandwich, pizza, and rice pilaf toppings. You may substitute frozen artichoke hearts for fresh ones, if necessary.*

1/4 cup extra virgin olive oil

2 medium yellow onions, cut into very thin slices

1 pound baby artichokes

1 tablespoon lemon juice

1 pint shiitake or other mushrooms, cut into very thin (1/8-inch) slices

8 basil leaves, hand torn

6 large eggs, beaten until foamy

1/4 cup grated pecorino Romano or parmigiano-reggiano cheese

1/4 teaspoon unrefined sea salt

Choices/Exchanges 4 Vegetable, 2 Lean Protein, 2 Fat
Calories 270 | Calories from Fat 140
Total Fat 16g | Saturated Fat 3.6g | Trans Fat 0.0g
Cholesterol 190mg
Sodium 420mg

Potassium 755mg
Total Carbohydrate 23g | Dietary Fiber 7g | Sugars 9g
Protein 13g
Phosphorus 325mg

1. Preheat oven to 350°F.

2. Heat the oil in a large, wide, ovenproof skillet over medium-high heat. Add the onions; sauté, stirring occasionally, until softened and very dark golden in color, 20–30 minutes.

3. Meanwhile, clean and trim the artichokes. Soak the artichokes in water to clean; drain, and repeat until water is clear. Peel away the outside leaves of the bottom half of the artichokes. Cut off the top quarter of the artichoke (at this point the artichoke should look like a flower, and the tough, dark leaves should all be removed, leaving only the lighter-colored, tenderer leaves). If tough, dark green leaves remain, peel those as well. Add lemon juice to a bowl full of cold water and place each artichoke inside once it's trimmed to avoid discoloration.

4. Bring a large pot of water to a boil and add cleaned artichokes. Bring back to boil over high heat. Reduce heat to medium-low and simmer 15–20 minutes or until artichokes are tender.

5. Add mushrooms to the skillet with the onions. Brown them for 4 minutes. Add the artichokes, and stir. Add basil leaves, beaten eggs, cheese, and salt. Mix well and reduce the heat to medium-low. Cook for 4–5 minutes, or until the eggs are cooked through.

6. Finish off the frittata by putting the skillet in the oven until the frittata top is golden. Cut into 6 pieces and serve.

Italian Living Tradition

Frittatas and other omelets are usually served as light dinners along with salad in Italy. I recommend serving this frittata with Tomatoes with Balsamic Vinegar in the summer and Cannellini Bean, Tuna, and Red Onion Salad in the winter.

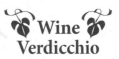

Wine
Verdicchio

CAMPANIA-STYLE RUSTIC VEGETABLE STEW (CIANFOTTA)

Serves: 6 | Serving Size: Approximately 1 cup
Prep Time: 15 minutes | Cooking Time: 45 minutes

This dish is a delicious, sweet-and-sour vegetarian hot pot from the Campania region of Italy. This recipe was introduced to me by fellow cookbook author and cooking instructor Alba Johnson, who hails from the region. Think of it as a Neapolitan spin on ratatouille. It is traditionally served as an appetizer or side dish in the summer, when all of the fruits and vegetables are in season. I think it makes a fantastic vegetarian main dish as well.

3 tablespoons extra virgin olive oil, divided

1 onion, diced

2 Chinese eggplants, diced

2 zucchini, diced

2 carrots, cut into 1/4-inch slices

2 small potatoes, diced

1/8 teaspoon unrefined sea salt

1 clove garlic, minced

1 red bell pepper, cut into small strips

4 ripe tomatoes, blanched, peeled, seeds removed, and crushed

2 Bosc pears, diced

1/8 cup golden raisins (or pitted dried plums)

15–20 fresh basil leaves, chiffonade

Choices/Exchanges 2 Starch, 1 Vegetable, 1 1/2 Fat
Calories 250 | Calories from Fat 70
Total Fat 8g | Saturated Fat 1.0g | Trans Fat 0.0g
Cholesterol 0mg
Sodium 130mg

Potassium 1270mg
Total Carbohydrate 44g | Dietary Fiber 12g | Sugars 21g
Protein 6g
Phosphorus 155mg

1. Preheat oven to 400°F. Line a large baking sheet with parchment paper.

2. In a bowl, add 2 tablespoons oil, the onion, eggplant, zucchini, carrots, and potatoes. Season with the salt and toss. Transfer to the baking sheet and bake until golden, about 25–30 minutes, turning once. When ready, set aside.

3. In a large skillet over medium-low heat, add the remaining 1 tablespoon oil. When oil is hot, add the garlic and bell pepper. Cook until the pepper is tender, and transfer to the baking sheet with baked vegetables.

4. Add the tomatoes and 1 cup hot water to the same skillet. Add the pears and raisins. Transfer the baked vegetables into the skillet and mix well. Cook about 15 minutes. Taste for doneness.

5. Transfer stew to a serving bowl and add fresh basil on top. Serve warm.

Italian Living Tradition

Each southern Italian region has its own version of and name for this stew. It is also called *ciambotta;* variations include *Ciambotta Lucana* from Basilicata, which is made with the region's famous sausages, peppers, onions, eggs, and tomatoes; and *Ciambotta Pugliese* from Puglia, which is made with fish.

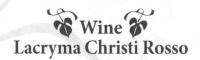

Wine
Lacryma Christi Rosso

SPICED CHICKPEA STEW
(STUFATO DI CECI ALLE SPEZIE)

Serves: 6 | Serving Size: 1 cup
Prep Time: 5 minutes | Cooking Time: About 30 minutes

Variations on this dish can be found throughout Italy. In Tuscany, it is usually prepared with cabbage and speck, a cured ham. In the Veneto region, it is prepared with radicchio. This is a flavorful and hearty recipe which both vegetarians and meat eaters will love. Pair with Whole-Wheat Fusilli with Pesto and Cherry Tomatoes (page 66) or Whole-Wheat Orecchiette Pasta with Broccoli and Garlic (page 68) for a meatless meal that can't be beat.

2 teaspoons extra virgin olive oil

1 medium yellow onion, diced

3 cloves garlic, minced

1 pound shredded cabbage or radicchio leaves

2 cups cooked chickpeas (see Dried Beans recipe on page 283) or reduced-sodium canned chickpeas

1/4 teaspoon saffron threads

1 teaspoon ground cloves

1 (28-ounce) can reduced-sodium diced or chopped tomatoes

1/4 teaspoon unrefined sea salt

1/4 teaspoon freshly ground black pepper

1/4 cup freshly chopped flat-leaf parsley

Choices/Exchanges 1 Starch, 1 Vegetable,
1 Lean Protein
Calories 140 | Calories from Fat 25
Total Fat 3g | Saturated Fat 0.5g | Trans Fat 0.0g
Cholesterol 0mg

Sodium 240mg
Potassium 590mg
Total Carbohydrate 23g | Dietary Fiber 8g | Sugars 8g
Protein 7g
Phosphorus 130mg

1. Heat olive oil in a large saucepan over medium heat. Add the diced onions and garlic, and cook until onions are soft.

2. Stir in the cabbage or radicchio, chickpeas, saffron, cloves, tomatoes, salt, and pepper. Increase heat to high and bring to a boil. Then reduce heat to low and cover the pot. Cook the stew for 15–20 minutes, or until cabbage or radicchio is very tender.

3. Garnish with parsley and serve.

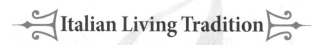

Italian Living Tradition

Legume-based second courses have been around since antiquity in Italy, but they are enjoying a resurgence in popularity. Easy on the wallet, waistline, and environment, beans and pulses are ingredients that everyone should take advantage of.

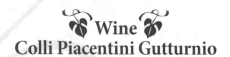

Wine
Colli Piacentini Gutturnio

EGGPLANT CROQUETTES
(POLPETTE DI MELANZANE)

Serves: 4 | Serving Size: 2 croquettes (4 ounces total)
Prep Time: 15 minutes | Cooking Time: 30 minutes

These eggplant "meatballs" are a delicacy of my ancestral homeland of Calabria, where they are known in the dialect as luminciana a pruppetta. *The name* Calabria *was given to the region by the Byzantines and means "fertile land." Eggplant is just one of the many prized agricultural crops that grows beautifully under the Calabrian sun. Some versions of this recipe include hard-boiled eggs and sausage, although I have never tried it that way. Eggplant croquettes are normally deep-fried in olive oil, but this is a more healthful baked version of the dish. Fresh bread crumbs make a huge difference in the final taste and texture of the dish.*

1 medium eggplant (approximately 1 pound), peeled and cubed

2 tablespoons pecorino Romano or pecorino Crotonese cheese (see Where to Buy Guide)

1/3 cup Fresh Bread Crumbs (page 291) or dried bread crumbs

1 egg, beaten

2 tablespoons water

2 tablespoons finely chopped fresh flat-leaf parsley

2 tablespoons finely chopped fresh basil

1 clove garlic, minced

1/4 teaspoon finely ground red chile flakes

1/2 teaspoon unrefined sea salt

1/8 teaspoon freshly ground black pepper

2 tablespoons extra virgin olive oil, divided

2 cups Fresh Tomato Sauce (page 228), for serving

Choices/Exchanges 1/2 Starch, 4 Vegetable, 3 Fat
Calories 290 | Calories from Fat 150
Total Fat 17g | Saturated Fat 2.9g | Trans Fat 0.0g
Cholesterol 50mg
Sodium 340mg

Potassium 1210mg
Total Carbohydrate 29g | Dietary Fiber 8g | Sugars 14g
Protein 8g
Phosphorus 180mg

1. Preheat oven to 350°F.

2. Place eggplant in a microwave-safe bowl and microwave on medium-high for 3 minutes. Turn eggplant over and microwave another 2 minutes. The eggplant should be tender; cook another 2 minutes if the eggplant is not tender. Drain any liquid from the eggplant, and mash.

3. Combine cheese, bread crumbs, egg, water, parsley, basil, garlic, chile flakes, salt, and pepper with the mashed eggplant. Mix well.

4. Shape the eggplant mixture into patties and place on a baking sheet greased with 1 tablespoon olive oil. Brush tops with remaining 1 tablespoon olive oil and bake until golden and crunchy, approximately 20–30 minutes.

5. Serve with tomato sauce.

Italian Living Tradition

Many of my cooking students are surprised to learn that not all eggplant dishes need to be salted and drained before cooking. This practice draws moisture out of the eggplants so that they absorb less oil while frying. If you're not frying your eggplant, you can skip the step. Disregard the old adage that salting the eggplant "draws out the bitter juices." Eggplant is actually very neutral in flavor to begin with.

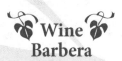

**Wine
Barbera**

ZUCCHINI AND HERB CROQUETTES (*POLPETTE DI ZUCCHINE*)

Serves: 6 | Serving Size: 2 (3-ounce) croquettes
Prep Time: 15 minutes | Cooking Time: 1 hour

These classic croquettes are served in various guises, not only throughout Italy, but also throughout the entire Mediterranean region. They may be served with pesto or tomato sauce in Italy or prepared with feta cheese in Greece and Turkey. I have incorporated quinoa into this recipe for a protein-packed, gluten-free alternative to the traditional recipes.

1/2 cup quinoa, soaked in water for 5 minutes

2 cups Homemade Vegetable Stock (page 287) or reduced-sodium vegetable stock

1/2 cup finely chopped fresh herbs (parsley, basil, and mint)

1 plum tomato, diced

1 cup shredded zucchini (from 1 medium zucchini)

2 tablespoons slivered almonds

1/4 teaspoon unrefined sea salt

1/8 teaspoon freshly ground black pepper

1 egg

1/4 cup bread crumbs or cornmeal

2 tablespoons extra virgin olive oil

2 cups Fresh Tomato Sauce (page 228), for serving

Choices/Exchanges 1 Starch, 2 Vegetable, 2 1/2 Fat
Calories 250 | Calories from Fat 130
Total Fat 14g | Saturated Fat 2.0g | Trans Fat 0.0g
Cholesterol 30mg
Sodium 240mg

Potassium 945mg
Total Carbohydrate 26g | Dietary Fiber 5g | Sugars 8g
Protein 9g
Phosphorus 210mg

1. Preheat oven to 375°F.

2. Drain and rinse the quinoa to remove the bitter flavors from the outer coating. Place quinoa in large saucepan. Add stock, herbs, tomato, zucchini, almonds, salt, and pepper, and bring to a boil over high heat. Reduce heat to low, cover tightly, and cook for 15 minutes. Let cool for about 15 minutes (so the egg doesn't cook when added).

3. Stir the egg and bread crumbs into the quinoa mixture. Form 12 patties (about 2 inches across and 1/4 inch thick), and refrigerate them for 15 minutes.

4. Grease a 9 × 13-inch baking dish with olive oil. Place patties in the dish and bake, uncovered, until golden and crunchy, approximately 20–30 minutes.

5. Serve with tomato sauce.

Italian Living Tradition

The Italian "locavore" style of eating (eating locally grown foods) evolved over centuries because farmers ate what they grew. Cooks needed to get crafty and create variations on the same types of vegetables in order to take advantage of large bumper crops. Shredded carrots would also work well in this recipe instead of or in addition to the zucchini.

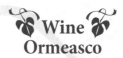

Wine
Ormeasco

PAN-SEARED SEA SCALLOPS (CAPESANTE IN PADELLA)

Serves: 4 | Serving Size: Approximately 1/4 pound scallops
Prep Time: 5 minutes (plus 1 hour marinating time) | Cooking Time: 10 minutes

These scallops are delicious on their own or tossed into a salad or pasta dish. If you don't have time to marinate the scallops, simply toss them with the marinade ingredients before frying. The recipe will still work well; the only difference is that the scallops will have a slightly less citrusy flavor at the end.

In the U.S., scallops are sometimes soaked in the preservative trisodium phosphate (TSP), which makes them weigh more, and consequently cost more. TSP also makes scallops exude moisture as they cook, thereby causing them to steam rather than sear properly. Look for scallops that are labeled "dry," meaning not soaked in TSP.

Juice and zest from 2 lemons
1 tablespoon extra virgin olive oil
1/4 teaspoon freshly ground black pepper
1 clove garlic, minced
1 pound dry scallops, cleaned
1 roasted red pepper, cut into tiny pieces

Choices/Exchanges 1/2 Carbohydrate, 2 Lean Protein, 1 Fat
Calories 160 | Calories from Fat 60
Total Fat 7g | Saturated Fat 1.0g | Trans Fat 0.0g
Cholesterol 30mg

Sodium 450mg
Potassium 330mg
Total Carbohydrate 9g | Dietary Fiber 1g | Sugars 2g
Protein 14g
Phosphorus 390mg

1. Make the marinade by combining lemon juice and zest, olive oil, pepper, and garlic in a large, shallow bowl or baking dish. Mix well to combine. Add scallops to the marinade, cover, and refrigerate 1 hour.

2. Heat a large skillet over medium-high heat. Drain scallops and place in skillet. Cook 4–5 minutes per side, until cooked through.

3. Arrange scallops on a serving platter or individual plates. Garnish with pieces of roasted peppers and serve.

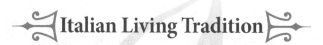

Italian Living Tradition

In Italy, scallops are often enjoyed raw in beautiful carpaccios. To make a carpaccio, simply place the scallops on a baking sheet lined with waxed paper. Cover with plastic wrap and place in the freezer for at least 1 hour. When the scallops are almost hard, remove them from the freezer and, using a sharp filleting knife, carefully cut the scallops width-wise into paper-thin slices. Place them on a platter. Drizzle with a vinaigrette and serve with greens. Note that consuming raw or undercooked seafood and shellfish may increase your risk of food-borne illness.

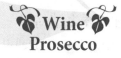

**Wine
Prosecco**

FISHERMEN KABOBS
(SPIEDINI ALLA MARINARA)

Serves: 4 | Serving Size: 1 skewer
Prep Time: 5 minutes | Cooking Time: 10 minutes

While this recipe could easily be prepared in any Italian coastal town, it is the Italian Riviera that comes to mind whenever I prepare it. Breathtaking Ligurian towns like Portofino, Santa Margherita, Rapallo, and Genoa have magical landscapes that are almost as sumptuous as the local cuisine. The region of Liguria is noted for a very fragrant variety of basil (Genoa, after all, is the birthplace of pesto), as well as wonderful produce and seafood.

Use whatever fresh fish, seafood, and herbs you have on hand in this recipe to come up with your own favorite combination. It's worth the effort to purchase "dry" scallops for this recipe—they are free of water-retaining additives—in order to ensure you're getting the real thing. Despite claims of being "natural, fresh, wild," etc., many scallops available on the market contain up to 80% water. Keep in mind that you will need four skewers for this dish. If you are using wooden skewers, you will need to soak them in water for a minimum of 20 minutes first. For additional flavor, use rosemary stems as skewers.

1 1/4 pounds skinless swordfish, cut into 1-inch cubes

24 grape tomatoes

1 cup lightly packed fresh basil

1/2 tablespoon extra virgin olive oil

1 clove garlic

1/4 teaspoon unrefined sea salt

1/4 teaspoon freshly ground black pepper

Crushed red chile flakes, to taste

Choices/Exchanges 1 Vegetable, 4 Lean Protein, 1/2 Fat
Calories 240 | Calories from Fat 100
Total Fat 11g | Saturated Fat 2.5g | Trans Fat 0.0g
Cholesterol 95mg
Sodium 220mg

Potassium 860mg
Total Carbohydrate 5g | Dietary Fiber 1g | Sugars 3g
Protein 29g
Phosphorus 390mg

1. Heat grill to high. Thread fish onto 4 skewers, alternating with tomatoes.

2. Place basil, oil, and garlic in a blender, and purée until smooth. Season with salt, pepper, and crushed red chile flakes. Reserve half the oil mixture in a separate container.

3. Brush kabobs with half of basil oil. Grill until fish is opaque, 6–10 minutes, turning occasionally.

4. With a clean brush, coat cooked kabobs with reserved basil oil. Serve immediately.

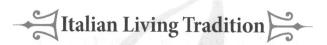

Italian Living Tradition

Even though the term *marinara* is often used to describe tomato sauce in the U.S., it actually means "in the way of the seafarer" in Italian—it's derived from the Italian word *mare,* which means "sea." Italians love to grill fish, and it's one of the healthiest and easiest ways to enjoy it.

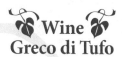

Wine Greco di Tufo

MUSSELS IN SAFFRON-TOMATO BROTH (COZZE IN BRODO DI ZAFFERANO)

Serves: 4 | Serving Size: 1 cup
Prep Time: 15 minutes | Cooking Time: 30 minutes

This elegant, restaurant-quality dish can be made in just a few minutes at home! The combination of seafood, tomatoes, and spices makes the dish sing. The secret ingredient in this recipe is saffron. The world's most expensive spice, saffron is cultivated from the stigmas of the crocus flower in the autumn. Its English name is derived from the feminine plural form of the Arabic word for yellow—saffra. Saffron provides a bright yellow pigment and unique flavor to drinks, savory dishes, and sweets.

Saffron originated in Central Asia, but it was introduced into Italy in the 8th century by the Spaniards. The Abruzzo region of Italy now produces some of the best saffron in the world, and it has DOP (Denominazione di origine protetta/Protected Designation of Origin) status under Italian law. Saffron is said to increase energy, suppress coughs, have diuretic properties, rejuvenate the heart, and ease labor pains.

4 tablespoons extra virgin olive oil

1/4 teaspoon saffron

1/2 teaspoon fennel seeds, crushed in a mortar to release aroma

2 cloves garlic, minced

1/2 teaspoon fresh orange zest

1 teaspoon fresh thyme

1 teaspoon fresh oregano

7 ounces fresh or canned reduced-sodium diced tomatoes

1 teaspoon tomato paste

2 cups Homemade Seafood Stock (page 288) or reduced-sodium seafood stock

1/8 teaspoon unrefined sea salt

1/4 teaspoon freshly ground black pepper

1/2 pound fresh mussels, scrubbed and beards removed (see Italian Living Tradition)

2 tablespoons finely chopped fresh flat-leaf parsley (for garnish)

Choices/Exchanges 1 1/2 Vegetable, 1 1/2 Lean Protein, 2 Fat

Calories 200 | Calories from Fat 140

Total Fat 16g | Saturated Fat 2.3g | Trans Fat 0.0g

Cholesterol 15mg

Sodium 290mg

Potassium 420mg

Total Carbohydrate 7g | Dietary Fiber 1g | Sugars 2g

Protein 10g

Phosphorus 165mg

1. Heat the olive oil in a large stock pot over medium heat. Add the saffron, fennel seeds, garlic, orange zest, thyme, and oregano, and cook for 2–3 minutes.

2. Stir in the tomatoes, tomato paste, stock, salt, and pepper, and bring to a boil over high heat. Reduce heat to low and simmer, covered, for 20 minutes.

3. Stir, add in mussels, cover, and cook for 7–10 minutes until mussels are open completely. (Resist the urge to open and close the lid often, as this causes steam to escape, making it harder for mussels to open and creating a firmer texture.) Discard any unopened mussels.

4. Pour into individual cups or bowls. Sprinkle with fresh parsley and serve.

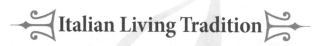

Italian Living Tradition

When choosing mussels, look for ones that are closed (this means they are alive and fresh) and completely smooth (not broken). It is best to purchase mussels from sources that sell them individually, so that you can be guaranteed of their freshness. Those sold in bags often seem fresh in the store, but when you take them home, you may realize that some are actually open (meaning they are dead) and need to be discarded.

To "scrub" mussels, wash them with a clean brush, and rinse them with cold water until the water runs clear and no sand or debris remains. You may need to do this multiple times.

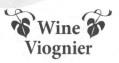

Wine
Viognier

BRAISED, STUFFED CALAMARI WITH TOMATO SAUCE (CALAMARI RIPIENI IN SALSA DI POMODORO)

Serves: 4 | Serving Size: 4 squid and 1/2 cup sauce
Prep Time: 10 minutes | Cooking Time: About 35 minutes

This traditional southern Italian recipe often uses a variety of calamari called totani—*which look like regular calamari except their fins are located near their tails. They are prepared in the same fashion as squid, so they are interchangeable in recipes. See Italian Living Tradition for squid-cleaning techniques.*

Because some supermarkets don't regularly stock squid, I suggest calling first to make sure it is available at your local market. Some stores stock frozen varieties year round. Note that they may need to be cleaned (tentacles and face removed) before proceeding with recipe.

2 tablespoons extra virgin olive oil, divided

1 medium yellow onion, finely chopped

10 ounces fresh baby spinach or kale

1/4 cup arborio rice

1/4 cup freshly chopped basil, parsley, or a combination of both

1/2 teaspoon unrefined sea salt

1/4 teaspoon freshly ground black pepper

Dash crushed red chile flakes

1 pound baby squid, cleaned and tentacles removed but reserved, divided

2 cups Fresh Tomato Sauce (page 228) or tomato purée

Choices/Exchanges 1 Starch, 2 Vegetable,
2 1/2 Lean Protein, 1 Fat
Calories 280 | Calories from Fat 100
Total Fat 11g | Saturated Fat 1.7g | Trans Fat 0.0g
Cholesterol 265mg

Sodium 370mg
Potassium 1000mg
Total Carbohydrate 23g | Dietary Fiber 4g | Sugars 4g
Protein 22g
Phosphorus 335mg

1. Heat 1 tablespoon olive oil in a very large, wide skillet over medium heat. Add onion and sauté until golden, about 5 minutes.

2. Add spinach or kale, rice, basil and/or parsley, salt, pepper, and red chile flakes, and sauté for 3–5 minutes. Take stuffing mixture off heat and allow to cool slightly.

3. Using your fingers, or a very small demitasse spoon, stuff calamari bodies 3/4 of the way full with stuffing. Secure top with a toothpick, leaving a little bit of room between the toothpick and the top of the stuffing for the rice to expand while cooking.

4. Heat remaining 1 tablespoon olive oil in a large frying pan over medium heat. Brown calamari on all sides. If you need to brown the squid in batches, simply brown half, transfer to a plate, and add the other half with additional olive oil.

5. Add Fresh Tomato Sauce or tomato purée and calamari tentacles to pan. Turn stuffed calamari over and spoon sauce over to coat. Cover, and simmer on low until cooked through, approximately 10–20 minutes. Serve warm.

Italian Living Tradition

To clean fresh, whole calamari, cut off the end with the tentacles and beak; remove and discard the beak and set the tentacles aside. Hold on to what is left of the head (the area with the eyes) and pull it out of the body, removing the internal organs. If you want the squid ink, carefully separate the ink sac and set it aside. Rinse the body cavity, reaching in with a finger and inverting the tube to make sure it is completely clean.

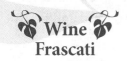

Wine
Frascati

SEA BASS WITH FENNEL BAKED IN PARCHMENT (BRANZINO CON FINOCCHIO AL CARTOCCIO)

Serves: 4 | Serving Size: 1 sea bass fillet and 1/2 cup vegetables
Prep Time: 10 minutes | Cooking Time: 20 minutes

Branzino *is a moist and flavorful Mediterranean fish that is becoming so popular in the U.S. that it is known just as well by its Italian name as it is by its English one (sea bass). The easy cooking method used in this recipe is popular all over Italy. The addition of fennel lends fresh, sweet notes to any type of white fish. A natural diuretic and digestive aid, fennel is also a popular addition to salads and after-dinner liqueur in both Italy and the entire Mediterranean region.*

3 cloves garlic, finely chopped

1/2 cup finely chopped fresh flat-leaf parsley

2 lemons, one juiced and zest reserved, and one cut into wedges, divided

1/3 cup extra virgin olive oil

1/2 teaspoon unrefined sea salt

1/4 teaspoon freshly ground black pepper

4 (4-ounce) sea bass fillets

1 cup cherry tomatoes, halved, divided

1 bulb fennel, trimmed and thinly sliced, divided

Choices/Exchanges 2 Vegetable, 3 1/2 Lean Protein, 2 1/2 Fat
Calories 320 | Calories from Fat 190
Total Fat 21g | Saturated Fat 3.2g | Trans Fat 0.0g
Cholesterol 55mg

Sodium 360mg
Potassium 720mg
Total Carbohydrate 9g | Dietary Fiber 3g | Sugars 4g
Protein 25g
Phosphorus 295mg

1. Preheat oven to 425°F.

2. Combine garlic, parsley, lemon zest and juice, olive oil, salt, and pepper in a small bowl.

3. Cut four pieces of parchment paper—each more than double the size of the sea bass.

4. Place 1 sea bass fillet, 1/4 cup cherry tomatoes, and 1/4 of fennel slices on top of half of each piece of parchment. Equally distribute 1/4 of garlic/herb mixture onto each piece of fish. Brush the mixture over the surface of the fish and fold the parchment over the fish. Fold and crimp the edges of the parchment packets to seal tightly. Place packets in a baking dish.

5. Bake about 15 minutes, until fish is cooked through. Remove from oven.

6. Serve with lemon wedges, allowing guests to open their own individual packages at the table.

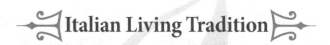

Italian Living Tradition

Al cartoccio, meaning "in parchment," is a popular Italian cooking method. Try cooking trout, tuna, vegetables, shrimp, and chicken breasts this way for great flavor and easy preparation.

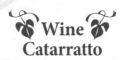

**Wine
Catarratto**

FRESH TUNA STEAKS WITH SAUTÉED ARTICHOKES
(TONNO CON CARCIOFI)

Serves: 4 | Serving Size: 1 (4-ounce) tuna steak
Prep Time: 10 minutes | Cooking Time: About 45 minutes

Fresh tuna and swordfish are plentiful around the shores of Sicily. This recipe combines many of Sicily's delicacies—olive oil, citrus, capers, anchovies, and mint—all in one delicious dish. This dish is impressive enough for guests, yet simple enough to make on the busiest of weeknights. Serve it with Marinated Eggplant Salad (page 202) and Sicilian olives for an authentic weeknight meal.

12 baby artichokes OR 4 regular-size artichokes

2 lemons, juiced

1/4 cup extra virgin olive oil

4 (4-ounce) tuna steaks

1 large yellow onion, thinly sliced

1 tablespoon capers packed in water, drained and rinsed well

8 oil-packed anchovy fillets, drained and rinsed well

3/4 cup freshly squeezed orange juice (2 oranges)

1/2 cup low-sodium chicken broth

1/4 teaspoon freshly ground black pepper

2 tablespoons freshly chopped mint

Choices/Exchanges 5 Vegetable, 4 Lean Protein, 2 Fat
Calories 390 | Calories from Fat 140
Total Fat 16g | Saturated Fat 2.4g | Trans Fat 0.0g
Cholesterol 60mg
Sodium 450mg

Potassium 1400mg
Total Carbohydrate 31g | Dietary Fiber 10g | Sugars 10g
Protein 36g
Phosphorus 425mg

1. Soak the artichokes in water to clean; drain and repeat until water is clear. Peel away the outside leaves of the bottom half of the artichokes. Cut off the top quarter of the artichoke (at this point the artichoke should look like a flower, and the tough, dark leaves should all be removed, leaving only the lighter-colored, tenderer leaves). If tough, dark green leaves remain, peel those as well.

2. Add juice of 2 lemons to a bowl full of cold water, and place artichokes inside to avoid discoloration. Bring a large pot of water to a boil, and add cleaned artichokes. Bring back to boil over high heat. Reduce heat to medium-low and simmer 15–20 minutes, or just until artichokes are fork tender. Drain artichokes. If using baby artichokes, set aside. If using regular-size artichokes, peel off leaves and reserve to serve as an appetizer; then dice the artichoke hearts and set aside.

3. Heat olive oil in a very large skillet over medium-high heat. Add tuna steaks and cook 2–3 minutes per side until golden. Remove tuna from pan and place on a platter. Set aside.

4. Add onions, capers, and anchovies to the skillet. Stir, and break up the anchovies with a wooden spoon. Sauté, uncovered, over medium heat until onions begin to caramelize (about 10–12 minutes). Add orange juice, chicken broth, and pepper. Stir well to combine, and cook, uncovered, for 3–4 minutes.

5. Add tuna steaks and artichokes back to the skillet, cover, and cook for 3 minutes per side until tuna is done.

6. Remove tuna from skillet to a serving platter. Pour sauce over tuna, and arrange onions around the top and sides of platter. Sprinkle fresh mint over the top of the dish. Serve warm.

⊰ Italian Living Tradition ⊱

While we're familiar with drizzling lemon juice over our seafood, orange juice is an often-overlooked condiment. In Sicily, however, orange juice is frequently paired with tuna, salmon, mussels, and other types of seafood. The sweet, floral notes of the juice pair well with rich, heavier types of seafood.

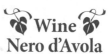

🍇 Wine 🍇
Nero d'Avola

TROUT FILLETS WITH SUN-DRIED TOMATO AND CURED-OLIVE CRUST
(FILETTI DI TROTA IMPANATI CON POMODORI SECCHI ED OLIVE CURATE)

Serves: 4 | Serving Size: 1 fillet
Prep Time: 5 minutes | Cooking Time: 15 minutes

Lake fish, such as trout, are popular in mountainous Italian regions. This recipe is very easy to put together with just a few pantry staples like olives and sun-dried tomatoes, which lend a piquant, sweet-and-savory flavor to the fish. Try serving this dish with Red Pepper and Sweet Potato Gnocchi (page 82) or Trapani-Style Almond Couscous (page 86) for a unique, easy, and delicious Italian feast.

3 cloves garlic, finely chopped
1/2 cup finely chopped fresh flat-leaf parsley
1/4 cup vacuum-sealed sun-dried tomatoes, chopped
1/4 cup oil-cured black olives, pitted and chopped
Zest and juice of 1 lemon
1 teaspoon extra virgin olive oil
4 (4-ounce) trout fillets
1/8 teaspoon unrefined sea salt
1/4 teaspoon freshly ground black pepper
1 lemon, quartered (optional)

Choices/Exchanges 1 Vegetable, 3 1/2 Lean Protein
Calories 170 | Calories from Fat 50
Total Fat 6g | Saturated Fat 1.1g | Trans Fat 0.0g
Cholesterol 60mg
Sodium 260mg

Potassium 735mg
Total Carbohydrate 5g | Dietary Fiber 1g | Sugars 2g
Protein 24g
Phosphorus 330mg

1. Preheat oven to 425°F.

2. Combine garlic, parsley, sun-dried tomatoes, olives, and lemon zest and juice in a small bowl.

3. Grease a baking dish with the olive oil. Place fish in the dish and brush the tomato/olive mixture over the fish. Bake for 10 minutes, until fish is cooked through.

4. Remove from oven, season with salt and pepper, and serve with lemon wedges if desired.

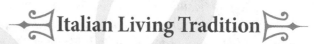

Italian Living Tradition

While this recipe celebrates sun-dried tomatoes and olives, sage and garlic are also commonly paired with trout in Italy. If you have fresh, whole trout, you can fill the cavities with chopped garlic, sage, and lemon slices. Drizzle with olive oil and sprinkle with salt and pepper. Roast at 425°F until fish flakes easily.

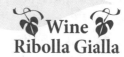

Wine
Ribolla Gialla

SWORDFISH WITH OLIVES, CAPERS, HERBS, AND TOMATOES (*PESCE SPADE ALLA GHIOTTA*)

Serves: 4 | Serving Size: 1 fillet
Prep Time: 5 minutes | Cooking Time: 25 minutes

Calabria is home to an annual swordfish festival, which draws locals and foreigners from all corners of the globe to pay tribute to the prized fish and the locals' ways of preparing it. Since swordfish is not always stocked in American supermarkets, it's a good idea to call ahead to find out when a shipment will be arriving and place an order. Pumpkin swordfish, tuna, haddock, and cod can all be substituted for swordfish when making this recipe. The swordfish also tastes great grilled with the sauce spooned over the top.

1 tablespoon extra virgin olive oil, divided

2 celery hearts, diced

2 cloves garlic, minced

2 cups boxed chopped tomatoes or reduced-sodium canned, diced tomatoes

3 tablespoons freshly chopped basil

1/8 teaspoon unrefined sea salt, divided

1/8 teaspoon freshly ground black pepper

Dash crushed red chile flakes

2 tablespoons capers, rinsed and well drained

1/4 cup green olives (such as sicilian colossal or Cerignola), rinsed, drained, pitted, and roughly chopped

4 (1/4-pound) boneless swordfish fillets

Choices/Exchanges 1 Vegetable, 3 1/2 Lean Protein, 1 Fat

Calories 230 | Calories from Fat 110

Total Fat 12g | Saturated Fat 2.5g | Trans Fat 0.0g

Cholesterol 75mg

Sodium 430mg

Potassium 770mg

Total Carbohydrate 7g | Dietary Fiber 2g | Sugars 3g

Protein 24g

Phosphorus 320mg

1. Heat olive oil in a large skillet over medium heat. Add celery and sauté until tender, approximately 5 minutes, stirring occasionally. Add garlic and cook until it releases its aroma—do not let garlic turn brown.

2. Stir in chopped tomatoes, basil, salt, pepper, chile flakes, capers, and olives. Mix well to combine, and cover. Reduce heat to low and simmer for 5 minutes.

3. Carefully remove lid from tomato sauce and add swordfish fillets into simmering sauce. Cover and cook for 10–15 minutes, or until fish is cooked through.

4. Transfer fish to a serving platter, top with sauce, and serve.

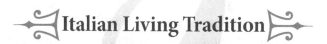

Italian Living Tradition

In Sicily and Calabria, the *ghiotta* style of cooking has been around for centuries. In addition to swordfish, stockfish is also prepared this way. Celery, onions, green olives, capers, and black pepper are essential to any *ghiotta* recipe. Red, high-quality onions from Tropea, along with capers from Salina, are traditionally considered the best to use in this recipe and can be ordered from some online sources (see the Where to Buy Guide on page 299). But you can substitute the red onions and capers of your choice.

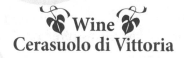

Wine
Cerasuolo di Vittoria

SICILIAN-STYLE FISH WITH VEGETABLES (DENTICE ALLA SICILIANA CON VERDURE AL FORNO)

Serves: 6 | Serving Size: 1 (2-ounce) piece fish and approximately 1 cup vegetables
Prep Time: 15 minutes | Cooking Time: 30 minutes

This recipe combines roasted fish with a Mediterranean vegetable medley and the sweet-and-sour flavors of onions, raisins, and pine nuts. Traditionally, this dish was made with red snapper, or dentice in Italian. Red snapper is a versatile Mediterranean fish that adapts well to many preparation styles; however, it has fallen prey to overfishing and unethical fishing practices, making it a non-environmentally friendly choice at this time. Sablefish from Alaska or Canada, mutton snapper, and yellowtail snapper are great substitutes.

12 ounces sablefish, mutton snapper, or yellowtail snapper fillets, cut into 6 (2-ounce) pieces

3 tablespoons extra virgin olive oil, plus more as needed

1 medium yellow onion, finely chopped

1 celery heart, finely chopped

1 carrot, peeled and finely chopped

1 cubanelle or green bell pepper, seeded and finely chopped

1 medium eggplant, cubed

6 ripe plum tomatoes, peeled, seeded, and finely chopped

1 tablespoon capers, rinsed well and drained

1 tablespoon golden raisins (preferably sultanas)

1 tablespoon pine nuts

1/8 teaspoon unrefined sea salt

1/4 teaspoon freshly ground black pepper

Choices/Exchanges 3 Vegetable, 2 Lean Protein, 1 1/2 Fat
Calories 220 | Calories from Fat 140
Total Fat 15g | Saturated Fat 2.5g | Trans Fat 0.0g
Cholesterol 30mg

Sodium 140mg
Potassium 670mg
Total Carbohydrate 14g | Dietary Fiber 5g | Sugars 7g
Protein 10g
Phosphorus 155mg

1. Preheat oven to 400°F.

2. Place the fish in a lightly oiled baking pan. Bake fish until the flesh flakes easily, about 20 minutes. Keep checking for doneness.

3. Heat 3 tablespoons olive oil in a large, wide skillet over medium heat; add the onion, celery, carrot, pepper, and eggplant, and cook until softer, about 6 minutes. Add the tomatoes, capers, raisins, pine nuts, salt, and pepper. Stir and cook until the sauce thickens, shaking the skillet, 7–8 minutes.

4. Remove the fish from the oven, cover with the sauce, and serve.

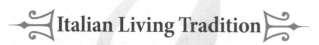

Italian Living Tradition

Roasting fish, poultry, or meat along with vegetables makes both the protein and vegetables even tastier. Try replacing the fish in this recipe with chicken or turkey breasts for a healthy meal the whole family will love.

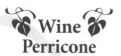

**Wine
Perricone**

SEA BREAM WITH DUCHESS-STYLE SWEET POTATOES (ORATA CON PATATE DOLCE ALLA DUCCHESSA)

Serves: 4 | Serving Size: 1 fish and 4 1/2 potato mounds
Prep Time: 5 minutes | Cooking Time: Approximately 1 hour 30 minutes

This elegant and nutritious meal is perfect for company. Sea bass or any medium white fish can be substituted for the sea bream, and regular potatoes or other root vegetables can be substituted for the sweet potatoes. If you don't like whole fish, you can substitute your favorite fillets. Rosemary adds an herbaceous perfume to the dish.

2 small sweet potatoes, washed and each cut into about 8 chunks

2 large egg whites, divided

3 tablespoons extra virgin olive oil, divided

1/8 teaspoon unrefined sea salt

1/4 teaspoon freshly ground black pepper

1/4 teaspoon freshly grated nutmeg

1/4 cup low-fat plain yogurt

4 whole sea bream (1 pound each), gutted, with scales still attached

4 cloves garlic

4 large sprigs rosemary

4 slices lemon

Choices/Exchanges 1/2 Starch, 4 Lean Protein, 1 1/2 Fat
Calories 300 | Calories from Fat 140
Total Fat 15g | Saturated Fat 2.7g | Trans Fat 0.0g
Cholesterol 75mg

Sodium 190mg
Potassium 585mg
Total Carbohydrate 10g | Dietary Fiber 1g | Sugars 4g
Protein 30g
Phosphorus 285mg

1. Preheat oven to 400°F.

2. Place sweet potatoes in the oven on a sheet of foil (to catch any drips while cooking) and bake for 45 minutes. Remove from oven and cool slightly. Peel off and discard skin. Reduce oven temperature to 375°F.

3. In the bowl of a standing mixer, add the cooked and cooled potatoes along with 1 egg white, 2 tablespoons olive oil, salt, pepper, nutmeg, and yogurt. Using whip attachment, whip until smooth.

4. Place potato mixture into a 16-inch pastry bag with a large star tip, and pipe mixture onto a parchment-lined sheet pan to make 18 little mounds, swirling pastry bag tip around as you build to the top of each mound. Mix the remaining egg white with a little water and gently brush on each mound without disturbing the nice swirl pattern. Set aside.

5. Place the 4 whole fish on a baking sheet. Add 1 garlic clove, 1 rosemary sprig, and 1 lemon slice into each cavity. Use the remaining 1 tablespoon olive oil to brush both sides of each fish.

6. Bake both the sheet of potatoes and the sheet of fish simultaneously, with the potatoes on top and the fish on the bottom, switching the position of the baking sheets halfway through, for 25–30 minutes, or until potatoes are slightly browned and fish is cooked through (flakes easily when cut into with a fork). Serve immediately.

Italian Living Tradition

There are many elaborate, decorative dishes in both France and Italy that boast the "Duchess style" title, including some risotto dishes, some desserts, and these potatoes. While we don't know the origins of all Duchess-style dishes, it is interesting to note that throughout the history of these cuisines, honorary recipes were created for noble women, and their legacies live on today through these recipes.

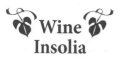
**Wine
Insolia**

VENETIAN-STYLE SOLE IN A SWEET-AND-SOUR SAUCE (SFOGI IN SAOR)

Serves: 4 | Serving Size: 1 fish fillet and 2 tablespoons onions
Prep Time: 15 minutes (plus 20 minutes raisin-soaking time)
Cooking Time: 15 minutes (plus refrigerating time)

This unique way of marinating fish in a sweet-and-sour sauce is Venetian. Recipes like this are a testament to the years of cross-cultural collaboration and synergy between Italy and the Middle East. Note that the recipe needs to marinate in the refrigerator for 24 hours before serving. Wheat flour makes a good coating, but you can use almond flour or cornmeal for a gluten-free alternative.

1/4 cup whole-wheat flour or almond flour

4 (4-ounce) sole or halibut fillets, skinned

1 tablespoon extra virgin olive oil

1/8 teaspoon unrefined sea salt

1/4 teaspoon freshly ground black pepper

2 large yellow onions (approximately 1 1/4 pounds total), thinly sliced

1/4 cup white wine

1/4 cup white wine vinegar

1 tablespoon sugar

1/4 cup raisins, soaked in warm water to cover for 20 minutes and drained

1/4 cup pine nuts or slivered almonds, toasted

1 tablespoon finely chopped flat-leaf parsley

Choices/Exchanges 1/2 Carbohydrate, 2 Vegetable, 3 1/2 Lean Protein, 1 Fat
Calories 300 | Calories from Fat 100
Total Fat 11g | Saturated Fat 1.3g | Trans Fat 0.0g
Cholesterol 55mg

Sodium 170mg
Potassium 850mg
Total Carbohydrate 26g | Dietary Fiber 3g | Sugars 14g
Protein 25g
Phosphorus 400mg

1. Spread flour on a plate. Coat fish fillets with flour, shaking off excess.

2. Heat oil in a large, wide skillet over medium heat. Add fish and cook until golden, about 2–3 minutes per side. Remove fish from heat and set on a plate. Season with salt and pepper, and set aside.

3. Add onions to the same skillet used for the fish, and stir. Sauté until golden, approximately 10 minutes, stirring occasionally. Increase heat, and add wine and vinegar. Bring mixture to a boil over high heat and cook, stirring constantly with a wooden spoon, until liquid condenses by approximately half. Add sugar, raisins, and pine nuts. Cook 1 minute longer.

4. Place fish in a shallow baking dish. Spoon onion mixture over fish, and allow for fish to cool to room temperature. Then cover with plastic wrap and refrigerate for 24 hours.

5. Remove fish from refrigerator and sprinkle with parsley before serving. Serve cold or at room temperature.

Italian Living Tradition

Il saor is a Venetian sauce containing onions, oil, and vinegar. It was originally used by fishermen to preserve seafood in terra-cotta dishes during long voyages. As trade increased, the addition of raisins and pine nuts became popular. Sardines are often prepared this way.

FISH STEW OVER POLENTA (PESCE IN UMIDO CON LA POLENTA)

Serves: 6 | Serving Size: Approximately 1/3 cup stew and 3 tablespoons polenta
Prep Time: 15 minutes (plus 1 hour marinating time) | Cooking Time: 30 minutes

Homey yet impressive dishes like this are popular in the Emilia-Romagna region. Often called the gastronomic capital of Italy, Emilia-Romagna is home to the cities of Modena (famous for balsamic vinegar) and Parma (famous for award-winning prosciutto) as well as parmigiano-reggiano cheese, rich ragus, and more. This dish combines many of the trademark, comfort-inducing flavors of the region without adding too many calories. This stew can be served cold; it is often preferred this way during the summer months.

2 medium yellow onions, diced, divided

1 celery heart, diced, divided

2 cloves garlic, minced

1 dried bay leaf

1 1/4 pounds halibut or swordfish fillet, boned, skinned, and cut into 3/4-inch cubes

1/2 teaspoon unrefined sea salt

1/8 teaspoon freshly ground black pepper

1/2 cup dry white wine, such as Trebbiano

2 oil-packed anchovy fillets, drained, rinsed, and chopped

1/3 cup extra virgin olive oil

2 tablespoons freshly chopped flat-leaf parsley

2 teaspoons Fresh Tomato Sauce (page 228) or tomato purée, stirred into 1/4 cup water

1 cup cooked Polenta (page 286)

Choices/Exchanges 1 Starch, 2 1/2 Lean Protein, 2 Fat
Calories 270 | Calories from Fat 130
Total Fat 14g | Saturated Fat 2.0g | Trans Fat 0.0g
Cholesterol 45mg
Sodium 310mg

Potassium 550mg
Total Carbohydrate 13g | Dietary Fiber 1g | Sugars 2g
Protein 20g
Phosphorus 260mg

1. Combine half of the onions and celery along with the garlic and bay leaf in a large glass bowl or baking dish. Arrange the fish cubes on top, season with salt and pepper, and top with the remaining onions and celery. Cover the vegetables and fish with the wine and anchovies. Allow to marinate, covered, for 1 hour in the refrigerator.

2. Drain the fish, reserving the marinade and anchovies, and discard the vegetables. Dry fish and set aside.

3. Heat the olive oil in a dutch oven or a large, wide skillet over medium heat. Add the anchovies, mashing them with a fork so that they dissolve into the oil. Add the parsley and stir to combine.

4. Add the fish pieces and cook for 1 minute on each side to brown. Pour in the leftover marinade. Increase the heat to high and allow the mixture to reduce by half.

5. Add the tomato sauce or purée, stir gently, and cover. Reduce heat to low and cook for 15–20 minutes, or until fish is cooked through and tender.

6. Serve over polenta.

Italian Living Tradition

Cornmeal is a staple all around Italy. Even though it was originally used as animal feed, cornmeal became a popular ingredient with the Jewish community in Venice and, afterwards, throughout Italy. Many people assume that polenta is strictly a northern Italian dish, but it is not. In southern Italy, it is very popular as well; it was once even a breakfast item eaten by farmers.

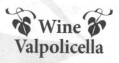

**Wine
Valpolicella**

CITRUS AND HERB–INFUSED SCALLOP STEW (CAPESANTE IN UMIDO CON ERBE ED AGRUMI)

Serves: 6 | Serving Size: Approximately 5 scallops
Prep Time: 10 minutes | Cooking Time: Approximately 10 minutes

The Italian name for scallops, capesante, *is a derivative of the French term for scallops—coquille Saint Jacques. The scallop shell is a symbol of the pilgrims who visited the famous cathedral of Saint James in Spain, and a symbol of Pope Benedict XVI. The scallop shell was also used in the infamous Botticelli painting of Venus. Regardless of scallops' symbolism, Italians love to cook them because they are both decadent and easy to prepare. When shopping, always choose "dry" scallops, which are free of chemical additives.*

3 tablespoons extra virgin olive oil

1 medium yellow onion, diced

1 cup diced fresh fennel

2 cloves garlic, minced

2 tablespoons all-purpose flour or cornmeal

Zest and juice of 1 orange

Zest and juice of 1 lemon

1/2 teaspoon unrefined sea salt

1/4 teaspoon finely ground black pepper

1 pound dry 20/30 scallops

1/4 cup finely chopped fresh flat-leaf parsley

2 tablespoons finely chopped fresh basil

Choices/Exchanges 2 Vegetable, 1 1/2 Lean Protein, 1 Fat

Calories 160 | Calories from Fat 60

Total Fat 7g | Saturated Fat 1.0g | Trans Fat 0.0g

Cholesterol 20mg

Sodium 310mg

Potassium 315mg

Total Carbohydrate 13g | Dietary Fiber 2g | Sugars 3g

Protein 10g

Phosphorus 280mg

1. Heat the olive oil in a dutch oven or a large, wide skillet over medium heat. Add the onion and fennel, and sauté until lightly golden, 5 minutes, stirring occasionally. Stir in garlic.

2. Sprinkle the mixture with the flour, stir, and cook for 1 minute, stirring constantly. Add the citrus juices and zest, salt, and pepper. Whisk the mixture to reach a smooth, sauce-like consistency.

3. Add the scallops and cook, covered, over medium heat until they are opaque, approximately 3–5 minutes. Remove from heat, gently stir in parsley and basil, and allow to rest, covered, for 1 additional minute.

4. Serve immediately.

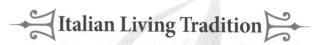

Italian Living Tradition

In Venice, and along the Adriatic coastline, a similar version of this dish (minus the fennel and orange) is served in the scallop shells for a dramatic presentation—plus it confirms the freshness and quality of the scallops.

HERB-MARINATED CHICKEN BREASTS (*PETTI DI POLLO MARINATE CON ERBE*)

Serves: 6 | Serving Size: Approximately 5 ounces chicken
Prep Time: 10 minutes (plus marinating time) | Cooking Time: 10 minutes

I make this recipe at least twice a month with whatever fresh herbs I happen to have on hand. It's quick, easy, lean, and delicious, and can also be quickly grilled or broiled. I often slice the leftovers and serve them over a salad made of spinach and arugula, cherry tomatoes, shredded carrots, fresh peas, and corn. The marinade in this recipe also works well with turkey breasts and firm-fleshed fish.

1/2 cup fresh lemon juice
1/4 cup extra virgin olive oil
4 cloves garlic, minced
1 medium yellow onion, sliced
1 bunch fresh flat-leaf parsley, finely chopped
1/4 cup fresh basil, finely chopped
2 pounds chicken breast tenders
1/8 teaspoon unrefined sea salt
1/4 teaspoon freshly ground black pepper

Choices/Exchanges 1 Vegetable, 5 Lean Protein, 1 Fat
Calories 280 | Calories from Fat 120
Total Fat 13g | Saturated Fat 2.1g | Trans Fat 0.0g
Cholesterol 110mg
Sodium 130mg

Potassium 680mg
Total Carbohydrate 5g | Dietary Fiber 1g | Sugars 2g
Protein 35g
Phosphorus 355mg

1. In a small bowl, whisk lemon juice, olive oil, garlic, onion, parsley, and basil well to combine.

2. Place the chicken tenders in a large, shallow bowl or glass baking pan and pour marinade over the top. Cover, place in the refrigerator, and allow to marinate for 1–2 hours. Remove from the refrigerator, and season with salt and pepper.

3. Heat a large, wide skillet over medium-high heat. Using tongs, spread out chicken tenders evenly on the bottom of the skillet. Pour the marinade over the chicken.

4. Cook chicken for 3–5 minutes on each side, or until chicken is golden, juices have been absorbed, and meat is cooked to an internal temperature of 160°F. Serve.

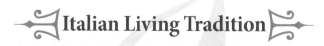

Italian Living Tradition

In addition to the flavor and moisture that the lemon juice adds to this recipe, lemons' antibacterial properties are coveted for killing bad bacteria in undercooked foods. So they are both beneficial and delicious to eat!

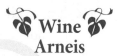

**Wine
Arneis**

CHICKEN STEW WITH MUSHROOMS AND ONIONS (*STUFATO DI POLLO CON FUNGHI E CIPOLLE*)

Serves: 4 | Serving Size: 1/2 cup
Prep Time: 15 minutes | Cooking Time: Approximately 1 hour

This dish reminds me of the rolling hills in Umbria—where mushroom foraging is taken seriously and rustic food is served in a charming way. If you usually overlook chicken meat when making stews, this is the perfect dish to change your mind. Chicken stew is healthful, light, and hearty all at the same time. The mushrooms and herb add a very autumnal touch to this dish. I recommend serving it with Calabrian-Style Roasted Potatoes (page 176) and/or Spinach Sautéed in Garlic and Oil (page 180).

2 tablespoons extra virgin olive oil
2 large yellow onions, thinly sliced
1 cup chanterelle, shiitake, or button mushrooms, cleaned and sliced
1 1/4 pounds boneless, skinless chicken breasts, cut into 1-inch cubes
1 cup canned low-sodium chopped or diced tomatoes
1 tablespoon freshly chopped thyme OR 1/2 teaspoon dried thyme
3/4 teaspoon kosher salt
1/4 teaspoon freshly ground black pepper

Choices/Exchanges 2 Vegetable, 4 Lean Protein, 1 Fat
Calories 280 | Calories from Fat 100
Total Fat 11g | Saturated Fat 1.8g | Trans Fat 0.0g
Cholesterol 105mg
Sodium 430mg

Potassium 770mg
Total Carbohydrate 11g | Dietary Fiber 3g | Sugars 5g
Protein 33g
Phosphorus 345mg

1. Heat oil in a large, wide skillet over medium heat. Add onions and sauté until golden, stirring occasionally, approximately 3 minutes. Add mushrooms and stir. Add chicken and brown on all sides, approximately 5 minutes total.

2. Add tomatoes, 1 cup water, thyme, salt, and pepper, and stir to combine. Increase the heat to high and bring stew to a boil, uncovered.

3. Reduce heat to low, cover, and simmer for 45 minutes–1 hour, or until chicken is tender and cooked through. Serve.

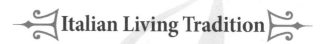

Italian Living Tradition

This recipe uses chicken breasts, which are lower in fat and quicker to cook than some other parts of the chicken. But in many Italian households, it would be the legs or the thighs *(cosce)* that would be used in this and other stewed chicken dishes such as *Pollo alla cacciatora*.

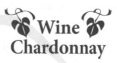

Wine
Chardonnay

CHICKEN BREASTS
WITH CITRUS, CAPERS, AND PINE NUTS
(PETTI DI POLLO AL LIMONE, CAPERI, E PINOLI)

Serves: 4 | Serving Size: 1 chicken breast half
Prep Time: 10 minutes | Cooking Time: 20 minutes

Scaloppine—an Italian weeknight staple—are thinly sliced pieces of chicken, beef, veal, or turkey. This dish is a classic in which the humble chicken breast is elevated by the addition of traditional Sicilian ingredients. You can substitute orange juice for the lemon juice, if desired. This recipe can also be used with veal scaloppini or thin fillets of fish such as tilapia or haddock.

2 tablespoons extra virgin olive oil

2 boneless, skinless chicken breasts, sliced in half width-wise and pounded thin

1 cup Homemade Chicken Stock (page 289) or reduced-sodium chicken stock

2 teaspoons capers, rinsed and drained

Zest of 1 lemon

1/2 cup freshly squeezed lemon juice

1/8 teaspoon unrefined sea salt

1/4 teaspoon freshly ground black pepper

2 tablespoons raisins

2 tablespoons pine nuts

1/4 cup finely chopped fresh flat-leaf parsley (for garnish)

Choices/Exchanges 2 Vegetable, 4 Lean Protein, 1 1/2 Fat

Calories 300 | Calories from Fat 130

Total Fat 14g | Saturated Fat 2.0g | Trans Fat 0.0g

Cholesterol 100mg

Sodium 200mg

Potassium 645mg

Total Carbohydrate 11g | Dietary Fiber 1g | Sugars 7g

Protein 33g

Phosphorus 350mg

1. Heat olive oil in a large, wide skillet over medium-high heat. Add chicken breasts and brown for approximately 5 minutes per side, or until slightly golden (turning only once).

2. In a medium bowl, stir together the chicken stock, capers, lemon zest, and lemon juice.

3. When the chicken is browned, pour stock mixture over the top. Reduce heat to low. Season with salt and pepper. Sprinkle raisins and pine nuts over chicken. Cover, and simmer for 10 minutes, or until sauce has reduced by about 3/4.

4. To serve, place chicken breasts on platter or individual plates, spoon sauce over the top, and garnish with parsley.

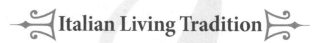

Italian Living Tradition

Scaloppine are usually pan-fried until golden and served with a slice of lemon (Milanese) or in a piccata sauce (lemon, white wine, and capers) or tomato sauce. They can also become the base for other dishes such as *Vitello alla parmigiana* (Veal Parmesan). Known as the housewife's best friend because they cook in minutes, *scaloppine* are also great for health-conscious cooks because they are relatively small portions of lean protein.

MARINATED CHICKEN WITH ROSEMARY AND BALSAMIC VINEGAR (POLLO MARINATO CON ROSMARINO ED ACETO BALSAMICO)

Serves: 4 | Serving Size: 1 (3-ounce) piece chicken
Prep Time: 15 minutes (plus marinating time) | Cooking Time: 45 minutes

This is one of the first recipes I learned to make as a child. It has a special place at my family's table even though it's a very easy and inexpensive dish. We refer to it as "Nonna Foti's Chicken" because my maternal great-grandmother served it this way. The Foti family originated in Reggio Calabria, which was a strong Greek outpost in antiquity. This dish is, in fact, very similar to one I have tasted on the Greek islands, where it is prepared with lemon juice instead of balsamic vinegar. The best thing about this dish is that it's a crowd pleaser and works all year round. During the warm weather, it pairs well with Whole-Wheat Fusilli with Pesto and Cherry Tomatoes (page 66). Or try it in the winter after a serving of Red Pepper and Sweet Potato Gnocchi (page 82).

1/2 cup balsamic vinegar

2 tablespoons finely chopped fresh rosemary or oregano

1/4 teaspoon unrefined sea salt

1/2 teaspoon freshly ground black pepper

Pinch crushed red chile flakes

12 ounces boneless, skinless chicken breasts, cut into 4 (3-ounce) pieces

1 tablespoon extra virgin olive oil

4 tablespoons freshly chopped flat-leaf parsley

Choices/Exchanges 1/2 Carbohydrate, 3 Lean Protein
Calories 170 | Calories from Fat 50
Total Fat 6g | Saturated Fat 1.0g | Trans Fat 0.0g
Cholesterol 60mg
Sodium 170mg

Potassium 385mg
Total Carbohydrate 7g | Dietary Fiber 1g | Sugars 5g
Protein 20g
Phosphorus 195mg

1. In a small bowl, combine vinegar, rosemary or oregano, salt, pepper, and crushed red chile flakes.

2. Place chicken in a baking dish greased with the olive oil and pour marinade over the top. Cover with plastic wrap and allow to marinate for 1 hour. Discard plastic wrap.

3. Preheat oven to 425°F.

4. Cover baking dish with aluminum foil and roast until chicken is cooked through, approximately 45 minutes.

5. Garnish with fresh parsley and serve.

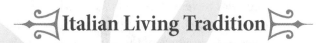

Italian Living Tradition

Fresh herbs are integral to the Italian kitchen. Even if they don't have a garden, many Italians grow herbs on their balcony, terrace, or windowsill. Having fresh herbs on hand is a great way to add more flavor and health benefits to your food without adding extra calories, fat, or sodium.

CACCIATORE-STYLE CHICKEN
(POLLO ALLA CACCIATORA)

Serves: 8 | Serving Size: 1 piece chicken and 1/4 cup sauce
Prep Time: 15 minutes | Cooking Time: 1 hour

Chicken was the centerpiece of many regal tables during the 15th century. In the 17th century, it became more commonplace, but still many families could only dream of eating it on a weekly basis. But by the 21st century, chicken had become a staple on Italian tables everywhere. Unlike many of the regional recipes in this book, this dish is made in various ways throughout Italy. For example, in Modena—famous for both its wine and vinegar production—a few tablespoons of wine vinegar are used in place of the wine. You can substitute 1/4 cup of balsamic vinegar or 1 cup of Homemade Chicken or Vegetable Stock (pages 289, 287) for the wine in this recipe.

3/4 cup whole-wheat flour or rice or almond flour

2 pounds boneless, skinless chicken breasts, cut into 8 pieces

1/4 cup extra virgin olive oil

1 tablespoon finely chopped fresh rosemary OR 1/2 teaspoon dried rosemary, crushed

1 medium onion, diced

3 cloves garlic, minced

1/4 cup dried porcini mushrooms, soaked in water for at least 20 minutes, drained, and chopped

1 cup dry marsala wine

2 cups reduced-sodium crushed or diced tomatoes

1/8 teaspoon unrefined sea salt

1/4 teaspoon freshly ground black pepper

1 dried bay leaf

Crushed red chile flakes (optional)

Choices/Exchanges 3 Vegetable, 4 Lean Protein, 1 Fat
Calories 300 | Calories from Fat 90
Total Fat 10g | Saturated Fat 1.6g | Trans Fat 0.0g
Cholesterol 80mg
Sodium 100mg

Potassium 600mg
Total Carbohydrate 17g | Dietary Fiber 2g | Sugars 4g
Protein 28g
Phosphorus 300mg

1. Place flour in a shallow dish. Coat the chicken liberally with flour and shake off excess.

2. Heat oil in large skillet over medium-high heat. Add the chicken, making sure not to crowd the skillet (work in batches if necessary). Cook until chicken is golden on all sides, 5–6 minutes. Transfer the chicken to a platter and set aside.

3. Reduce the heat under the skillet to medium, and add the rosemary and onion. Cook, stirring, until the mixture begins to color and onion softens, 4–5 minutes. Stir in the garlic and mushrooms, and cook for 1 more minute.

4. Return the chicken to the skillet, raise the heat to high, and add the wine. Cook and stir until the wine is almost all reduced, 5–6 minutes.

5. Add the tomatoes, and season with salt, pepper, bay leaf, and crushed red chile flakes (if using). Bring the tomatoes to a boil, then reduce the heat to medium-low and cover the skillet, leaving the lid slightly askew. Cook until the chicken is tender, 40–50 minutes. Stir and turn the chicken a few times during cooking.

6. When chicken is cooked, discard bay leaf and serve.

Italian Living Tradition

Recipes for stews like this one were created with older, tougher meats, like stewing hens, in mind. Dousing the meat with wine and then slowly simmering it in tomatoes created a tender texture and deep flavor that compensated for the tough meat.

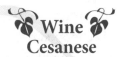 **Wine Cesanese**

CLASSIC ROASTED CHICKEN
(POLLO AL FORNO)

Serves: 6 | Serving Size: 1 piece chicken and 1/2 cup vegetables
Prep Time: 15 minutes | Cooking Time: 45 minutes

Many Italian cooks, myself included, don't bother roasting one thing at a time. As long as you've got the ingredients out and the oven heated, you might as well roast a few items to save time and energy. If I'm roasting chicken, I always make extra and use the leftover chicken to make Monday Salad (page 196). Sometimes I roast chicken and a whole fish, which can be dressed in the same way as the chicken and needs only one third of the time to cook. The fish and the chicken can be served later in the day or the following day—with leftovers on the third day. That way, you've got dinner for three nights made in the same time it takes to make one recipe.

1 1/2 pounds raw, boneless, skinless chicken breasts, cut into 6 pieces

1 tablespoon extra virgin olive oil

1 teaspoon unrefined sea salt

1/4 teaspoon freshly ground black pepper

2 tablespoons finely chopped fresh rosemary

1 tablespoon finely chopped fresh sage

1 head garlic, stem sliced off, left intact

1 lemon, cut in half and one half sliced

3/4 pound yukon gold or other potatoes, peeled and cut into 1-inch pieces

1 1/2 pounds carrots, cut into 2-inch pieces on the diagonal

Choices/Exchanges 1 Starch, 1 Vegetable,
4 1/2 Lean Protein
Calories 300 | Calories from Fat 60
Total Fat 7g | Saturated Fat 1.6g | Trans Fat 0.0g
Cholesterol 130mg

Sodium 440mg
Potassium 1220mg
Total Carbohydrate 25g | Dietary Fiber 5g | Sugars 6g
Protein 40g
Phosphorus 390mg

1. Preheat oven to 425°F.

2. Place chicken pieces in a roasting pan and drizzle olive oil over the chicken, turning to make sure both the pan and chicken are coated. Season with salt, pepper, rosemary, and sage by rubbing them into the top and sides of the chicken.

3. Place garlic and the lemon slices on top of chicken, and squeeze remaining lemon half over the chicken. Scatter the potatoes and carrots around the chicken, turning to coat in olive oil.

4. Bake for 30–45 minutes, or until chicken is done and potatoes are tender. (Chicken is done when clear juices run from the thickest part after being pierced with a fork.)

5. Cover chicken and allow to rest 10 minutes. Discard garlic and lemon before serving.

Italian Living Tradition

Carrots and potatoes are classic vegetables that work year round in this dish. I suggest changing the vegetables you include according to the season. For example, asparagus and fennel are delicious in the spring, and eggplant, zucchini, and tomatoes work best in the summer. For fall, try a mix of cauliflower and broccoli or fresh mushrooms.

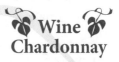

Wine
Chardonnay

ROASTED CHICKEN WITH GRAPES AND CHESTNUTS
(POLLO CON LE UVE E CASTAGNE)

Serves: 6 | Serving Size: 1 piece chicken and approximately 2 ounces chestnut/grape mixture
Prep Time: 15 minutes | Cooking Time: 40 minutes

In Italy, it is quail, not chicken, that is normally served with this grape and chestnut combination. I absolutely love the flavor and texture of that classic dish. It was my original intention to include it in this book. Unfortunately, while I was testing the recipe, none of the specialty stores that I contacted in Washington, D.C., had quail available; it is now only sold for the holidays in most areas. I figured that if I couldn't source quail in Washington, D.C., it would be difficult for many readers to find. So I decided to substitute chicken for the quail, and the dish is still delicious!

1 1/4 pounds raw, boneless, skinless chicken breasts, cut into 6 pieces

3/4 teaspoon unrefined sea salt

1/4 teaspoon freshly grated black pepper

2 tablespoons extra virgin olive oil, divided

1 teaspoon dried thyme, finely crushed

4 whole cloves garlic

2 cups Homemade Chicken Stock (page 289) or low-sodium chicken broth, divided

1 bay leaf

1 medium carrot, finely chopped

2 celery hearts, finely chopped

1 medium onion, finely chopped

8 ounces (1/2 pound) seedless green grapes, half sliced in half, rest left whole

14 roasted chestnuts (either prepackaged or peeled and roasted fresh)

Choices/Exchanges 1 Carbohydrate, 2 Vegetable, 4 Lean Protein
Calories 300 | Calories from Fat 80
Total Fat 9g | Saturated Fat 1.9g | Trans Fat 0.0g
Cholesterol 110mg

Sodium 380mg
Potassium 700mg
Total Carbohydrate 23g | Dietary Fiber 2g | Sugars 10g
Protein 33g
Phosphorus 300mg

1. Put oven rack in middle position and preheat oven to 425°F.

2. Sprinkle chicken all over with salt and pepper. Grease a large baking or roasting pan with 1 tablespoon olive oil. Add chicken and turn to coat. Sprinkle thyme, crushing with your fingers, over chicken. Place garlic cloves in pan.

3. Pour 1 1/2 cups stock around sides of chicken and add bay leaf to the liquid. Place in oven and roast, uncovered, until chicken is cooked through and clear liquid runs from the meat when pierced with a fork (30–40 minutes).

4. While chicken is cooking, heat the remaining 1 tablespoon olive oil in a large, wide skillet over medium heat. Add carrot, celery, and onion, and stir to combine. Cook, uncovered, stirring occasionally, for approximately 20 minutes, or until vegetables are very tender. Add grapes and chestnuts, and stir to combine. Pour in the remaining 1/2 cup stock and stir. Cook, stirring occasionally, until liquid is mostly absorbed and grapes have plumped up (approximately 20 minutes).

5. Remove chicken from oven and place in the skillet with the grape/chestnut mixture. Cook for 1 minute to allow flavors to come together, and serve.

Italian Living Tradition

"Spaghetti, pollo, insalatina, e una tazzina di caffè" are lyrics to a song by Italian singer Fred Bongusto. They translate to "spaghetti, chicken, a little salad, and a cup of coffee (espresso)," and refer to a typical Italian 4-course lunch. Low in fat and high in protein and B vitamins, chicken meat is an excellent protein source for diners everywhere.

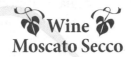

Wine
Moscato Secco

VEGETABLE-STUFFED TURKEY BREAST
(PETTO DI TACCHINO RIPIENO DI VERDURE)

Serves: 8 | Serving Size: 1 slice turkey breast and approximately 2 tablespoons sauce
Prep Time: 15 minutes | Cooking Time: 1 hour

Stuffed breasts of veal, chicken, lamb, and turkey are very popular main courses for Sunday dinners in Italy. While they are elegant to serve and present, they are also relatively easy to make. Breast meat is lower in fat than many other cuts of meat and poultry, and filling the roast with healthful vegetables can increase the nutrient quotient of the meal as well.

6 ounces fresh baby spinach

2 tablespoons extra virgin olive oil, divided

1 yellow onion, minced, divided

1 clove garlic, minced

1/2 cup (2 ounces) shredded carrots

1/4 cup parmigiano-reggiano or pecorino Romano cheese

1 tablespoon dry bread crumbs or ground almonds

1 teaspoon dried rosemary, crushed

1/2 teaspoon dried sage

3/4 teaspoon unrefined sea salt, divided

3/8 teaspoon freshly ground black pepper, divided

1 large egg white, lightly beaten

1 (1 3/4-pound) boneless turkey breast half, butterflied

1/2 cup dry white wine

3/4 cup Homemade Chicken Stock (page 289) or reduced-sodium chicken stock

1 1/2 teaspoons cornstarch

Fresh rosemary sprigs (for garnish; optional)

Choices/Exchanges 1 Vegetable, 3 1/2 Lean Protein, 1/2 Fat

Calories 210 | Calories from Fat 50

Total Fat 6g | Saturated Fat 1.4g | Trans Fat 0.0g

Cholesterol 60mg

Sodium 430mg

Potassium 460mg

Total Carbohydrate 7g | Dietary Fiber 1g | Sugars 2g

Protein 27g

Phosphorus 255mg

1. Heat a large saucepan over medium-high heat. Add 1 tablespoon water and spinach. Cover, reduce heat to low, and cook 5 minutes or until spinach wilts, stirring occasionally. Place spinach in a colander and press until barely moist.

2. Heat 1 tablespoon olive oil in a small saucepan over medium-high heat. Add half of the onion, 2 tablespoons water, and garlic. Cover and cook 3 minutes, or until moisture evaporates. Spoon mixture into a small bowl. Add the spinach, carrot, cheese, bread crumbs, rosemary, sage, 1/4 teaspoon salt, 1/8 teaspoon pepper, and egg white, and combine.

3. Place turkey breast between 2 sheets of plastic wrap. Pound to an even 1/2-inch thickness using a meat mallet or rolling pin. Remove top layer of plastic wrap. Spread spinach mixture over the turkey, leaving a 1-inch border. Roll up breast, jelly-roll fashion, starting with one short side. Secure the roll at 2-inch intervals with twine. Rub 1/2 teaspoon salt and 1/4 teaspoon pepper evenly over turkey.

4. Preheat oven to 350°F.

5. Heat 1 tablespoon oil in a large dutch oven over medium-high heat. Add the turkey and cook 5 minutes, browning on all sides. Remove turkey from pan. Add remaining onion to pan, stir, and sauté 30 seconds. Stir in wine, scraping pan to loosen browned bits. Add turkey back to pan with the stock. Increase the heat to high and bring to a boil.

6. Cover and carefully transfer to the oven. Bake for 40 minutes, or until a thermometer inserted in thickest portion of turkey registers 170°F. Remove turkey from pan and keep warm.

7. Place pan back on stovetop over high heat. Combine cornstarch and 1 tablespoon water, stirring with a whisk. Add cornstarch mixture to pan and bring to a boil. Cook 1 minute or until slightly thick, stirring constantly. Remove from heat.

8. Remove and discard twine from turkey. Cut turkey into 8 slices. Serve sauce with the turkey. Garnish with rosemary sprigs, if desired.

❖ Italian Living Tradition ❖

If you cannot find a turkey breast already butterflied, you can do it yourself by cutting horizontally through the center of the breast. You should cut to, but not through, the other side using a sharp knife, then open flat as you would a book.

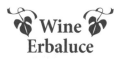

Wine
Erbaluce

HERB-ROASTED TURKEY
(TACCHINO AL FORNO)

Serves: 8 | Serving Size: Approximately 1/3 pound turkey meat
Prep Time: 10 minutes | Cooking Time: Approximately 1 hour 20 minutes

Even though turkey isn't usually the first meat that comes to mind when we think of the Italian kitchen, it is actually quite popular in Italy. I once served this dish on May Day (May 1) in Italy to my Roman friends. They decided that it might be fun to have a traditional American-style Thanksgiving meal like they had seen in so many movies. Whole turkeys are hard to come by in Italy in the spring, but luckily, we knew a butcher who had a friend in Perugia (2 hours away) who was willing to get one for us.

I prepared an Italian-style bird, along with homemade cranberry sauce (I had to go to a specialty grocer in the center of the city to get the cranberries), mashed potatoes, homemade stuffing, and a spinach, cheese, and artichoke casserole, along with a cake for dessert! This recipe is an even easier version of the turkey I made for my friends—I've substituted turkey breasts for the whole bird.

2 tablespoons extra virgin olive oil, divided

4 pounds skinless turkey breasts

1/4 teaspoon freshly ground black pepper

1 tablespoon dried rosemary, crushed

1 teaspoon dried sage

1 head garlic, top chopped off

2 lemons, halved

Choices/Exchanges 7 Lean Protein
Calories 300 | Calories from Fat 60
Total Fat 7g | Saturated Fat 1.1g | Trans Fat 0.0g
Cholesterol 130mg
Sodium 260mg

Potassium 585mg
Total Carbohydrate 2g | Dietary Fiber 1g | Sugars 1g
Protein 54g
Phosphorus 460mg

1. Preheat oven to 425°F.

2. Use 1 tablespoon olive oil to grease the bottom of a large roasting pan. Wash and dry the turkey breasts thoroughly. Season them with pepper on the top.

3. Place turkey meat side up in the pan. Brush the turkey with the remaining 1 tablespoon olive oil. Sprinkle rosemary and sage on turkey breasts and rub in with your hands. Place whole garlic head and 2 lemon halves in the pan.

4. Place turkey in the oven, add 1 cup water to the bottom of the pan, and roast for 1 hour, uncovered. Baste turkey after 1 hour of cooking. Roast until the internal temperature of the thickest part of the turkey breast meat reads 180°F on a meat thermometer. If the meat has not reached 180°F after the first hour, return to the oven and check the temperature every 10 minutes.

5. Remove turkey breasts from the oven and place on a carving board. Let rest for 10 minutes before cutting or serving.

6. Strain the liquid from the bottom of the pan into another saucepan. Add lemon juice from the remaining lemon halves to the saucepan and stir. Bring to a boil over high heat and cook for 10 minutes, or until sauce has reduced. Serve sauce in a gravy boat next to turkey.

⤜Italian Living Tradition⤐

Much leaner than red meat, turkey doesn't need to be saved for Thanksgiving. It was first introduced to Europe by the Spanish; Italians now eat whole turkeys for holidays like Christmas and New Year's Day, and they eat other cuts, such as ground turkey and turkey *scallopine,* often. Turkey is appreciated for its protein content and versatility in the kitchen.

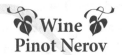

Wine
Pinot Nerov

VEAL, POTATO, AND PEPPER STEW (*SPEZZATINO DI VITELLO*)

Serves: 4 | Serving Size: Approximately 3/4 cup
Prep Time: 15 minutes | Cooking Time: 1 hour 30 minutes

This stew tastes even better the following day!
You can use beef, lamb, or even goat instead of the veal, if you choose.

1/4 cup plus 2 tablespoons extra virgin olive oil, divided

1 large yellow onion, diced

1 pound boneless veal shoulder, cut into 1-inch cubes

4 cloves garlic, minced

1 pound crushed or diced tomatoes

1/2 teaspoon unrefined sea salt

1/8 teaspoon freshly ground black pepper

Pinch crushed red chile flakes (preferably Calabrian; see Where to Buy Guide)

1 large red bell pepper, cut into 1-inch cubes

1 large green bell pepper, cut into 1-inch cubes

2 Yukon gold potatoes, peeled and cut into 1-inch cubes

2 tablespoons finely chopped fresh flat-leaf parsley

2 tablespoons finely chopped fresh basil

Choices/Exchanges 1 Starch, 1 1/2 Vegetable,
2 1/2 Lean Protein, 2 Fat
Calories 300 | Calories from Fat 140
Total Fat 16g | Saturated Fat 2.5g | Trans Fat 0.0g
Cholesterol 65mg

Sodium 410mg
Potassium 930mg
Total Carbohydrate 24g | Dietary Fiber 4g | Sugars 7g
Protein 19g
Phosphorus 250mg

1. Heat 1/4 cup olive oil in a large, deep skillet over medium heat. Add onion and sauté for 3–4 minutes, or until light golden brown. Add veal and brown on all sides. Stir in garlic, tomatoes, salt, pepper, and chilies. Cover, reduce heat to low, and simmer for 1 hour, or until veal is almost tender.

2. Meanwhile, in a dutch oven or large, wide saucepan, heat 2 tablespoons olive oil over medium heat. Add in red and green peppers, potatoes, and parsley. Stir and sauté, uncovered, just until vegetables are tender, approximately 12–15 minutes. Stir in basil.

3. Once veal has cooked for an hour, add in pepper/potato mixture and stir. Cover and cook until all ingredients are tender and flavors have blended, approximately 15 minutes. Serve hot.

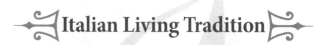

Italian Living Tradition

Most American stews are made by combining everything in one pot. Many Italians use this two-step process—sautéing the vegetables in olive oil before adding them to the stew— for additional flavor and unique texture. Leftover sautéed vegetables can be added into stews as well.

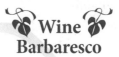

Wine
Barbaresco

ABRUZZESE-STYLE ROASTED BABY GOAT WITH PEPPERS (*CAPRETTO ALLA NERETESE*)

Serves: 8 | Serving Size: Approximately 1 cup
Prep Time: 15 minutes | Cooking Time: 3 hours

Many Italian-Americans hail from the Abruzzo region in Italy, known for its lush national parks and waterfalls as well as its wheat and other agricultural products. With a geographic location that boasts the presence of different types of Mediterranean ecosystems, Abruzzo is home to a wide variety of vegetation that is a part of its unique cuisine. This recipe represents the typical Abruzzese way of preparing goat meat, which is popular in the spring, and for Easter and other special occasions in Italy. See the Where to Buy Guide (page 299) to learn where to find goat meat. Beef, veal, or lamb can also be used in this recipe; just remember that cooking times will need to be adjusted accordingly.

1/4 cup extra virgin olive oil

1/2 pound yellow onions, peeled and diced

1/2 pound carrots, peeled and diced

1 stalk celery, diced

6 cloves garlic, sliced

2 1/2 pounds goat meat cubes (from the thigh or shoulder), about 1 1/2-inch each

1/2 cup dry white wine

1/8 teaspoon unrefined sea salt

1 clove

4 cups Homemade Chicken Stock (page 289), reduced-sodium chicken stock, or water

1 pound red bell peppers, cored and cut into 1-inch pieces

1 cup peeled crushed tomatoes

1 teaspoon crushed red chile flakes

Choices/Exchanges 3 Vegetable, 4 1/2 Lean Protein, 1/2 Fat

Calories 300 | Calories from Fat 100

Total Fat 11g | Saturated Fat 2.2g | Trans Fat 0.0g

Cholesterol 80mg

Sodium 280mg

Potassium 1040mg

Total Carbohydrate 14g | Dietary Fiber 3g | Sugars 7g

Protein 34g

Phosphorus 340mg

1. Heat olive oil in a large, heavy-bottomed saucepan or dutch oven over medium-high heat.

2. Add the onions, carrots, and celery, and turn to coat in oil. Reduce heat to medium-low and sauté vegetables until tender. Add the garlic, stir, and cook for 1 minute, or until it releases its aroma.

3. Add the goat meat and cook 3–5 minutes, until browned on all sides. Pour in the wine and increase heat to high.

4. When liquid is almost completely evaporated, season with salt. Add the clove and stock or water. Increase heat to high and bring to a boil. Stir, reduce heat to low, cover, and simmer for 2 hours, stirring occasionally.

5. After 2 hours have passed, add peppers, tomatoes, and chile flakes. Stir, and cover. Cook for 1 more hour, or until meat is very tender. Remove clove, if desired, and serve.

❧ Italian Living Tradition ❧

The unique Abruzzese climate makes it a great place to grow spices that many people don't associate with central or southern Italy, such as saffron. These award-winning spices give the local cuisine and the region's economy a much-needed boost. Many southern Italian regions have special goat recipes similar to this one, but the addition of clove (usually associated with savory Middle Eastern cooking) makes this recipe uniquely Abruzzese.

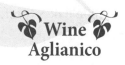

Wine
Aglianico

CLASSIC MEATBALLS
(POLPETTE)

Serves: 6 | Serving Size: 5 meatballs
Prep Time: 15 minutes | Cooking Time: 40 minutes

Meatballs are one of the first foods that Calabrese children learn to make. Called purpette *in the local dialect, they are part of the traditional Sunday meal in Calabria. Instead of serving them on top of spaghetti, as is done in many Italian-American restaurants in the U.S., the meatballs are served either as a second course, in a rich traditional lasagna called* sagne chine *prepared on holidays, or in Calabrian Wedding Soup (page 50). Many people use a combination of beef, veal, and pork to make their meatballs. You can also use turkey or chicken if you'd like.*

1/2 cup dried Italian bread or gluten-free bread cubes, drizzled with 1/4 cup skim milk, drained, and squeezed of excess liquid

3/4 pound very lean ground beef (95% lean)

1 egg, lightly beaten

2 tablespoons fresh flat-leaf parsley or basil, finely chopped

1/2 teaspoon salt

1/4 teaspoon freshly ground black pepper

Pinch crushed red chile flakes (preferably Calabrian; see Where to Buy Guide)

2 cups Fresh Tomato Sauce (page 228)

Choices/Exchanges 1 Carbohydrate, 1 Lean Protein, 1/2 Fat

Calories 130 | Calories from Fat 50

Total Fat 6g | Saturated Fat 1.2g | Trans Fat 0.0g

Cholesterol 40mg

Sodium 300mg

Potassium 675mg

Total Carbohydrate 13g | Dietary Fiber 3g | Sugars 7g

Protein 6g

Phosphorus 115mg

1. Combine all of the ingredients except for the tomato sauce in a large bowl. Mix well with hands.

2. Shape mixture into uniform 1/2-inch meatballs and set on a clean baking sheet or cutting board.

3. Bring tomato sauce to a light boil in a large saucepan over medium heat. Add the meatballs, stir, and cover. Reduce heat to medium-low and simmer for 30 minutes, or until meatballs are cooked through and tender.

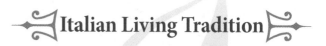

Italian Living Tradition

These meatballs are sometimes fried in pure olive oil or baked at 350°F until cooked. Then they can be added to sauces, soups, or other recipes.

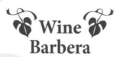

**Wine
Barbera**

SIDE DISHES
(CONTORNI)

161   Carrot and Zucchini Ribbons/*Nastri di carote e zucchine*

162   Pan-Fried Fennel with Parmesan/*Finocchi con parmigiano*

163   Sweet-and-Sour Cabbage/*Cavoli acidi*

164   Artichokes with Garlic and Oil/*Carciofi all'aglio e olio*

166   Mixed Grilled Vegetables/*Verdure miste alla griglia*

168   Venetian-Style Beans with Swiss Chard/*Fagioli alla Veneziana con bietole*

170   Kale Sautéed in Garlic, Oil, and Hot Chile Peppers/*Ravizzone con aglio, olio, e peperoncino*

171   Marinated Eggplant/*Melanzane al funghetto*

172   Mixed Mushroom and Herb Medley/*Funghi in padella con erbe*

173   Sautéed Zucchini with Vinegar and Mint/*Zucchine in padella con aceto e menta*

174   Pepper, Potato, and Eggplant Medley/*Peperoni, patate, e melanzane al forno*

175   Haricots Verts with Hazelnuts/*Fagiolini alle nocciole*

176   Calabrian-Style Roasted Potatoes/*Patate Calabrese al forno*

178   Chargrilled Asparagus with Balsamic and Parmesan/
      Asparagi grigliati con balsamico e parmigiano

180   Spinach Sautéed in Garlic and Oil/*Spinaci all'aglio e olio*

"La patata dà più forza quando è cotta con la scorza."
"Potatoes give more strength when they're cooked with the peel."
—Italian proverb

Italian-style side dishes are among the most delectable, simplest to prepare, and healthiest in the world. In order to fully appreciate these vegetable-centric recipes, we must take a look at the agricultural history of Italy. Italians have worked the land since prehistoric times. Many Italian *contorni* recipes were originally created to take advantage of the abundance of various harvests. Before modern times, food was preserved in salt or olive oil, but it was most often consumed when it was fresh and in season.

For the sake of variety, different recipes using the same vegetables were created. One ancient Italian custom that is still in practice today allows Italians to celebrate the vegetable harvest and learn multitudes of ways to prepare these vegetables: the agricultural festivals known as *sagre*. The word *sagre*, meaning "sacred," descends from the Latin word *sacrum*, which referred to the gods or anything in their power. In ancient Rome, there were 182 "sacred" days, and many of them had their own foods!

In pre-Christian times, the *sagre* were held to pay tribute to the Agrarian gods—namely Saturn, who was the god of both agriculture and commerce (which is fitting since food was used as currency back then). With the advent of Christianity, the festivals were held on saints' days or Christian holidays, especially if they coincided with the harvest. *Sagre* are celebrated not only for the vegetable harvest, but also for the harvest of various types of fruits, legumes, beans, nuts, animal products, fish, seafood, and, of course, the grape or wine harvest.

Because Italians attend these cultural food festivals from a young age, it is second nature for them to incorporate fresh produce into their daily meals. Seasonal produce is incorporated into appetizers, first courses (pasta, soup, gnocchi, and risotto dishes), second courses, if possible, and these straightforward side dishes.

Italian *contorni* can be served on the same plate as the second course (if it is a large dinner plate), on a separate small plate, or family style in the middle of a table. In the Italian kitchen, as with other cuisines, careful consideration of the second course determines which side dish will pair best. For best results, use only the freshest vegetables possible.

During the colder months, Pan-Fried Fennel with Parmesan (page 162), Sweet-and-Sour Cabbage (page 163), Mixed Mushroom and Herb Medley (page 172), and Pepper, Potato, and Eggplant Medley (page 174) are the perfect accompaniments for roasted or braised poultry/meat dishes.

In the spring, Artichokes with Garlic and Oil (page 164), Carrot and Zucchini Ribbons (page 161), and Haricots Verts with Hazelnuts (page 175) pair perfectly with pan-fried, roasted, and stewed main courses.

During the summer, Mixed Grilled Vegetables (page 166), Sautéed Zucchini with Vinegar and Mint (page 173), Marinated Eggplant (page 171), and Chargrilled Asparagus with Balsamic and Parmesan (page 178) will add flavor and dimension to a second course consisting of grilled or pan-fried seafood, chicken, or meat.

When entertaining casually, I sometimes like to serve a buffet of these vegetable side dishes as main courses, along with aged cheeses and freshly made bread. It's a fun way to eat a nutritious, vegetarian meal that many of my friends and family appreciate. It's wholesome recipes like these which prove that, when it comes to food, "Italian" and "healthful" don't have to be mutually exclusive. By adding a few of these simple recipes to your repertoire, you'll increase your vitamin, mineral, and antioxidant intake—and enjoy every minute of it!

CARROT AND ZUCCHINI RIBBONS
(NASTRI DI CAROTE E ZUCCHINE)

Serves: 4 | Serving Size: 1/2 cup
Prep Time: 5 minutes | Cooking Time: 10 minutes

One of the keys to making simple, nutritious foods more appealing is presentation. Cutting zucchini into thin ribbons instead of thick rounds takes its appeal to new heights. Serve this pretty contorno *with Swordfish with Olives, Capers, Herbs, and Tomatoes (page 120), Sicilian-Style Fish with Vegetables (page 122), or Sea Bream with Duchess-Style Sweet Potatoes (page 124) for an impressive and nutritious dinner.*

3 medium carrots, peeled
1 large zucchini
Juice of 1/2 lemon
2 tablespoons extra virgin olive oil
1/4 teaspoon unrefined sea salt
1/8 teaspoon freshly ground black pepper
1/4 cup finely chopped fresh flat-leaf parsley

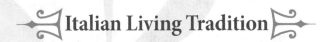

Italian Living Tradition

Pairing the Italian *contorno,* or side dish, with a second course is a delicate balancing act of flavors, textures, and appearance. If the second course has a tomato-based sauce or strong flavors, for example, a simple side dish like this one work best.

1. Using a vegetable peeler, cut carrots into long ribbons. Stop peeling when you reach the core, and discard it. With a mandoline or cheese grater, shave zucchini into ribbons. Stop peeling when you reach seeds; discard the core. Cut all ribbons in half.

2. In a large saucepan fitted with a steamer basket, bring 2 inches water to a boil. Add the carrots, cover, and steam for 2 minutes. Place the zucchini over the carrots, cover, and steam until the vegetables are just tender, 2–3 more minutes. Transfer the vegetables to a large bowl.

3. Pour lemon juice into a small bowl. Whisk in olive oil, salt, and pepper until emulsified. Drizzle lemon mixture over the vegetables, add parsley, and toss to combine. Serve immediately.

Choices/Exchanges 1 1/2 Vegetable, 1 1/2 Fat
Calories 90 | Calories from Fat 60
Total Fat 7g | Saturated Fat 1.0g | Trans Fat 0.0g
Cholesterol 0mg
Sodium 190mg

Potassium 385mg
Total Carbohydrate 8g | Dietary Fiber 2g | Sugars 4g
Protein 2g
Phosphorus 50mg

PAN-FRIED FENNEL WITH PARMESAN (*FINOCCHI CON PARMIGIANO*)

Serves: 6 | Serving Size: 1/2 cup
Prep Time: 5 minutes | Cooking Time: 30 minutes

Fennel is an herbaceous plant that originated in the Mediterranean region (where it has been used since circa 3000 BCE). The ancient Romans used dried fennel seeds to preserve foods. A single cup of fennel is a significant source of vitamin C and potassium. All across the Mediterranean region, fennel is celebrated for its mildly sweet flavor, culinary versatility, nutritional benefits, and budget-friendly price. In some regions, such as Emilia-Romagna, thinly sliced fennel is battered and fried. This healthier version of that fried dish makes a great side to accompany roasted meats.

2 tablespoons extra virgin olive oil

4 medium heads fennel, bulbs cored and cut into 1/2-inch-thick slices, stalks reserved for another dish

1 cup freshly chopped flat-leaf parsley

1/8 teaspoon unrefined sea salt

1/2 teaspoon freshly ground black pepper

1 cup Homemade Vegetable Stock (page 287) or reduced-sodium vegetable stock

1/4 cup grated parmigiano-reggiano cheese

⟡ Italian Living Tradition ⟡

In Italy, many people munch on raw fennel the way Americans enjoy crunchy celery sticks. Fennel bulbs can be eaten raw, pickled, or cooked. The fennel stalks, which resemble celery, can be added into slow-simmering stocks or stews for additional flavor. Don't overlook fennel for your next crudité platter or salad.

1. Heat olive oil in a large, wide skillet over medium heat. Add fennel slices and turn to coat. Sauté, stirring occasionally, until fennel is golden, approximately 5–7 minutes.

2. Stir in the parsley, salt, pepper, and stock. Increase heat to high and bring to a boil. Reduce heat to low, cover, and simmer for 10–20 minutes, or until fennel is tender and most of the liquid has reduced.

3. Transfer fennel to a serving platter or individual plates, and sprinkle with parmigiano-reggiano cheese. Serve warm.

Choices/Exchanges 2 1/2 Vegetable, 1 Fat
Calories 120 | Calories from Fat 50
Total Fat 6g | Saturated Fat 1.5g | Trans Fat 0.0g
Cholesterol 5mg
Sodium 200mg

Potassium 745mg
Total Carbohydrate 13g | Dietary Fiber 5g | Sugars 6g
Protein 5g
Phosphorus 125mg

SWEET-AND-SOUR CABBAGE
(CAVOLI ACIDI)

Serves: 4 | Serving Size: Approximately 1 cup
Prep Time: 10 minutes | Cooking Time: 30 minutes

The German and Austrian influences in northern Italy are undeniable. The Italian equivalent of sauerkraut, this recipe is typical of the Emilia-Romagna, Alto Adige, Veneto, and Friuli-Venezia Giulia regions, as are strudel and rye breads. This dish is traditionally served in the fall or winter, alongside grilled meats and polenta. I would also recommend serving it with Tyrolean Rye Bread with Fennel and Cumin (page 212) when possible.

3 tablespoons extra virgin olive oil

1 small yellow onion, finely chopped

1 medium head savoy cabbage

1 cup Homemade Vegetable or Chicken Stock (pages 287, 289)

1/4 cup good-quality red wine vinegar

1 tablespoon organic honey

1/8 teaspoon unrefined sea salt

1/4 teaspoon freshly ground black pepper

◀ Italian Living Tradition ▶

Although the Tyrolean regions now belong to Italy, they have often been under foreign control over the course of their history. Many natives, especially the older ones, spoke German or a Geman-based dialect at home before learning Italian in schools. This cultural mix has created a unique regional cuisine that is unlike any other in Italy.

1. Heat the oil in a large skillet over medium heat. Add the onions and sauté, stirring occasionally, until tender and lightly golden. Add the cabbage and stir. Add the stock, stir, and bring the mixture to a boil over high heat. Reduce heat to low, cover, and simmer until cabbage is soft and reduced by half its original volume, approximately 20–25 minutes.

2. Add in vinegar, increase heat to high, and cook until most of liquid evaporates, about 3–5 minutes.

3. Reduce heat to low, stir in honey, and season with salt and pepper. Cook for a few more minutes to allow flavors to combine. Serve warm or at room temperature.

Choices/Exchanges 2 Vegetable, 2 Fat
Calories 150 | Calories from Fat 90
Total Fat 10g | Saturated Fat 1.5g | Trans Fat 0.0g
Cholesterol 0mg
Sodium 190mg

Potassium 265mg
Total Carbohydrate 12g | Dietary Fiber 3g | Sugars 7g
Protein 3g
Phosphorus 55mg

ARTICHOKES WITH GARLIC AND OIL
(CARCIOFI ALL'AGLIO E OLIO)

Serves: 4 | Serving Size: 1 artichoke (or 2 baby artichokes)
Prep Time: 15 minutes | Cooking Time: About 35 minutes

In addition to their creamy texture and buttery flavor, artichokes contain healthful antioxidants. If you've never worked with fresh artichokes before, don't be intimidated. The steps to prepare them are simple, and after cooking them once, you'll be a pro. When baby artichokes are in season, try using those—they cook in only half the time. When fresh artichokes are not in season, substitute canned, reduced-sodium artichoke hearts or frozen hearts.

4 small or 8 baby artichokes
2 lemons, juiced, divided
3 tablespoons extra virgin olive oil
4 cloves garlic, minced
1/4 teaspoon unrefined sea salt
1/8 teaspoon freshly ground black pepper
Pinch crushed red chile flakes
1 tablespoon finely chopped fresh flat-leaf parsley

Choices/Exchanges 2 Vegetable, 2 Fat
Calories 150 | Calories from Fat 90
Total Fat 10g | Saturated Fat 1.4g | Trans Fat 0.0g
Cholesterol 0mg
Sodium 210mg

Potassium 420mg
Total Carbohydrate 14g | Dietary Fiber 6g | Sugars 2g
Protein 4g
Phosphorus 95mg

1. Soak the artichokes in water to clean; drain and repeat until water is clear. Peel away the outside leaves of the bottom half of the artichokes. Cut off the top quarter of the artichoke (at this point the artichoke should look like a flower, and the tough, dark leaves should all be removed, leaving only lighter-colored, tenderer leaves). If tough, dark green leaves remain, peel those as well. Add juice of 1 lemon to a bowl full of cold water, and place cleaned artichokes inside to avoid discoloration.

2. Bring a large pot of water to a boil, and add cleaned artichokes. Bring back to a boil on high heat. Reduce heat to medium-low and simmer artichokes 25–30 minutes, or until tender. Drain artichokes well, pat dry with a paper towel, and set aside.

3. In a large skillet, heat olive oil over medium heat. Add garlic and sauté until garlic begins to release its aroma, approximately 1 minute. Add artichokes, turn to coat in oil, and season with salt, pepper, and crushed red chile flakes. Sprinkle with parsley and serve warm.

Italian Living Tradition

In Rome, freshly sautéed artichokes, like these, are tossed into hot spaghetti and garnished with finely chopped fresh mint. It's a simple yet divine combination!

MIXED GRILLED VEGETABLES
(VERDURE MISTE ALLA GRIGLIA)

Serves: 10 | Serving Size: 1 cup
Prep Time: 15 minutes (plus 1 hour eggplant-resting time) | Cooking Time: 15 minutes

Grilling is one of the least fattening ways of preparing vegetables. Grilled vegetables are used in a multitude of ways in the Italian kitchen; from antipasti to pastas to accompaniments for second courses, you'll find them everywhere. This dish works very well for buffets.

1 small, firm eggplant, cut into 1/2-inch-thick slices
1/8 teaspoon unrefined sea salt
1/4 cup balsamic vinegar
1/2 cup extra virgin olive oil
2 cloves garlic, finely minced
1/4 teaspoon freshly ground black pepper
1/4 cup fresh basil, finely chopped
2 large red bell peppers
4 small zucchini, trimmed and cut in half lengthwise
1 pint cherry tomatoes
1 bulb fennel, cored and quartered

Choices/Exchanges 2 Vegetable, 2 Fat
Calories 150 | Calories from Fat 100
Total Fat 11g | Saturated Fat 1.5g | Trans Fat 0.0g
Cholesterol 0mg
Sodium 80mg

Potassium 555mg
Total Carbohydrate 12g | Dietary Fiber 5g | Sugars 7g
Protein 2g
Phosphorus 65mg

1. Place eggplant on a large baking tray and sprinkle with salt. Let the eggplant stand at room temperature for 1 hour to draw out moisture. Drain, rinse well, and pat dry.

2. Combine balsamic vinegar, olive oil, garlic, pepper, and basil in a small bowl and set aside.

3. Hold (with tongs) whole peppers over an open flame of a gas grill, or broil under the broiler, until blackened and blistered. Place peppers in paper lunch bags and seal shut. In a few minutes, open the bags carefully (steam will escape), remove peppers, peel off the skin, and cut into slices.

4. Preheat broiler (to high) or grill. Place eggplant, zucchini, cherry tomatoes, and fennel on a large baking tray and broil or grill until golden and tender on all sides. Remove grilled vegetables to a large bowl.

5. Stir in peppers, pour balsamic dressing over all, and mix together. Serve hot or at room temperature.

Italian Living Tradition

Try grilling vegetables in large batches and storing them in the refrigerator in individual containers. Use them throughout the week to top pizzas, add to pastas and soups, or serve as fast side dishes.

VENETIAN-STYLE BEANS WITH SWISS CHARD (*FAGIOLI ALLA VENEZIANA CON BIETOLE*)

Serves: 8 | Serving Size: Approximately 1/2 cup
Prep Time: 10 minutes | Cooking Time: 10 minutes

Italians are masters at creating innovative bean-and-greens dishes, the benchmark of the true Mediterranean diet. Those interested in achieving optimal health would be wise to add all of these dishes to their repertoire. The mere mention of Venice might bring more glamourous culinary creations such as bellinis and carpaccios to mind, but Venetian residents are no strangers to nutritious home-style cooking.

Many cooks prepare this dish in advance because it has more flavor once the ingredients have spent the night together. To do that, let the dish cool to room temperature after cooking, transfer to an airtight container, and refrigerate overnight. The next day, transfer to a serving dish and serve at room temperature.

3 tablespoons extra virgin olive oil, divided

1 pound swiss chard leaves, stems trimmed and leaves cut into 2-inch-wide pieces

2 tablespoons minced garlic

1 oil-packed anchovy fillet, drained, rinsed, and mashed (optional)

3/4 cup Homemade Vegetable Stock (page 287), reduced-sodium vegetable stock, or water

3 cups cooked borlotti (cranberry) beans (see Dried Beans recipe on page 283)

2 tablespoons chopped fresh basil

2 teaspoons chopped fresh mint OR 1 teaspoon dried mint

2 teaspoons fresh marjoram leaves OR 1 teaspoon dried marjoram

1 1/2 tablespoons red wine vinegar

2 tablespoons finely chopped fresh flat-leaf parsley

Choices/Exchanges 1 Starch, 1 Lean Protein, 1/2 Fat
Calories 150 | Calories from Fat 50
Total Fat 6g | Saturated Fat 1.0g | Trans Fat 0.0g
Cholesterol 0mg
Sodium 150mg

Potassium 515mg
Total Carbohydrate 20g | Dietary Fiber 8g | Sugars 1g
Protein 8g
Phosphorus 130mg

1. Warm 2 tablespoons olive oil in a large, wide skillet over medium heat. Add the swiss chard and sauté until almost limp, 3–4 minutes. Add the remaining 1 tablespoon olive oil and garlic, and sauté until fragrant, about 30 seconds; do not allow garlic to brown. Add the anchovy, if using, and stir. Add the stock, increase heat to high, and bring to a boil.

2. Reduce heat to medium, add the beans, and allow beans to heat through, 2–3 minutes.

3. Add the basil, mint, and marjoram, and stir until blended. Add the vinegar and stir for a few seconds, allowing some of the liquid to evaporate. Remove from heat.

4. Garnish with parsley and serve at room temperature.

◆ Italian Living Tradition ◆

Many people shy away from adding anchovies to their dishes. However, they are extremely popular in Italy. This is because salt was heavily taxed by the Romans in ancient times. One way for people to get around the tax was to import salt-cured fish, such as anchovies, instead of plain salt. Once they began using the cured fish as a condiment, the fish added a depth of flavor to recipes that couldn't be obtained with salt alone. Nowadays, even though salt is widely available, many people still prefer the addition of preserved anchovies.

KALE SAUTÉED IN GARLIC, OIL, AND HOT CHILE PEPPERS (*RAVIZZONE CON AGLIO, OLIO, E PEPERONCINO*)

Serves: 4 | Serving Size: 1 cup
Prep Time: 3 minutes | Cooking Time: 7 minutes

Kale, the superfood that keeps gaining media attention, has always been popular in Italy. Named one of the world's healthiest foods, it has been known to lower cholesterol and reduce the risk of various kinds of cancer. Researchers have found 45 different flavonoids (antioxidant and anti-inflammatory benefits) in kale, which makes it one of the smartest additions to a diet.

Even if you think you don't like kale, I urge you to try this recipe. It's fast, easy, and full of flavors you might just come to love. This recipe tastes great with Braised, Stuffed Calamari with Tomato Sauce (page 112), Fish Stew over Polenta (page 128), and Cacciatore-Style Chicken (page 140).

2 tablespoons extra virgin olive oil

4 cloves garlic, finely chopped

Crushed red chile flakes, to taste

2 bunches kale (8 cups total), stems trimmed and torn into bite-size pieces

1/8 teaspoon unrefined sea salt

1/4 teaspoon freshly ground black pepper

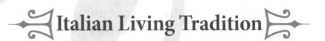
Italian Living Tradition

This dish is just one of the many ways to incorporate the health benefits of kale into your lifestyle. You can also use baby kale in salads or add kale into soups and stews.

1. Heat the olive oil in a large skillet over medium heat. Add the garlic and chile flakes and cook just until they begin to release their aroma, approximately 1 minute.

2. Add the kale and cook until the kale is bright green and wilted, approximately 5 minutes.

3. Taste, season with salt and pepper, and serve.

Choices/Exchanges 3 Vegetable, 1 1/2 Fat
Calories 140 | Calories from Fat 70
Total Fat 8g | Saturated Fat 1.0g | Trans Fat 0.0g
Cholesterol 0mg
Sodium 200mg

Potassium 710mg
Total Carbohydrate 14g | Dietary Fiber 5g | Sugars 4g
Protein 6g
Phosphorus 135mg

MARINATED EGGPLANT (MELANZANE AL FUNGHETTO)

Serves: 10 | Serving Size: Approximately 3–4 tablespoons
Prep Time: 10 minutes (plus marinating time) | Cooking Time: 10 minutes

The picture-perfect Sicilian town of Taormina, where this recipe comes from, is famous for its natural springs and serene spas—and its plethora of vegetable-based appetizers. The local lifestyle is one of the healthiest in the world.

I've tweaked this recipe just a bit from the traditional version; since eggplant skin contains antioxidants, potassium, magnesium, and fiber, I've chosen to leave it on in this recipe. In addition, I've replaced the traditional white wine vinegar with balsamic vinegar, which comes from northern Italy.

1/4 cup balsamic vinegar

4 baby eggplants (about 1 pound total), trimmed and diced into 1-inch pieces

1/4 cup extra virgin olive oil

4 cloves garlic, finely minced

2 tablespoons finely chopped fresh mint

2 tablespoons finely chopped fresh oregano

2 tablespoons finely chopped fresh flat-leaf parsley

1/8 teaspoon unrefined sea salt

1/4 teaspoon freshly ground black pepper

⊰ Italian Living Tradition ⊱

Fresh, in-season eggplant is one of the most healthful and versatile vegetables of all. When shopping, choose shiny, smooth-skinned eggplants that are free of bruises. The fresher the eggplant, the less bitter it will taste.

1. Bring a large pot of water to a boil over high heat and add the vinegar. Add the eggplant to the pot and boil for 5 minutes. Drain and rinse with cold water.

2. Place the eggplant in a large bowl and refrigerate for 1 hour or overnight.

3. In a small bowl, combine olive oil, garlic, mint, oregano, parsley, salt, and pepper. Add eggplant and toss. Serve cold or at room temperature.

Choices/Exchanges 1 Vegetable, 1 Fat
Calories 70 | Calories from Fat 50
Total Fat 6g | Saturated Fat 0.8g | Trans Fat 0.0g
Cholesterol 0mg
Sodium 60mg

Potassium 135mg
Total Carbohydrate 4g | Dietary Fiber 2g | Sugars 2g
Protein 1g
Phosphorus 15mg

MIXED MUSHROOM AND HERB MEDLEY
(FUNGHI IN PADELLA CON ERBE)

Serves: 4 | Serving Size: 1/2 cup
Prep Time: 5 minutes | Cooking Time: 20 minutes

Both the Alps and Apennine mountain ranges provide many varieties of mushrooms for Italians to cook with. In order to flourish, mushrooms need the perfect amount of sun, rain, warmth, and humidity. Just as the vintage year of a wine is often deemed good or bad, Italians in mushroom-growing communities will label a year as "good" when there are a lot of mushrooms to be found. This quick side dish is easy and lends a fragrant, fall-like flavor to meals. Feel free to use your favorite mushroom varieties in this recipe. Serve with Vegetable-Stuffed Turkey Breast (page 146) or Veal, Potato, and Pepper Stew (page 150) for an amazing meal.

2 tablespoons extra virgin olive oil

2 cloves garlic, sliced

1 1/2 pounds mushrooms (a mix of chanterelles, shiitake, or other mushrooms)

1/4 teaspoon unrefined sea salt

1/4 teaspoon freshly ground black pepper

1/2 teaspoon dried thyme
OR leaves from 2 fresh thyme sprigs

3 fresh sage leaves, finely chopped

1/4 cup balsamic vinegar

4 teaspoons chopped fresh flat-leaf parsley

❖ Italian Living Tradition ❖

Foraging for mushrooms is an important fall ritual that many Italians look forward to. Wild mushrooms are both delicious and healthful, and the experience is fun. Many Americans are passionate about mushroom foraging as well. In fact, there are several societies in the U.S. devoted to mycology (the study of fungi).

1. Heat olive oil in a large, wide skillet over medium heat. Add garlic and cook until it releases its aroma. Add the mushrooms, salt, pepper, thyme, and sage. Sauté for approximately 5–10 minutes, or until mushrooms are tender.

2. Increase the heat to high, add balsamic vinegar, and cook until vinegar is reduced by one quarter.

3. Transfer to a serving platter, and garnish with parsley.

Choices/Exchanges 2 Vegetable, 1 1/2 Fat
Calories 120 | Calories from Fat 60
Total Fat 7g | Saturated Fat 1.0g | Trans Fat 0.0g
Cholesterol 0mg
Sodium 160mg

Potassium 805mg
Total Carbohydrate 11g | Dietary Fiber 2g | Sugars 5g
Protein 5g
Phosphorus 210mg

SAUTÉED ZUCCHINI WITH VINEGAR AND MINT (*ZUCCHINE IN PADELLA CON ACETO E MENTA*)

Serves: 4 | Serving Size: 1/2 cup (equivalent of 1 zucchini)
Prep Time: 5 minutes | Cooking Time: 10 minutes

While zucchini are treated as a vegetable, they are considered to be a fruit by botanists. This is another super-simple recipe that takes a few straightforward ingredients to new heights. This side can be served hot, warm, or at room temperature. Cooked artichokes also taste delicious when prepared this way. These zucchini can be tossed into hot pasta, if desired.

2 tablespoons extra virgin olive oil

4 small zucchini, very thinly sliced

2 cloves garlic, diced

Small bunch fresh mint, leaves finely chopped and stems discarded

1/4 cup white wine vinegar

1/8 teaspoon unrefined sea salt

1/4 teaspoon freshly ground black pepper

1. Heat olive oil in a large skillet over medium heat. Add zucchini and garlic, and sauté until golden and slightly tender, approximately 7 minutes.

2. Transfer zucchini and garlic to a serving bowl and toss with mint and vinegar. Taste, and season with salt and pepper. Serve.

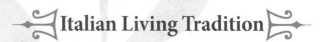

Italian Living Tradition

The first step of this recipe can also be the base of a great frittata: Instead of taking the zucchini out of the skillet, arrange them in an attractive pattern on the bottom. Whisk together 6 large eggs, salt, pepper, and some pecorino or parmigiano-reggiano cheese. Pour egg mixture over the top of the zucchini and cook over medium-low heat until set. Then transfer the frittata to a 350°F oven and bake until the eggs are cooked through, about 10–15 minutes.

Choices/Exchanges 1 1/2 Vegetable, 1 1/2 Fat
Calories 100 | Calories from Fat 60
Total Fat 7g | Saturated Fat 1.0g | Trans Fat 0.0g
Cholesterol 0mg
Sodium 95mg

Potassium 455mg
Total Carbohydrate 7g | Dietary Fiber 3g | Sugars 2g
Protein 3g
Phosphorus 65mg

PEPPER, POTATO, AND EGGPLANT MEDLEY (*PEPERONI, PATATE, E MELANZANE AL FORNO*)

Serves: 4 | Serving Size: 1/2 cup
Prep Time: 15 minutes | Cooking Time: 40 minutes

Even though potatoes, peppers, and tomatoes are "New World" ingredients, you'll be hard pressed to find a traditional Calabrian recipe that doesn't contain this holy trinity of produce. It's no accident that the combination is so popular. This side dish serves up a healthy dose of flavor and health benefits, and it's easy to prepare. This is a great recipe to make while preparing a roasted chicken or fish in the oven. I like to pair it with Cacciatore-Style Chicken (page 140), Trout Fillets with Sun-Dried Tomato and Cured-Olive Crust (page 118), and Herb-Roasted Turkey (page 148).

1 medium eggplant, cubed

1 large yukon gold potato, peeled and cut into
1-inch slices

1 yellow onion, peeled and cut into eighths

1 red bell pepper, cut into 1-inch pieces

1/2 cup cherry tomatoes, halved

1/4 teaspoon unrefined sea salt

1/4 teaspoon freshly ground black pepper

Crushed red chile flakes, to taste

1 tablespoon finely chopped fresh rosemary

1/4 cup extra virgin olive oil

Italian Living Tradition

There is no need to salt eggplant when roasting it. Many people salt eggplant prior to cooking it in order to "draw out the bitter juices." But eggplant generally has a neutral taste, which is why it is used in such a wide range of recipes in Italy. Salting is necessary, however, when deep-frying eggplant. By salting it and removing the excess moisture, the eggplant fries more quickly and evenly, ensuring that it won't be soggy.

1. Preheat oven to 425°F. Line a baking sheet with aluminum foil.

2. In a large bowl, toss together eggplant, potato, onion, pepper, and tomatoes. Season with salt, pepper, chile flakes, rosemary, and olive oil. Toss well to coat. Transfer vegetables to the baking sheet.

3. Bake until vegetables are tender and golden brown, approximately 40 minutes. Serve.

Choices/Exchanges 1 1/2 Carbohydrate, 1 Vegetable, 2 1/2 Fat
Calories 250 | Calories from Fat 130
Total Fat 14g | Saturated Fat 2.0g | Trans Fat 0.0g
Cholesterol 0mg

Sodium 160mg
Potassium 880mg
Total Carbohydrate 30g | Dietary Fiber 8g | Sugars 7g
Protein 4g
Phosphorus 110mg

HARICOTS VERTS WITH HAZELNUTS
(FAGIOLINI ALLE NOCCIOLE)

Serves: 6 | Serving Size: 1/2 cup
Prep Time: 5 minutes | Cooking Time: 15 minutes

The classic combination of green beans and hazelnuts is as healthful as it is tasty. Variations of this dish can be found throughout Italy during the appropriate season. Hazelnuts are one of the oldest cultivated crops in Europe; records of them being traded from the ports of Genoa go back to the 11th century. Currently, Turkey and Italy produce the majority of the world's hazelnuts.

1 1/2 pounds haricots verts (green beans), stem ends trimmed

2 tablespoons extra virgin olive oil, divided

1 yellow onion, diced

1/2 teaspoon unrefined sea salt, divided

1/8 teaspoon freshly ground black pepper

1/3 cup hazelnuts, blanched

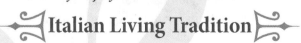

Italian Living Tradition

Skin hazelnuts by spreading them in a single layer on a baking sheet and toasting in a 375°F oven until skins are mostly split and nuts are light golden brown (the skins will look darker) and fragrant, about 10 minutes. Place the hot nuts in a clean dishtowel and, once cool enough to handle, vigorously rub them against themselves in the towel to remove most of the skins.

1. Preheat oven to 375°F.

2. Bring a pot of water to a boil. Add haricots verts. Reduce heat to medium and cook until just tender, 3–4 minutes. Drain, and plunge haricots verts into an ice-water bath to chill. Drain, and set aside. (This can be done up to a day in advance.)

3. Heat 1 tablespoon oil in a large, wide skillet over medium heat Add onion, salt, and pepper, and cook, stirring occasionally, until onions are light golden brown, 4–5 minutes.

4. Meanwhile, place hazelnuts in a baking pan and toast in the oven until they darken, 5–7 minutes. Chop roughly and set aside.

5. In a large skillet, heat the remaining 1 tablespoon olive oil over medium-high heat. Add haricots verts and cook, stirring occasionally, until heated through, about 3 minutes. Add cooked onions and hazelnuts and cook 1 additional minute. Transfer to a serving dish, and serve.

Choices/Exchanges 2 Vegetable, 2 1/2 Fat
Calories 160 | Calories from Fat 110
Total Fat 12g | Saturated Fat 1.2g | Trans Fat 0.0g
Cholesterol 0mg
Sodium 200mg

Potassium 350mg
Total Carbohydrate 13g | Dietary Fiber 6g | Sugars 3g
Protein 4g
Phosphorus 85mg

CALABRIAN-STYLE ROASTED POTATOES (*PATATE CALABRESE AL FORNO*)

Serves: 8 | Serving Size: 1/2 cup
Prep Time: 10 minutes | Cooking Time: 45 minutes

Since the southern Italian region of Calabria is known for its pepperoncino, *or hot chile peppers, many American or other recipes are called "Calabrese" simply because someone has sprinkled crushed red chile flakes over the dish. This recipe is actually an authentic Calabrian dish known in the region as* Patate raganate. *The word* raganate, *meaning "gratin," is a dialect word from the neighboring Basilicata region that is now used throughout Calabria.*

1/4 cup extra virgin olive oil, divided
2 pounds yukon gold potatoes, peeled and cut into 1/3-inch slices
2 medium red onions, thinly sliced
1 teaspoon finely chopped fresh oregano OR 1/2 teaspoon dried oregano
Pinch crushed red chile flakes
1 teaspoon unrefined sea salt
1/4 teaspoon freshly ground black pepper
1/3 cup Fresh Bread Crumbs (page 291) or almond flour
1/2 cup grated pecorino Crotonese, ricotta salata, or pecorino Romano cheese

---

Choices/Exchanges 1 1/2 Carbohydrate, 2 Fat
Calories 200 | Calories from Fat 80
Total Fat 9g | Saturated Fat 2.1g | Trans Fat 0.0g
Cholesterol 5mg
Sodium 140mg

Potassium 540mg
Total Carbohydrate 26g | Dietary Fiber 3g | Sugars 2g
Protein 6g
Phosphorus 135mg

1. Preheat oven to 425°F.

2. Grease a 8 ×12-inch baking dish with 1 table-spoon olive oil. Add potatoes, onions, oregano, chile flakes, salt, and pepper. Drizzle with 2 tablespoons olive oil and toss well to combine. Sprinkle bread crumbs and cheese over the top. Drizzle with remaining 1 tablespoon olive oil.

3. Bake, uncovered, until potatoes are tender and topping is golden, approximately 45 minutes. Serve.

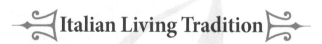

Italian Living Tradition

Try experimenting with different types of pecorino (sheep's milk) cheese if they are available in your area. While pecorino Romano cheese is the most widely available variety outside of Italy, pecorino Crotonese is delicious, with a strong herbal flavor reminiscent of the Calabrian fields. A little goes a long way, and you'll be surprised at how much this cheese can brighten an otherwise humble dish.

CHARGRILLED ASPARAGUS WITH BALSAMIC AND PARMESAN (ASPARAGI GRIGLIATI CON BALSAMICO E PARMIGIANO)

Serves: 4 | Serving Size: 6 asparagus spears, 1 tablespoon sauce, and 1/2 tablespoon cheese
Prep Time: 5 minutes | Cooking Time: 5 minutes

Freshly grilled asparagus with sweet balsamic vinegar and shards of freshly shaved parmigiano-reggiano cheese makes for a simple yet dramatic side dish. The health benefits of eating asparagus are many. The herbaceous plant is a great detoxifier, and asparagus is also a good source of vitamins A, B12, C, E, and K, along with chromium, fiber, and folate. Asparagus is believed to help fight and prevent certain forms of cancer, and its antioxidant content is said to help slow the aging process. Its B12 content may help reduce cognitive impairment. Asparagine, a natural diuretic found in asparagus, is believed to help with high blood pressure, edema, and other heart-related diseases.

24 asparagus spears, trimmed
2 tablespoons extra virgin olive oil
2 tablespoons balsamic vinegar (preferably Aceto Balsamico di Modena)
2 tablespoons grated or shaved parmigiano-reggiano cheese

Choices/Exchanges 1 Vegetable, 1 1/2 Fat
Calories 100 | Calories from Fat 70
Total Fat 8g | Saturated Fat 1.4g | Trans Fat 0.0g
Cholesterol 0mg
Sodium 40mg

Potassium 220mg
Total Carbohydrate 6g | Dietary Fiber 2g | Sugars 3g
Protein 3g
Phosphorus 75mg

1. Preheat a grill or griddle to high heat (you should be able to hold your hand above the grates for just 1–2 seconds).

2. On a large platter or baking sheet, brush asparagus with olive oil to coat easily. Place on grill, cover, and cook for 4 minutes. Lift lid, turn, and continue to cook until al dente, approximately 4–5 more minutes, turning often.

3. Remove from grill, drizzle with balsamic vinegar, and sprinkle with parmigiano-reggiano cheese to serve.

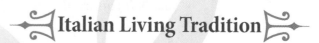

Italian Living Tradition

You can peel away the tough outer layers of asparagus by grasping the base of the asparagus in one hand and, using a vegetable peeler in the other hand, *carefully* peeling toward (but stopping short of) your hand, and rotating the asparagus as you peel. You'll end up with a short piece of unpeeled stalk, which can easily be snapped off at the point where the peeling stops.

SPINACH SAUTÉED IN GARLIC AND OIL
(SPINACI ALL'AGLIO E OLIO)

Serves: 4 | Serving Size: Approximately 1/2 cup
Prep Time: 5 minutes | Cooking Time: 5 minutes

This dish is so simple that it's almost a crime to call it a recipe. But I included it in this book because it is easy, healthful, and tasty. Over the years I've noticed that many of my cooking students don't know how to cook fresh spinach. They are surprised at how easy it is. Delicious and healthful dishes like this one should be the base of our diet.

2 tablespoons extra virgin olive oil

2 1/4 pounds spinach, trimmed, well washed, and dried

3 cloves garlic, minced

Pinch crushed red chile flakes

1/8 teaspoon kosher salt

1/4 teaspoon freshly ground black pepper

1 lemon, halved

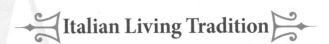

Italian Living Tradition

Vegetables of any kind—cauliflower, broccoli, peppers, potatoes, and/or green beans—can be blanched until just tender, and prepared the same way.

1. Heat the oil over high heat in a very large skillet until very hot. Add the spinach (you may need to work in batches) and cook, stirring, for about 1–2 minutes; the spinach should turn bright green and wilt slightly. Add the garlic and red chile flakes and continue to cook, stirring constantly, until the garlic begins to release its aroma, approximately 30 seconds.

2. Remove the spinach from the heat, and season with salt and and pepper. Toss well to combine, and serve with lemon on the side (for squeezing juice over the spinach).

Choices/Exchanges 2 1/2 Vegetable, 1 1/2 Fat
Calories 130 | Calories from Fat 70
Total Fat 8g | Saturated Fat 1.0g | Trans Fat 0.0g
Cholesterol 0mg
Sodium 250mg

Potassium 1450mg
Total Carbohydrate 11g | Dietary Fiber 6g | Sugars 1g
Protein 8g
Phosphorus 130mg

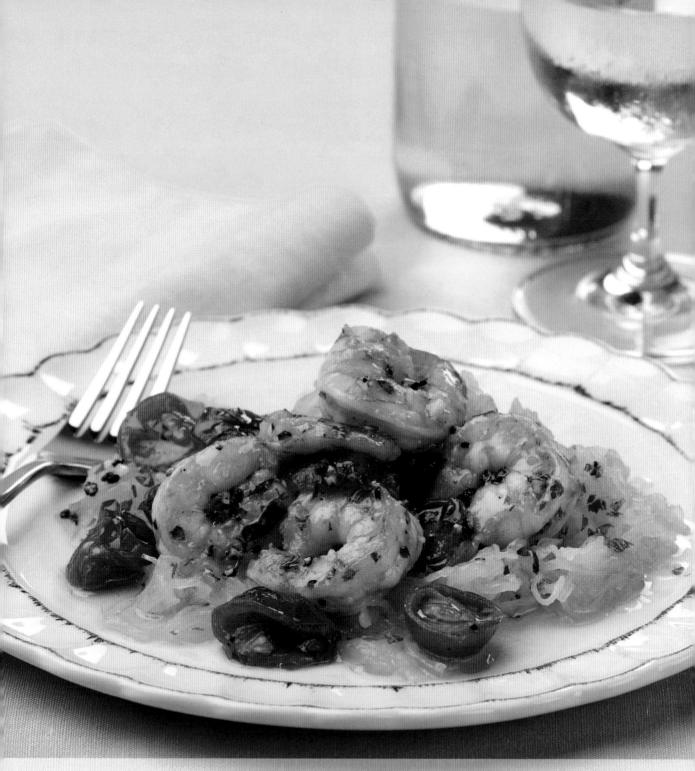

Spaghetti Squash "Pasta" with Shrimp, Tomatoes, and Basil, p. 62

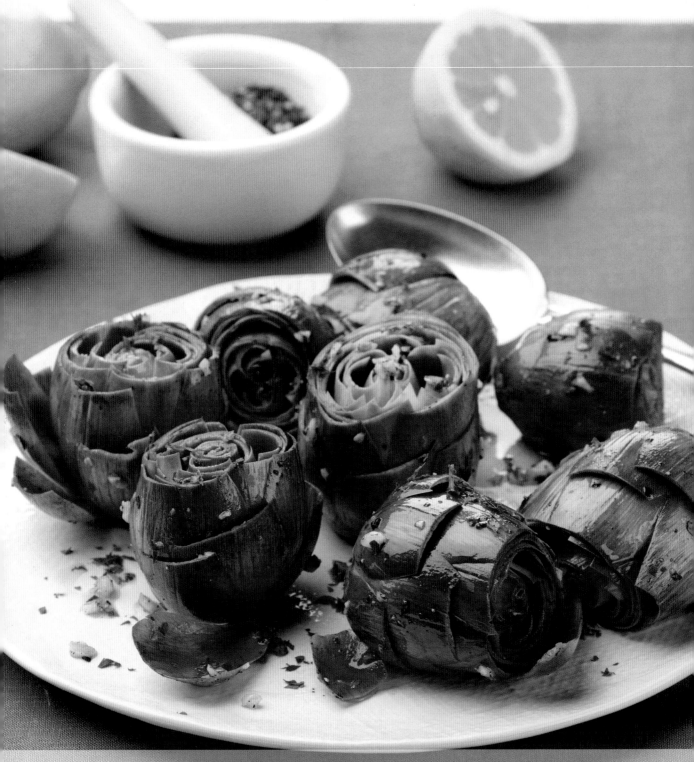

Artichokes with Garlic and Oil, p. 164

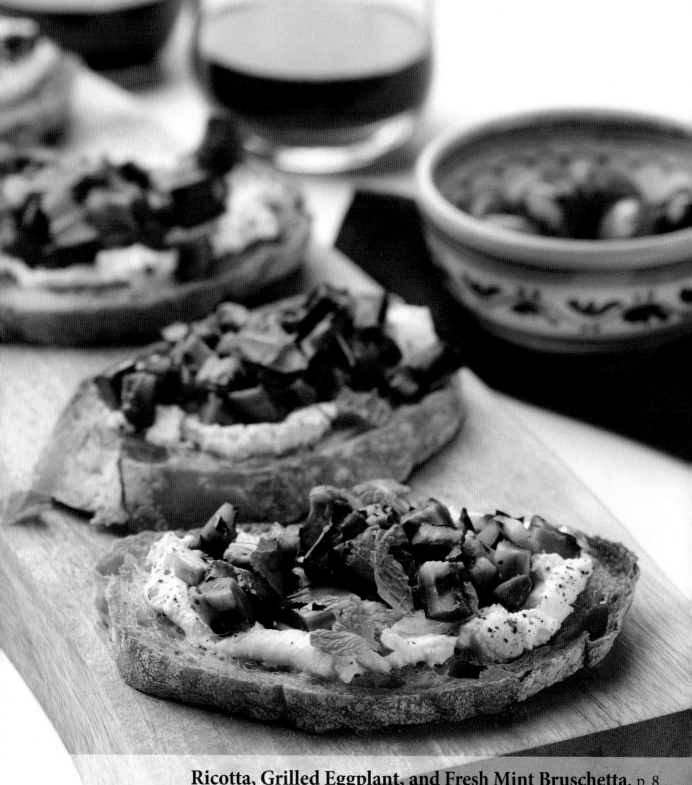

Ricotta, Grilled Eggplant, and Fresh Mint Bruschetta, p. 8

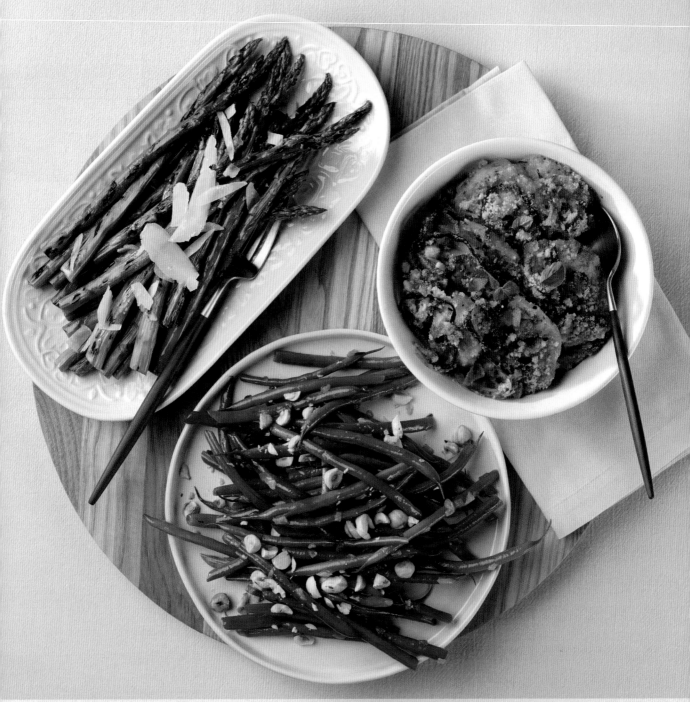

Chargrilled Asparagus with Balsamic and Parmesan, p. 178
Haricots Verts with Hazelnuts, p. 175 / **Calabrian-Style Roasted Potatoes,** p. 176

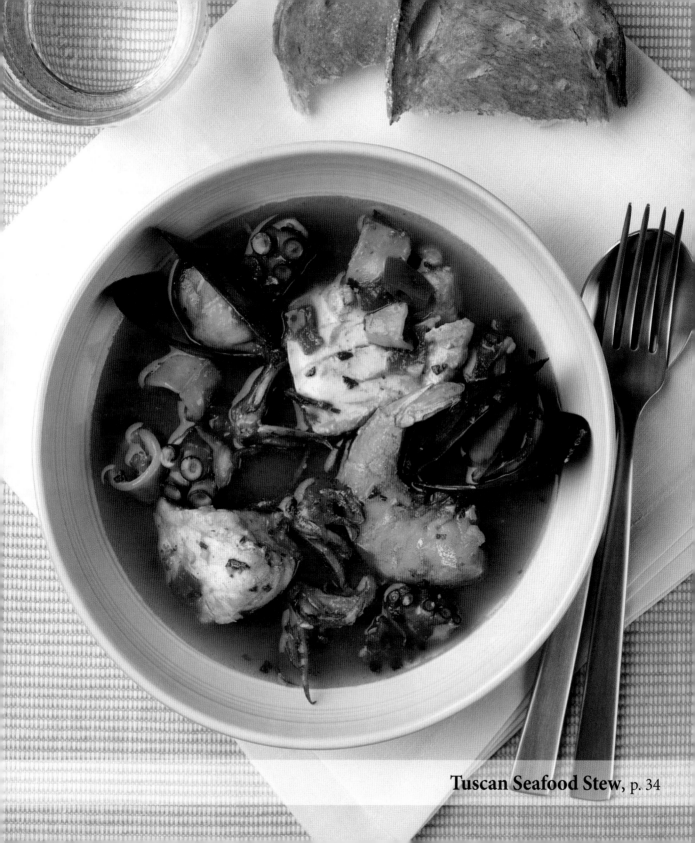

Tuscan Seafood Stew, p. 34

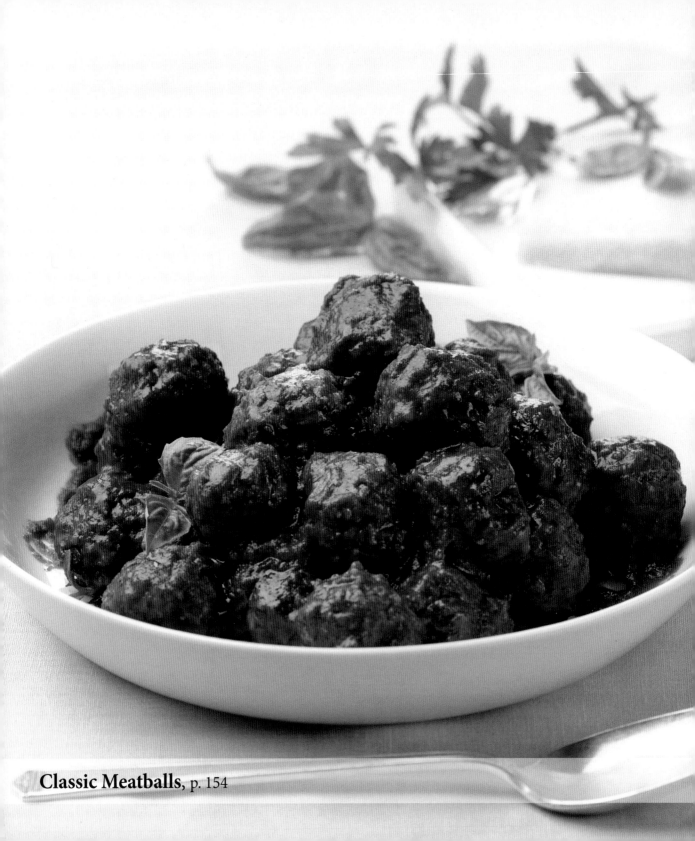

Classic Meatballs, p. 154

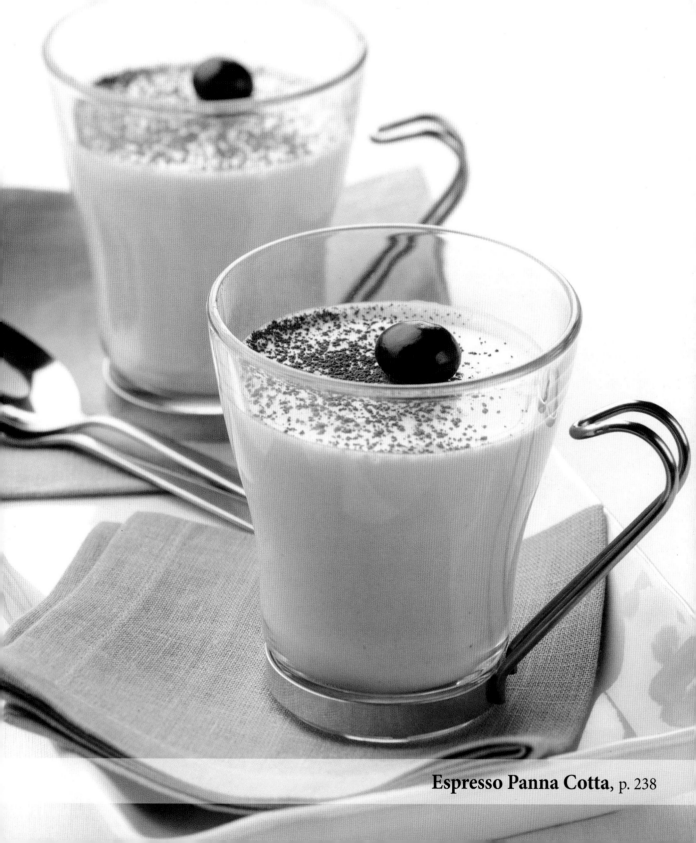

Espresso Panna Cotta, p. 238

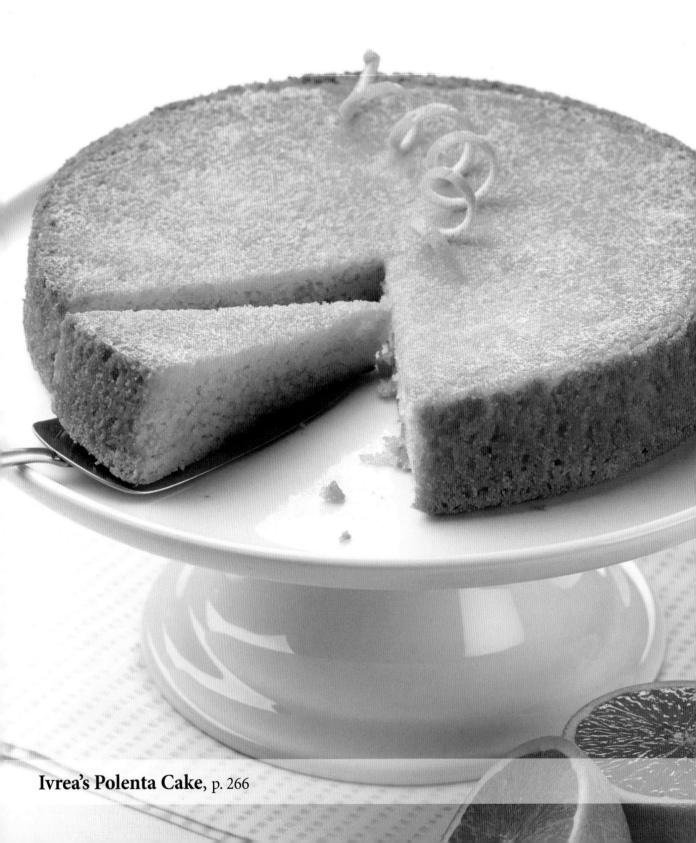

Ivrea's Polenta Cake, p. 266

SALADS
(INSALATE)

185 Beet, Quinoa, and Arugula Salad/*Insalata di barbabietole, quinoa, e rucola*

186 Cannellini Bean, Tuna, and Red Onion Salad/*Insalata di cannellini, tonno, e cipolle rosse*

187 Red Pepper, Yellow Tomato, and Artichoke Salad/
       Insalata di peperoni rossi, pomodori gialli, e carciofi

188 Asparagus, Orange, and Fennel Salad/*Insalata di asparagi, arance, e finocchi*

190 Tomatoes with Balsamic Vinegar/*Insalata di pomodori all'aceto balsamico*

191 Belgian Endive, Radicchio, and Grapefruit Salad/*Insalata d'indivia, radicchio, e pompelmo*

192 Arugula Salad with Pears, Parmesan, and Cocoa Nibs/
       Insalata di rucola con pere, parmigiano, e pennini di cacao

193 Val d'Aosta–Style Dandelion Salad/*Insalata di dente di leone Valdostana*

194 Smoked Fish, Orange, and Radicchio Salad with Olives/
       Insalata di pesce affumicato, arance, e radicchio

196 Monday Salad/*Insalata del lunedi*

198 Blood Orange Salad/*Insalata d'arance sanguose*

199 Cauliflower and Herb Salad from Le Marche/*Insalata di cavolfiore alla Marchigiana*

200 Seafood Salad/*Insalata di pesce*

202 Marinated Eggplant Salad/*Melanzane in insalata alla Calabrese*

203 Chickpea Salad/*Insalata di ceci*

204 Tuscan Farro Salad/*Insalata di farro alla Toscana*

"Con patate e cipolle dentro l'orto, mai di fame nessuno è morto."
"With potatoes and onions in the garden, no one has ever died hungry."
—Italian proverb

While there are many classic Italian salads to choose from, most Italians (myself included) eat an *insalata verde* (a mixture of fresh greens drizzled with olive oil and vinegar) or an *insalata mista* (a lettuce-based salad with tomatoes, carrots, and maybe a few other vegetables, drizzled with olive oil and vinegar) at the end of their meals. The salad course always follows the second course and side dish in Italy. Salads are not paired with wine because the vinegar used to dress salads clashes with the flavor of the wine.

During Roman times, salads were eaten before and during meals, much as they are in the U.S. today. Lettuce was actually believed to be an aphrodisiac by the Romans, but not all Italian salads are lettuce based. Some are made up of legumes, grains, rice, and a variety of cooked vegetables. For summer entertaining, try preparing a variety of salads from this chapter and serving them with artisan bread, aged Italian cheeses, and olives.

It is a sad fact that salads are an afterthought in many homes and restaurants today. The average American eats only 57% of the recommended daily amount of vegetables. Only 6% of Americans eat the amount of vegetables they should. This is a shame, because eating vegetables is one of the easiest ways to stay healthy and in shape. We should be consuming 4–5 different types of fresh vegetables daily, preferably of different colors, to ensure the widest range of nutrients. The greatest benefit of creating a variety of salads is that it is an easy and tasty way to "eat the rainbow." Medical experts agree that by eating a wide variety of brightly colored fresh fruits and vegetables, we increase our nutrient intake greatly (since each color generally represents a different nutrition profile).

Vegetables naturally have high water content, making them virtually fat-free and low in calories. Consuming vegetables helps to maintain blood pressure levels and promotes health of the digestive, skeletal, and excretory systems. The antioxidants in vegetables help keep cancer, cardiovascular problems, and strokes at bay and deliver vitamins A, K, B6, folate, and carotenoids—like beta carotene from carrots, zeaxanthin from greens, and lutein from spinach and collard greens.

It's important to try to eat vegetables when they are in season locally; it is at those times of year that our bodies especially require the nutrients they possess. When ripe, in-season, organic vegetables are cooked to perfection—with their natural sugars coaxed out of them and combined with other savory ingredients—eating healthfully becomes a joy! I recommend eating the salads in this chapter seasonally, so I've provided a list of the salad recipes organized by the best time of year to enjoy them.

Salads by Season

Spring
Asparagus, Orange, and Fennel Salad (page 188)
Val d'Aosta–Style Dandelion Salad (page 193)
Blood Orange Salad (page 198)

Summer
Red Pepper, Yellow Tomato, and Artichoke Salad
    (page 187)
Tomatoes with Balsamic Vinegar (page 190)
Marinated Eggplant Salad (page 202)

Fall
Arugula Salad with Pears, Parmesan, and Cocoa
    Nibs (page 192)
Cauliflower and Herb Salad from Le Marche
    (page 199)

Winter
Belgian Endive, Radicchio, and Grapefruit Salad
    (page 191)
Cannellini Bean, Tuna, and Red Onion Salad
    (page 186)

All Year
Beet, Quinoa, and Arugula Salad (page 185)
Smoked Fish, Orange, and Radicchio Salad with
    Olives (page 194)
Monday Salad (page 196)
Seafood Salad (page 200)
Chickpea Salad (page 203)
Tuscan Farro Salad (page 204)

BEET, QUINOA, AND ARUGULA SALAD
(INSALATA DI BARBABIETOLE, QUINOA, E RUCOLA)

Serves: 8 | Serving Size: Approximately 3/4 cup
Prep Time: 5 minutes | Cooking Time: 45 minutes

This Mediterranean-inspired salad combines nutritious quinoa with arugula and bright, beautiful beets. The citrus dressing makes this salad sing! For quicker prep, use leftover beets or cook the beets a day in advance.

2 whole beets, trimmed
1/2 cup extra virgin olive oil
Juice of 1 orange
1/4 teaspoon unrefined sea salt
1/4 teaspoon freshly ground black pepper
4 cups cooked quinoa
6 ounces baby arugula

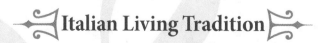
Italian Living Tradition

Adding healthful whole grains, such as farro and barley, to salads is very popular in Italy. Originally from Latin America, quinoa is relatively new to Italy. Due to the rise in gluten intolerance, however, it is becoming more popular.

1. Preheat oven to 425°F.

2. Pierce holes in beets with a fork and wrap them in aluminum foil. Place on a baking sheet and bake until tender, approximately 45 minutes. Allow beets to cool slightly, then peel and dice.

3. Whisk olive oil, orange juice, salt, and pepper together to make a vinaigrette.

4. Place quinoa in a large bowl and lightly fluff with a fork. Add the vinaigrette. Gently stir in the arugula and beets. Serve immediately.

Choices/Exchanges 1 1/2 Starch, 2 Vegetable, 4 Fat
Calories 330 | Calories from Fat 190
Total Fat 21g | Saturated Fat 2.8g | Trans Fat 0.0g
Cholesterol 0mg
Sodium 135mg

Potassium 435mg
Total Carbohydrate 32g | Dietary Fiber 5g | Sugars 5g
Protein 7g
Phosphorus 215mg

CANNELLINI BEAN, TUNA, AND RED ONION SALAD (*INSALATA DI CANNELLINI, TONNO, E CIPOLLE ROSSE*)

Serves: 8 | Serving Size: 3/4 cup

Prep Time: 10 minutes (plus 1 hour onion-soaking time) | Cooking Time: 0 minutes

With the addition of bread, this salad can become a light lunch or dinner. Keep in mind that this recipe is a great way to use up leftover beans. If you're using dried beans, they need to be soaked overnight before cooking. But they can be soaked and cooked up to a week in advance, so this salad can be assembled quickly at the last minute. Try bringing this salad to your next summertime picnic.

4 cups Braised Cannellini Beans (page 284), drained and cooled

4 tablespoons red wine vinegar

1/3 cup good-quality extra virgin olive oil (preferably first cold-pressed and unfiltered)

1 small red onion, thinly sliced, soaked in a bowl of cold water for 1 hour (see Italian Living Tradition)

14 ounces white tuna packed in olive oil, drained, and broken into small pieces with a fork

1/4 cup finely chopped fresh flat-leaf parsley

2 tablespoons finely chopped basil

1/8 teaspoon unrefined sea salt

1/4 teaspoon freshly ground black pepper

Italian Living Tradition

Soaking onions in water is a trick that helps to remove the strong bitter flavors, making onions more palatable even when eaten raw. Many older people in Italy like to eat raw onions with dinner for a better night's sleep.

1. Place cannellini beans in a large salad bowl.

2. In a small bowl, whisk vinegar and olive oil together until emulsified.

3. Add onions and dressing to the beans, and stir to combine. Add in tuna, parsley, and basil, and stir well to combine. Taste and season with salt and pepper. Serve at room temperature.

Choices/Exchanges 1 1/2 Starch, 3 Lean Protein, 1 1/2 Fat
Calories 350 | Calories from Fat 130
Total Fat 14g | Saturated Fat 2.0g | Trans Fat 0.0g
Cholesterol 15mg

Sodium 240mg
Potassium 1100mg
Total Carbohydrate 32g | Dietary Fiber 8g | Sugars 2g
Protein 25g
Phosphorus 290mg

RED PEPPER, YELLOW TOMATO, AND ARTICHOKE SALAD
(INSALATA DI PEPERONI ROSSI, POMODORI GIALLI, E CARCIOFI)

Serves: 6 | Serving Size: Approximately 3/4 cup
Prep Time: 15 minutes | Cooking Time: 0 minutes

Italians do not typically eat large salads for a meal the way that Americans do. Instead, salads are usually served at the end of a meal to cleanse the palate, or as part of a series of appetizers when dining out to whet the appetite. Some traditional Italian salads, however, are so satisfying when prepared with fresh, seasonal produce that they could almost be eaten alone. And this one is no exception. If I ever have any of this salad left over, I toss it with hot pasta the following day.

1 pound artichokes, cooked and roughly chopped

12 ounces Roasted Peppers (page 282)

1 pint yellow grape tomatoes

1/3 cup extra virgin olive oil

1/4 cup balsamic vinegar (preferably Aceto Balsamico di Modena) or red wine vinegar

2 tablespoons finely chopped fresh basil or flat-leaf parsley

1/4 teaspoon unrefined sea salt

1/4 teaspoon freshly ground black pepper

⊰ Italian Living Tradition ⊱

When making this salad, prepare a double batch of vegetables and save the extras to be tossed into pasta or a stew the following day. If you're not sure how to cook artichokes, see the cooking instruction in the Artichokes with Garlic and Oil recipe on page 164.

1. Combine artichokes, roasted peppers, and grape tomatoes in a large salad bowl or on a platter. Stir.

2. In a small bowl, whisk olive oil into vinegar until emulsified and stir in basil or parsley.

3. Drizzle dressing over vegetables. Taste, and season with salt and pepper. Serve.

Choices/Exchanges 3 1/2 Vegetable, 2 1/2 Fat
Calories 190 | Calories from Fat 120
Total Fat 13g | Saturated Fat 1.8g | Trans Fat 0.0g
Cholesterol 0mg
Sodium 150mg

Potassium 535mg
Total Carbohydrate 18g | Dietary Fiber 8g | Sugars 7g
Protein 4g
Phosphorus 90mg

ASPARAGUS, ORANGE, AND FENNEL SALAD (INSALATA DI ASPARAGI, ARANCE, E FINOCCHI)

Serves: 6 | Serving Size: 1/2 cup
Prep Time: 10 minutes | Cooking Time: 5 minutes

Fresh fennel, while relatively "new" to many American palates, is very common in Italy. It has been used for both culinary and medicinal purposes since antiquity. Fresh fennel is a diuretic and contains many healthful properties. Dried fennel seeds have been used to freshen breath and aid digestion, from the Mediterranean region all the way to India. Fennel tea is made by boiling a teaspoon of fennel seeds, and straining the tea; it is usually enjoyed at night, after a meal. It's best to make this vegan salad in the spring and fall when freshly harvested asparagus and fennel are easy to find.

1 (1-pound) bunch fresh asparagus, trimmed

2 large bulbs fennel (about 1 1/2 pounds total)

2 large oranges (about 1 pound total), peeled and sliced into segments

4 tablespoons chopped fresh flat-leaf parsley

1/4 cup black olives (such as gaeta or kalamata), pitted and halved

1/3 cup orange juice

Juice of 1 lemon

2 tablespoons extra virgin olive oil

1/4 teaspoon unrefined sea salt

1/4 teaspoon freshly ground black pepper

Choices/Exchanges 1/2 Carbohydrate, 3 Vegetable, 1 Fat
Calories 150 | Calories from Fat 50
Total Fat 6g | Saturated Fat 0.9g | Trans Fat 0.0g
Cholesterol 0mg

Sodium 210mg
Potassium 825mg
Total Carbohydrate 26g | Dietary Fiber 9g | Sugars 7g
Protein 4g
Phosphorus 115mg

1. Bring a large pot of water to a boil. Add asparagus and boil until just tender, approximately 5 minutes. Drain and place asparagus in a bowl of ice-cold water.

2. Cut stalks off of fennel and remove bruised leaves. Slice off the end of bases, cut the bulbs into quarters, and slice into thin slices horizontally. Place fennel in a salad bowl. Add oranges and parsley, and lightly toss to combine.

3. Drain asparagus and add to salad with the olives.

4. In a mixing bowl, whisk orange juice, lemon juice, and olive oil together, and season with salt and pepper. Pour dressing over the salad and serve immediately.

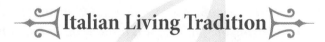

Italian Living Tradition

Look for the sweetest oranges possible for this recipe. When available, use Sicilian blood oranges.

TOMATOES WITH BALSAMIC VINEGAR (INSALATA DI POMODORI ALL'ACETO BALSAMICO)

Serves: 4 | Serving Size: 1/2 cup
Prep Time: 5 minutes | Cooking Time: 0 minutes

When ripe tomatoes are plentiful, this sumptuous salad is the perfect thing to make. When I was growing up, this dish was a staple on our summer table—although my mother prepared it with wine vinegar and oregano instead of balsamic and basil. Feel free to experiment and use whichever flavor profile you prefer. Serve this salad alongside grilled and roasted meats, poultry, and fish, or toss it into cooked pasta, barley, or farro for a different type of delicious salad.

2–3 ripe beefsteak tomatoes, sliced

2 teaspoons good-quality balsamic vinegar

2 teaspoons extra virgin olive oil
   (preferably first cold-pressed and unfiltered)

1/4 teaspoon unrefined sea salt

1/8 teaspoon freshly ground black pepper

1/2 cup fresh basil leaves, finely chopped

1. Arrange tomato slices on a plate. Drizzle with vinegar and olive oil. Sprinkle salt and pepper. Top with basil, and serve.

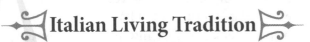
Italian Living Tradition

It's no secret that for the last few centuries tomatoes have held a special place on the Italian table. Prized for their flavor, culinary versatility, and high antioxidant and lycopene content, fresh tomatoes are an easy addition to meals. For another variation on this recipe, dress the tomatoes with the ingredients as indicated and then place them on a parchment paper–lined baking sheet. Roast in a 425°F oven until tender and slightly golden, approximately 20 minutes.

Choices/Exchanges 1 Vegetable, 1/2 Fat
Calories 50 | Calories from Fat 25
Total Fat 3g | Saturated Fat 0.4g | Trans Fat 0.0g
Cholesterol 0mg
Sodium 150mg

Potassium 335mg
Total Carbohydrate 6g | Dietary Fiber 2g | Sugars 4g
Protein 1g
Phosphorus 35mg

BELGIAN ENDIVE, RADICCHIO, AND GRAPEFRUIT SALAD
(INSALATA D'INDIVIA, RADICCHIO, E POMPELMO)

Serves: 6 | Serving Size: Approximately 1 cup
Prep Time: 15 minutes (plus 1 hour onion-soaking time) | Cooking Time: 0 minutes

In Italy, the most prized variety of radicchio—Treviso—comes from the northern Italian town of the same name. It has elongated, red leaves that are slightly sweeter in taste than the round types that are more readily available in the U.S. Use whichever type of radicchio you can find for this recipe. If you need a substitute for the radicchio, red cabbage or red leaf lettuce, although very different, work well.

Segments and juice of 1 grapefruit
(see Italian Living Tradition), divided

3 tablespoons extra virgin olive oil
(preferably first cold-pressed and unfiltered)

1/8 teaspoon unrefined sea salt

1/4 teaspoon freshly ground black pepper

1 head radicchio or Treviso, leaves separated and
torn into bite-size pieces

1 head endive, torn into spears

1/2 small red onion, thinly sliced, soaked in
cold water for 1 hour, and drained

1/4 cup toasted almonds or hazelnuts,
roughly chopped

Italian Living Tradition

To section grapefruit: Begin by cutting away both ends of the grapefruit and setting the fruit on a work surface. With a sharp knife, cut away the skin and white pith in wide bands. Hold the peeled fruit over a bowl and begin cutting each segment away from the membrane by sliding the knife between the membrane and flesh on one side of each segment and then on the other side, cutting the segment free. Once you've removed all the segments, squeeze the membranes over a strainer into a bowl to get any remaining juice.

1. In a small bowl, whisk the grapefruit juice with the olive oil. Season with salt and pepper.

2. Arrange the radicchio, endive, and grapefruit sections on a platter. Garnish with the onion and drizzle with the dressing. Sprinkle nuts on top, and serve.

Choices/Exchanges 2 Vegetable, 2 Fat
Calories 120 | Calories from Fat 80
Total Fat 9g | Saturated Fat 1.2g | Trans Fat 0.0g
Cholesterol 0mg
Sodium 100mg

Potassium 255mg
Total Carbohydrate 10g | Dietary Fiber 2g | Sugars 6g
Protein 2g
Phosphorus 50mg

ARUGULA SALAD WITH PEARS, PARMESAN, AND COCOA NIBS (INSALATA DI RUCOLA CON PERE, PARMIGIANO, E PENNINI DI CACAO)

Serves: 4 | Serving Size: Approximately 1 1/3 cups
Prep Time: 10 minutes | Cooking Time: 0 minutes

This delicious and healthful salad combines peppery arugula with sweet pears, rich parmesan and pistachios, and crunchy cocoa nibs.

Cocoa nibs are usually sold in small packages at specialty stores and markets to be used for cooking and snacking and in chocolate dishes. Since nibs come directly from the cocoa tree, they contain high amounts of theobromine, which has diuretic, stimulant, and relaxing effects and can lower blood pressure.

4 cups baby arugula, washed well

2 pears, peeled, cored, and sliced into sixths

1/4 cup slivered almonds, toasted

1/8 cup cocoa nibs

1 tablespoon good-quality balsamic vinegar

4 tablespoons extra virgin olive oil

1/8 teaspoon unrefined sea salt

1/4 teaspoon freshly ground black pepper

1 ounce shaved parmigiano-reggiano cheese

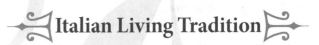

Italian Living Tradition

Many people don't associate chocolate with traditional Italian cooking, but the town of Modica in Sicily is actually famous for their chocolate, which is made using an ancient Aztec recipe introduced by the Spaniards. Their unsweetened chocolate is a secret ingredient in the local *caponata* recipe (see Sicilian Sweet-and-Sour Vegetable Medley on page 6).

1. Divide arugula between 4 salad plates. Arrange pear slices on top of arugula and sprinkle almonds and cocoa nibs over the top.

2. To make the dressing, pour balsamic vinegar in a small bowl. Whisk in the olive oil until blended, and season with salt and pepper.

3. Pour dressing over the salad, top with cheese, and serve.

Choices/Exchanges 1 Fruit, 1 Vegetable, 4 1/2 Fat
Calories 300 | Calories from Fat 200
Total Fat 22g | Saturated Fat 5.0g | Trans Fat 0.0g
Cholesterol 0mg
Sodium 190mg

Potassium 300mg
Total Carbohydrate 21g | Dietary Fiber 5g | Sugars 12g
Protein 6g
Phosphorus 130mg

VAL D'AOSTA–STYLE DANDELION SALAD (*INSALATA DI DENTE DI LEONE VALDOSTANA*)

Serves: 6 | Serving Size: Approximately 1 cup
Prep Time: 5 minutes | Cooking Time: 15 minutes

The Latin name for dandelion translates as "official disease remedy." Widely used in Italy, dandelion is praised for its pronounced flavor and health benefits. The "dressing" for this salad is actually a lighter version of a bagna cauda *(literally translated as "hot bath"), which is usually served in Piedmont and Val d'Aosta in a fondue dish to keep it warm.*

1/2 cup finest-quality extra virgin olive oil
   (preferably unfiltered)

1 tablespoon unsalted butter, room temperature

6 oil-packed anchovy fillets, drained and rinsed

3 large cloves garlic, chopped

6 cups roughly chopped or baby dandelion greens

1/4 cup chopped walnuts, toasted

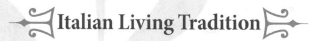

Italian Living Tradition

While this dressing uses olive oil, it is believed that original versions of *bagna cauda* used walnut oil, since walnut groves were plentiful in Piedmont and Val d'Aosta. Once deforestation occurred, the locals began to import olive oil from the Liguria region. Typically butter is added to the sauce, and it is served warm in a fondue or traditional clay pot; it is used as a dip for raw vegetables and bread.

1. Add olive oil, butter, anchovies, and garlic to a food processor, and blend until smooth.

2. Transfer oil mixture to heavy-bottomed, medium saucepan. Cook, uncovered, over low heat for 15 minutes, whisking occasionally. (Sauce will separate.) Set aside.

3. Place dandelion greens in a salad bowl. Add walnuts and dressing, and toss. Serve immediately.

Choices/Exchanges 1 Vegetable, 1 Lean Protein, 4 Fat
Calories 240 | Calories from Fat 220
Total Fat 24g | Saturated Fat 4.2g | Trans Fat 0.0g
Cholesterol 10mg
Sodium 190mg

Potassium 270mg
Total Carbohydrate 6g | Dietary Fiber 2g | Sugars 1g
Protein 4g
Phosphorus 65mg

SMOKED FISH, ORANGE, AND RADICCHIO SALAD WITH OLIVES
(INSALATA DI PESCE AFFUMICATO, ARANCE, E RADICCHIO)

Serves: 4 | Serving Size: 1/2 cup
Prep Time: 10 minutes | Cooking Time: 15 minutes

Smoked white fish, more commonly associated with Eastern European cooking, is actually very popular in the Italian regions of Calabria and Sicily. In this recipe, it is paired with bright citrus and crispy radicchio for an additional Mediterranean touch. If you've never tried orange with seafood before, you don't know what you're missing! It's a common Italian pairing that makes the flavors of fish sing! Leeks and cheese such as caciotta *or* provolone *are other common additions which transform this simple salad into a full meal.*

1 1/4 pounds whole smoked white fish, such as trout or chub

2 large juice oranges, peeled and supremed (see Italian Living Tradition)

2 tablespoons oil-cured black olives, pitted and halved

2 tablespoons finely chopped fresh oregano or mint

2 tablespoons extra virgin olive oil

1/4 teaspoon freshly ground white pepper

1 small head radicchio, leaves separated and torn into bite-size pieces

---

Choices/Exchanges 2 Vegetable, 2 1/2 Lean Protein, 2 Fat
Calories 270 | Calories from Fat 130
Total Fat 14g | Saturated Fat 2.1g | Trans Fat 0.0g
Cholesterol 60mg

Sodium 290mg
Potassium 630mg
Total Carbohydrate 13g | Dietary Fiber 3g | Sugars 9g
Protein 22g
Phosphorus 275mg

1. Preheat oven to 300°F.

2. Wrap the fish in aluminum foil and place on a baking sheet in the center of the oven. Bake until warmed through, about 15 minutes. Remove from the oven and from the foil.

3. Transfer the fish to a cutting board and let cool briefly. Using a sharp knife, make 2 crosswise slashes, one below the gills and the other at the narrow part of the fish at the tail end, just deep enough to reach the spine of the fish. Then, using the tip of the knife, make a lengthwise slash down the center of the fish, following the spine. Working from the middle of the fish, lift off the skin and discard. Using the knife and a fork, lift one side of the fish fillet from the spine and transfer to a bowl. Lift the other side from the spine and transfer to the bowl. Turn the fish over and repeat with the other side. Flake the fish into bite-size pieces.

4. Add orange pieces to the bowl along with the olives, oregano or mint, and olive oil. Toss well. Season with white pepper.

5. Place radicchio leaves on the bottom of a large platter and scoop the fish mixture into the center. Serve at room temperature.

Italian Living Tradition

To supreme an orange: Begin by cutting away both ends of the orange and setting the fruit on a work surface. With a sharp knife, cut away the skin and white pith in wide bands. Hold the peeled fruit over a bowl and begin cutting each segment away from the membrane by sliding the knife between the membrane and flesh on one side of each segment and then on the other side, cutting the segment free. Select the neatest orange segments for this recipe.

MONDAY SALAD
(INSALATA DEL LUNEDI)

Serves: 6 | Serving Size: Approximately 1 cup
Prep Time: 15 minutes | Cooking Time: 0 minutes

Sunday is the traditional day when families congregate in Italy. On the day of rest, families would combine their best culinary ingredients and begin preparing slow-cooked meals early in the morning. After Mass, large extended families often gathered, and the Sunday meal would take place. This ritual is so deeply imbedded in Italian culture that it spawned a separate type of cooking, known as "Sunday cooking." Even today, as more and more stores are open 24 hours, and restaurants are serving clientele "nonstop" (without the traditional break between lunch and dinner), a reported 70% of Italians still enjoy the Sunday meal at home with family.

This salad was traditionally served on Mondays by housewives trying to use up the leftovers from Sunday dinner. Leftovers often included roasted or grilled meats or seafood, bread, beans, and vegetables, and the tastiest and most creative way to repurpose these ingredients was in salads—hence the origin of the Monday Salad, which was always eaten for dinner.

1 head romaine lettuce, washed, dried, and cut into bite-size pieces

2 ripe tomatoes, diced

1 baby cucumber OR 1/3 English cucumber, sliced thinly on the diagonal

1/4 pound fresh mozzarella balls

1/4 cup black olives, pitted

1 cup Braised Cannellini Beans (page 284) or other cooked beans

1/2 pound shredded (leftover) roasted chicken

2 cups Homemade Croutons (page 292; optional)

3 tablespoons red wine vinegar or lemon juice

1/8 teaspoon unrefined sea salt

1/4 teaspoon freshly ground black pepper

1/2 cup extra virgin olive oil (preferably unfiltered)

Choices/Exchanges 1 Starch, 1 Vegetable, 3 Lean Protein, 3 1/2 Fat
Calories 400 | Calories from Fat 230
Total Fat 26g | Saturated Fat 5.5g | Trans Fat 0.0g
Cholesterol 50mg

Sodium 330mg
Potassium 715mg
Total Carbohydrate 22g | Dietary Fiber 6g | Sugars 3g
Protein 22g
Phosphorus 255mg

1. Place the lettuce on a large platter. Add tomatoes and cucumber, and toss to combine.

2. Scatter mozzarella, olives, beans, chicken, and croutons over the top in an attractive pattern.

3. Pour wine vinegar or lemon juice into a small bowl. Add salt and pepper. Slowly pour in the olive oil while whisking vigorously.

4. Once dressing is emulsified, pour it over the salad and serve immediately.

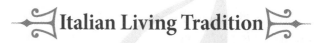

Italian Living Tradition

As if recycling Sunday's leftovers into this delicious salad isn't frugal enough, leftovers of this salad can be added to a soup on Tuesday!

BLOOD ORANGE SALAD
(INSALATA D'ARANCE SANGUOSE)

Serves: 6 | Serving Size: 1/2 cup
Prep Time: 5 minutes | Cooking Time: 0 minutes

Sicily is known for its beautiful, lush orange groves, which produce some of the world's most fragrant oranges. First introduced by the Arabs during their rule of the island, orange trees flourished in the ashes along the base of Mt. Etna. Look for the sweetest oranges possible for this recipe. If you can, use Sicilian blood oranges; their red color imparts festive flair to this sumptuous salad.

4 blood oranges (about 1 pound total),
 peeled and sliced into rounds

2 green onions, finely chopped

Juice of 1 orange

2 tablespoons extra virgin olive oil
 (preferably first cold-pressed and unfiltered)

1/4 teaspoon unrefined sea salt

1/4 teaspoon freshly ground black pepper

Pinch crushed red chile flakes

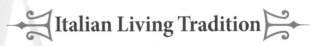

Italian Living Tradition

Because citrus fruits originally grew only in southern Italy, they were expensive and hard to come by in northern regions. Recipes like Duck in Orange Sauce, which were developed by the Florentine courts under the auspices of Caterina de Medici, were extremely lavish for their time. But you will find hints of citrus in holiday and special occasion recipes all over the peninsula.

1. Place orange slices on a large platter and scatter green onions over the top.

2. In a small bowl, whisk orange juice and olive oil together, and season with salt, pepper, and crushed red chile flakes. Drizzle over the salad, and serve immediately.

Choices/Exchanges 1 Fruit, 1 Fat
Calories 80 | Calories from Fat 45
Total Fat 5g | Saturated Fat 0.6g | Trans Fat 0.0g
Cholesterol 0mg
Sodium 100mg

Potassium 175mg
Total Carbohydrate 11g | Dietary Fiber 2g | Sugars 8g
Protein 1g
Phosphorus 15mg

CAULIFLOWER AND HERB SALAD FROM LE MARCHE (INSALATA DI CAVOLFIORE ALLA MARCHIGIANA)

Serves: 4 | Serving Size: 1/2 cup
Prep Time: 10 minutes | Cooking Time: 10 minutes

Located in northeastern Italy, the Le Marche region has a cuisine that is relatively unknown to people who have never travelled there. Le Marche is nestled between lush fields and the Adriatic Sea, and both fresh seafood and first-rate produce combine to form the local culinary landscape of this region. This straightforward recipe dresses up cauliflower with typical Italian finesse.

1 (1 1/4-pound) cauliflower, trimmed into florets

4 oil-packed anchovy fillets, drained, rinsed, and cut into small pieces

1/4 cup black olives, drained, pitted, and chopped

2 tablespoons capers, rinsed and drained

1/4 cup extra virgin olive oil (preferably first cold-pressed and unfiltered)

1/8 teaspoon unrefined sea salt

1/4 teaspoon freshly ground black pepper

1/4 cup finely chopped fresh flat-leaf parsley

2 tablespoons finely chopped fresh mint or basil

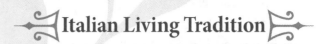

Italian Living Tradition

Prepare a double amount of this cauliflower and save half for the next day. What is left over can be simmered in stock and puréed to make a creamy cauliflower soup.

1. Bring a medium-size saucepan 3/4 full of water to a boil over high heat. Add cauliflower and cook, uncovered, just until fork tender, approximately 5–7 minutes. Drain and transfer cauliflower to a bowl of ice water. When cauliflower is cool to the touch, drain very well.

2. In a large salad bowl, combine anchovy fillets, olives, and capers. Stir in olive oil. Add cauliflower, and stir in salt, pepper, and herbs. Serve at room temperature.

Choices/Exchanges 1 Vegetable, 1 1/2 Fat
Calories 90 | Calories from Fat 60
Total Fat 7g | Saturated Fat 1.0g | Trans Fat 0.0g
Cholesterol 0mg
Sodium 220mg

Potassium 240mg
Total Carbohydrate 4g | Dietary Fiber 2g | Sugars 2g
Protein 2g
Phosphorus 40mg

SEAFOOD SALAD
(INSALATA DI PESCE)

Serves: 8 | Serving Size: Approximately 1 cup
Prep Time: 10 minutes | Cooking Time: 10 minutes

Reserve this recipe for a time when the freshest seafood and produce possible are available to you. The simplicity of the preparation allows the natural flavors of the dish to shine through. This salad embodies the soul of the true Italian kitchen. Feel free to improvise and use your favorite combination of seafood—this recipe is only a guide.

4 vine-ripened tomatoes, chopped

1 carrot, thinly sliced

1/4 teaspoon unrefined sea salt

1/8 teaspoon freshly ground black pepper

Juice and zest from 1 large lemon, divided

1 pound dry scallops

3/4 pound shrimp, peeled and deveined

1 pound boneless, skinless snapper, mahi mahi, orange roughy, or monkfish, cut into 1-inch pieces

1 pound baby squid tubes, cleaned and sliced into small rings

1/2 cup extra virgin olive oil

1/2 cup finely chopped fresh flat-leaf parsley

Choices/Exchanges 2 Vegetable, 5 Lean Protein, 2 Fat
Calories 360 | Calories from Fat 180
Total Fat 20g | Saturated Fat 4.2g | Trans Fat 0.0g
Cholesterol 240mg
Sodium 410mg

Potassium 855mg
Total Carbohydrate 9g | Dietary Fiber 2g | Sugars 3g
Protein 36g
Phosphorus 545mg

1. Place the tomatoes, carrot, salt, pepper, and lemon zest in a large bowl, and mix well.

2. Bring a medium-size pot 3/4 full of water to boil over high heat.

3. Lower the heat to medium and add the scallops. Cook, uncovered, until scallops are opaque, approximately 1 minute. Remove scallops with a slotted spoon to a dish lined with paper towels. Add the shrimp and fish and cook until opaque, 1–2 minutes. Transfer to another dish lined with paper towels. Add the squid and cook for approximately 40 seconds, until rings begin to slightly tighten up. Remove with a slotted spoon into a colander. Immediately transfer squid to a bowl of very cold water to stop the cooking.

4. In a small bowl, make the dressing by whisking the olive oil and the lemon juice together until emulsified.

5. Add the seafood to a salad bowl and stir to combine. Drizzle with dressing and stir. Sprinkle with parsley, and serve immediately.

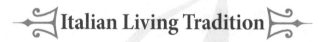

Italian Living Tradition

Squid is very high in copper, a trace mineral that helps the body with nutrient absorption. A great source of complete protein, squid is good for burning fat and building muscle. Squid is also high in vitamin B2 (among other vitamins), which can be an effective pain reliever for migraine symptoms.

MARINATED EGGPLANT SALAD
(MELANZANE IN INSALATA ALLA CALABRESE)

Serves: 8 | Serving Size: 1/2 cup
Prep Time: 10 minutes | Cooking Time: 10 minutes

When making this recipe, many people boil the eggplants as you would potatoes. In Calabria, heating an oven is frowned upon in warm weather, which is when eggplant is in season; however, I prefer the taste of roasted eggplant over boiled. This salad can be eaten immediately, or it can sit at room temperature for up to 1 hour. If you like to prepare food in advance, keep in mind that this recipe tastes even better next day.

3 small (5- or 6-inch-long) eggplants
2 medium tomatoes, chopped
1/4 cup finely chopped fresh flat-leaf parsley
2 tablespoons finely chopped oregano
1 clove garlic, minced
1/4 cup extra virgin olive oil
   (preferably first cold-pressed)
2 tablespoons red wine vinegar
1/8 teaspoon kosher salt
1/4 teaspoon freshly ground black pepper
1 head romaine lettuce, washed, trimmed, and chopped into bite-size pieces

⫷ Italian Living Tradition ⫸

Eggplant fits well into a diabetes-friendly diet. It is low in carbohydrate and full of calcium, phosphorous, potassium, and thiamine, so it can become a healthful staple for people with diabetes to rely upon. Southern Italian cuisine is full of delicious eggplant recipes that were developed to take advantage of large bumper crops.

1. Preheat broiler to high.

2. Prick eggplants all over with a fork. Place eggplants on a baking sheet and broil for 5–10 minutes, or until soft. Cool eggplants until cool enough to handle.

3. Meanwhile, combine tomatoes, parsley, oregano, garlic, olive oil, vinegar, salt, and pepper in a salad bowl.

4. Peel eggplants, cut off tops, and chop into bite-size pieces. Add eggplant to salad bowl with the dressing. Mix well to coat, cover, and refrigerate overnight, if desired.

5. To serve, place romaine lettuce on the bottom of a serving platter (or on individual plates). Spoon eggplant mixture on top of the lettuce.

Choices/Exchanges 2 1/2 Vegetable, 1 1/2 Fat
Calories 130 | Calories from Fat 60
Total Fat 7g | Saturated Fat 1.0g | Trans Fat 0.0g
Cholesterol 0mg
Sodium 65mg

Potassium 695mg
Total Carbohydrate 15g | Dietary Fiber 9g | Sugars 6g
Protein 3g
Phosphorus 80mg

CHICKPEA SALAD
(INSALATA DI CECI)

Serves: 4 | Serving Size: 1/2 cup
Prep Time: 5 minutes | Cooking Time: 0 minutes

Salads don't always contain lettuce. One of my favorite "salad" experiences in Italy is sampling from antipasto bars in trattorias. Instead of offering individual ingredients for people to construct their own salad, antipasto bars offer various dressed salads, such as this one, carrot salads, roasted vegetable salads, and pasta salads.

2 cups cooked dried chickpeas
   or canned reduced-sodium chickpeas

1/4 cup finely chopped fresh flat-leaf parsley

1 carrot, trimmed and grated

2 teaspoons extra virgin olive oil

Juice of 1 lemon

1/8 teaspoon kosher salt

1/4 teaspoon freshly ground black pepper

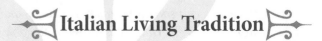
Italian Living Tradition

To make a meal out of this salad, add leftover shredded turkey or chicken, arugula, and croutons (see Homemade Croutons recipe on page 292), or toss it with quinoa, rice, barley, or pasta along with Tomatoes with Balsamic Vinegar (page 190).

1. Combine chickpeas, parsley, and carrot in a medium bowl.

2. In a small bowl, whisk together olive oil and lemon juice until emulsified. Stir in salt and pepper.

3. Add dressing to vegetables, toss, and serve at room temperature.

Choices/Exchanges 1 1/2 Starch, 1 Lean Protein, 1/2 Fat
Calories 170 | Calories from Fat 35
Total Fat 4g | Saturated Fat 0.5g | Trans Fat 0.0g
Cholesterol 0mg

Sodium 220mg
Potassium 335mg
Total Carbohydrate 26g | Dietary Fiber 7g | Sugars 5g
Protein 8g
Phosphorus 145mg

TUSCAN FARRO SALAD
(INSALATA DI FARRO ALLA TOSCANA)

Serves: 6 | Serving Size: 3/4 cup
Prep Time: 20 minutes (plus farro-soaking time) | Cooking Time: 45 minutes

Farro, which is becoming more and more popular by the minute, is an ancient grain similar to spelt. Full of protein and vitamins, it's a nutritious whole grain that will add fiber to your diet. It is believed that farro was cultivated in 7000 BCE near the Tuscan town of Lucca. Farro can be served in many ways—with chicken or shrimp as a main course, with milk and fruit as a breakfast cereal, or in pastries for special occasions. You can buy presoaked farro that cooks in only 18 minutes and does not need to be soaked overnight, or you can soak it yourself. I usually soak more farro than I need and store the excess in the refrigerator for a week. That way, if I want to cook with it, I don't have to wait until the following day.

Basil Pesto

1/4 cup extra virgin olive oil (preferably first cold-pressed and unfiltered)
1 1/2 cups fresh basil leaves
1 clove garlic
1/8 cup pine nuts
1/8 cup grated parmigiano-reggiano cheese
1/8 cup pecorino Romano cheese

Salad

1 1/4 cups farro, soaked 6–8 hours
1/2 pound green beans
1 small red onion, thinly sliced
1/4 cup Basil Pesto (prepared in step 1)
1 cup cherry tomatoes
2 tablespoons extra virgin olive oil
1/2 teaspoon unrefined sea salt
2 tablespoons pine nuts, toasted

Choices/Exchanges 1 1/2 Starch, 1 Vegetable, 3 Fat
Calories 280 | Calories from Fat 140
Total Fat 16g | Saturated Fat 2.3g | Trans Fat 0.0g
Cholesterol 0mg
Sodium 210mg

Potassium 340mg
Total Carbohydrate 31g | Dietary Fiber 6g | Sugars 4g
Protein 8g
Phosphorus 220mg

1. Add all pesto ingredients except cheeses into a food processor and pulse until thoroughly combined. You may use less oil if you would like a thicker consistency. (If you do not have a food processor, a pestle can be used to grind the ingredients together.) Add the cheeses and stir. Measure out 1/4 cup pesto for the salad and set aside. Save any remaining pesto for another recipe.

2. Drain and rinse the soaked farro, and place in a medium saucepan with 2 1/2 cups water. Place saucepan over medium-high heat, cover, and bring to a boil. Reduce the heat to low and simmer for 45 minutes, or until the farro is tender but chewy and the water is absorbed.

3. While the farro is cooking, bring 2 inches water to a boil in a large saucepan fitted with a steamer basket. Add the green beans, cover, and steam until just tender, 2 minutes. Set green beans aside until cool.

4. Transfer the cooked farro and green beans to a large bowl. Add 1/4 cup pesto and all the remaining ingredients, and toss well to coat. Serve warm, at room temperature, or chilled.

Italian Living Tradition

"Farrotto" is a type of dish that involves preparing farro in the same manner that you would prepare risotto—instead of using rice, you substitute farro. Try using farro in your favorite risotto recipe!

BREAD
(PANE)

212   Tyrolean Rye Bread with Fennel and Cumin/*Ur-Paarl della Val Venosta*

214   No-Knead Italian "Baguettes"/*Filoni (senza impanare)*

216   Homemade Bread with Mother Yeast from Molise/*Pane spiga*

218   Whole-Wheat Rolls/*Panini di San Giovanni*

220   Whole-Wheat Country Loaves/*Pane casareccio integrale*

222   Whole-Wheat Cracker Rings with Black Pepper and Fennel Seeds/
      Taralli integrali con pepe e finocchio

"E' meglio pane e cepolla 'a casa toja ca galline e fassano 'n casa d'autre."

"It's better to have bread and onions in your own home than hens and pheasants in the home of another."

—Italian proverb

One of my greatest hopes for this book is that it changes the way non-Italians think about "Italian" bread. There isn't just one kind of bread in Italy—there are thousands. Like all other authentic traditional foods in the country, each town, region, and province claims its own types of bread. Some of Italy's historic bread recipes are so interwoven with the culture at large that they are considered part of the nation's intangible cultural heritage and are protected by organizations such as Slow Food.

The bread traditions in each Italian region do a fantastic job of representing the various cultural influences that exist in particular areas. Take the Tyrolean Rye Bread with Fennel and Cumin recipe (page 212), for example; this recipe reveals northern Italy's Austrian influence, and it is very different from the stereotypical "Italian bread." This rye bread is so special that it is now protected by Slow Food, an international movement that strives to preserve traditional and regional cuisines and local food cultures. Whole-Wheat Cracker Rings with Black Pepper and Fennel Seeds (page 222), on the other hand, strongly embody the more Mediterranean-inspired traditions of the south.

In order to understand Italian bread, one must know a little bit about the way it has been artisanally prepared for millennia. In the Italian language, there are two words for bakeries. The first is *panifici*, which refers to bread bakeries that make the traditional breads of the area along with festival and holiday fruit-and-nut–studded breads, crack-ers, savory pies, crunchy bread sticks, and simple biscotti recipes. Some members of my family in Crotone, Italy, run a *panificio*.

Whenever the term *artigiano* (meaning "crafts-man") accompanies the word *bakery* in Italian, it means that the establishment has met specific, government-mandated criteria for using particular ingredients, preparation methods, and techniques that are in accordance with Italian culinary standards. In short, if you buy bread baked in one of these bakeries, you are getting the real thing. Unfortunately, the newer generation of Italians is not as enthusiastic about getting up in the middle of the night to follow in the baking footsteps of their forefathers.

Italians eat more bread per capita than any other nation in Europe. It is an integral part of Italian culture. However, if artisanal bakeries continue to fall out of fashion, the appeal and healthfulness of traditional Italian cuisine will suffer. Luckily, Italians from north to south celebrate *sagre* (see Side Dishes/*Contorni,* page 157), or food festivals, for bread just as they do for produce. These festivals are a great way to highlight the specialties of the various regions and prevent traditional recipes from becoming extinct.

One of the practices that distinguishes artisan bread from other breads is the use of "natural fermentation of yeast." Instead of beginning with chemical yeast, artisan bread bakers and pizza makers in Italy use (sometimes centuries-old) yeast starters made from grapes, figs, dates, or other fruits that were left to ferment naturally. Some of the most important bakers in Italy are actually chemists who have perfected the ancient yeast-fermenting technique into an art form. Nothing compares to the flavor, aroma, and texture of bread prepared with natural yeast.

When you break open a loaf of bread made the traditional way, it does not have a strong "yeasty" odor. It usually has a dense, tender crumb and a crunchy exterior. Although they contain only a few ingredients, artisan breads seem like a meal in themselves; they are so satisfying, comforting, and filling. Try the Homemade Bread with Mother Yeast from Molise recipe (page 216) if you would like to give a natural starter a shot in your own kitchen. It's easier than you may think—and you'll be delighted with the results. If you don't like to knead, the No-Knead Italian "Baguettes" (page 214) will be a welcome addition to your repertoire.

When deciding which bread to serve with a meal, there are two factors to consider. First, consider how "heavy" the meal is and how much carbohydrate it already contains, and then take into account the region from which your first and/or second courses come. If you are making a meal that contains both a filling pasta dish and second course, you may want to forgo bread. In this sense, Italian cultural sensibilities fit well with a diabetes-friendly lifestyle. If, on the other hand, you are serving a soup and salad, or a second course and salad, then healthy, homemade bread would help to complete the meal. Considering the region that your recipe comes from is also important. It is not advisable to serve Tyrolean Rye Bread with Fennel and Cumin (a northern recipe) with a tomato-based first course and seafood second course from the south. It would, however, taste great with a hearty, legume-based *minestra* or a roasted dish.

TYROLEAN RYE BREAD WITH FENNEL AND CUMIN (*UR-PAARL DELLA VAL VENOSTA*)

Makes: 8 (8-inch) loaves | Serves: 24 | Serving Size: 1/3 loaf
Prep Time: 5 minutes (plus 3 1/2 hours rising time) | Cooking Time: 25–40 minutes

The full German name of this bread is Ur-Paarl nach Klosterart, *which means "the original double rye bread in the manner of the convent." It is the oldest variety of Vinschger Paarl bread, which is common in northeastern Italy—where strong German and Austrian influences prevail. This bread is so special that the Slow Food Movement in Italy is preserving the recipe as part of the region's culinary heritage. Luckily, this recipe is easily adaptable to modern kitchens, and it's a unique addition to anyone's repertoire.*

Sourdough Starter

2 cups rye flour

3/4 cup lukewarm water

1 teaspoon active dry yeast

Dough

2 cups rye flour

3 cups wheat flour or gluten-free flour, plus extra for work surface

4 teaspoons active dry yeast, dissolved in 3 cups lukewarm water

1 teaspoon unrefined sea salt

2 tablespoons fennel seeds

1 tablespoon cumin seeds

Choices/Exchanges 1 1/2 Starch
Calories 110 | Calories from Fat 10
Total Fat 1g | Saturated Fat 0.0g | Trans Fat 0.0g
Cholesterol 0mg
Sodium 100mg

Potassium 140mg
Total Carbohydrate 24g | Dietary Fiber 4g | Sugars 0g
Protein 4g
Phosphorus 100mg

1. Combine all the starter ingredients in a small bowl. Stir slowly for 5 minutes, and then use your knuckles to knead the mixture for 5 minutes. Cover with a clean kitchen towel and allow to rest for 2 hours.

2. After 2 hours have elapsed, mix the starter with the remaining bread ingredients to form a smooth dough. Turn out onto a lightly floured work surface and knead for 10–15 minutes. Place in bowl, cover with a clean kitchen towel, and allow to rise for 1 hour.

3. On a lightly floured work surface, punch down the dough and divide into 8 equally sized balls.

4. Line 2 baking sheets with parchment paper. Place 4 balls on each sheet. Press the center of the balls down to form flattened disks with 2 disks side by side, touching, so that they will puff up and stay connected while baking. This will give them their signature double shape.

5. Cover with a clean kitchen towel and allow to rise for another 30 minutes.

6. Preheat oven to 400°F.

7. Bake for 25–40 minutes, or until bread is lightly golden on top and sounds hollow when tapped on the bottom.

❖ Italian Living Tradition ❖

This bread is now baked daily in bakeries of the Alpine region, but it was once baked only two to three times a year in wood-burning ovens by farmers. Before industrialization in the 1950s, many local farmers grew rye, which flourished in the dry climate. Nowadays, the Slow Food Movement has begun initiatives to reintroduce the heritage varieties of the grain, and about a dozen farmers have begun planting rye again on their farms.

NO-KNEAD ITALIAN "BAGUETTES" (FILONI [SENZA IMPANARE])

Makes: 1 long baguette | Serves: 14 | Serving Size: 1 (3/4-inch) slice
Prep Time: 15 minutes (plus 2 hours rising time) | Cooking Time: 30 minutes

Kneading bread is one of the activities that provides a great deal of pleasure in my life. I realize, however, that not everyone feels this way. If you've never made bread before, you'll be astounded by how easy it is to prepare this delicious loaf, which has a crunchy crust and tender interior. Filoni is the Italian word for "baguettes," and they are the type of bread that we often refer to as "Italian" in the U.S. These baguettes can be made in advance, wrapped in plastic, and frozen until needed.

1 tablespoon active dry yeast

1 1/2 cups warm water (110–115°F), divided

1 tablespoon sugar

4 cups all-purpose flour OR 2 cups corn flour and 2 cups gluten-free flour, divided

1 teaspoon unrefined sea salt

2 tablespoons olive oil, divided

1/2 ounce cornmeal

Choices/Exchanges 2 Starch
Calories 160 | Calories from Fat 20
Total Fat 2g | Saturated Fat 0.5g | Trans Fat 0.0g
Cholesterol 0mg
Sodium 170mg

Potassium 50mg
Total Carbohydrate 30g | Dietary Fiber 1g | Sugars 1g
Protein 4g
Phosphorus 45mg

1. In the bowl of a mixer (or a large mixing bowl), mix yeast into 1/2 cup warm water. Mix well until combined. Let the mixture sit in the bowl for 4–5 minutes, until yeast is dissolved.

2. Add sugar, 2 cups flour (or the gluten-free flour), and remaining 1 cup water to the bowl; mix with mixer (or with wooden spoon) until smooth. The dough will resemble a batter. Let stand for 10 minutes or so, until mixture rises and bubbles a little in the bowl.

3. Add in salt, 1 tablespoon oil, and 1/2 cup flour (or corn flour); mix. Continue adding flour or corn flour, 1/2 cup at a time, and mixing it in until it is all added. Mix until the dough forms a ball. Dump the ball of dough on the countertop, and gather it into a ball.

4. Grease another mixing bowl with the remaining 1 tablespoon olive oil. Place the dough into the bowl and turn to coat. Cover with a kitchen towel and place in an oven set to the proof setting (about 100°F), or cover with additional towels and set in a warm place. Allow dough to rise until it doubles in size, about 1 hour.

5. Turn risen dough onto a floured surface, and roll and pull until you've shaped a 16-inch-long loaf. (You can also make two 8-inch loaves.) Place the loaf on a greased baking sheet sprinkled with the cornmeal.

6. Cover the loaf with a clean kitchen towel and let rise until it doubles in size, about 45 minutes.

7. Make 6–8 diagonal slashes in the top of the loaf using a very sharp knife. Bake at 400°F for 25–30 minutes, or until nicely browned. Cool on wire rack.

Italian Living Tradition

Each Italian region has dozens of types of artisanal breads that are sold in *panifici*—or bread bakeries. Good-quality bread is highly appreciated in Italy, and many people still prefer to buy their bread from an artisan bakery that has been making bread with the same high-quality ingredients for centuries, rather than buying something at a supermarket. *Panifici* can be found in almost every shopping center in urban and residential areas in Italy.

HOMEMADE BREAD
WITH MOTHER YEAST FROM MOLISE
(PANE SPIGA)

Makes: 1 large (14–16-inch) loaf | Serves: 18 | Serving Size: 1 (3/4-inch) slice
Prep Time: 15 minutes (plus 4 days rest for starter yeast and dough rising time) | Cooking Time: 40 minutes

The region of Molise is known for its wonderful variety of high-quality grains. This recipe makes flattened bread that was traditionally prepared in a communal oven. The bread takes its Italian name from the v-shaped slits that are traditionally made down the sides of the bread before baking. These slits cause the bread to resemble wheat sheaves, which are called "ears" (spiga) in Italian.

Keep in mind that in order to create a mother yeast from scratch, you will need to begin making this bread 4 days in advance. I suggest starting on a Wednesday so you can enjoy the bread on Sunday. Making the yeast couldn't be easier, but it needs time to rest and "refresh," as we say in the baking world. The result is a highly perfumed bread with a crisp crust and a tender, hole-studded crumb that is so complex it barely needs an accompaniment.

Mother Yeast

1 1/4 cups 00 flour (such as Antimo Caputo brand)
    or all-purpose flour, divided

2 tablespoons plain, organic yogurt

1 tablespoon honey

1/4 cup lukewarm water (or as much as necessary
    to create a unified yet soft, batter-like dough)

Bread

4 cups bread flour,
    plus extra for work surface and dusting

1/2–1 cup tepid water

1 tablespoon extra virgin olive oil

1 teaspoon unrefined sea salt

1. Begin making the mother yeast by combining 3/4 cup 00 flour, yogurt, honey, and water in a medium bowl. Mix well to combine. The goal is to achieve a batter-like dough. (If your batter is too thick, add more water, 1 tablespoon at a time, mixing after each addition, until it looks like a light cookie dough.) Cover the bowl with plastic wrap and then seal with aluminum foil. Allow the mixture to sit at room temperature for 48 hours. During that time, it will begin to ferment, and you will notice bubbles at the top.

Choices/Exchanges 2 Starch
Calories 160 | Calories from Fat 10
Total Fat 1g | Saturated Fat 0.0g | Trans Fat 0.0g
Cholesterol 0mg
Sodium 110mg

Potassium 45mg
Total Carbohydrate 30g | Dietary Fiber 1g | Sugars 1g
Protein 5g
Phosphorus 40mg

2. Once the 48 hours have passed, add an additional 1/2 cup 00 flour and 2 tablespoons water. This is called "refreshing" the dough. Mix well to combine. Cover with plastic wrap and aluminum foil, and allow to rest for another 48 hours.

3. When the mother yeast is ready, combine it with the 4 cups bread flour, 1/2 cup water, olive oil, and salt. Mix well to combine. Add more water, 1 tablespoon a time, if needed, in order to make a moist dough. (The amount of water required will depend on the moisture level in your kitchen.) Once the dough forms a ball, you can stop adding water.

4. Sprinkle a clean work surface with 1–2 tablespoons bread flour. Turn the dough out onto the work surface and knead vigorously for 10 minutes, or until dough is smooth and elastic. If dough seems too heavy and is difficult to work, add more water, 1 tablespoon at a time, kneading after each addition, until it is easier to work.

5. Once the dough is smooth, supple, and almost shiny in appearance, stop kneading. Sprinkle another tablespoon flour on the work surface and place the dough on top. Sprinkle the top with 1/2 teaspoon flour, and place a clean kitchen towel over the top. Cover with 2 additional clean kitchen towels and allow to rise overnight, or for a minimum of 6 hours. The dough should be almost doubled in size.

6. Punch the dough down and shape it into an oblong baguette, approximately 14–16 inches long. Cover with a clean kitchen towel and allow to rest for 1 more hour.

7. Line a baking sheet with parchment paper. Heat oven to 425°F. Working from the center of the loaf to the edges, and making sure not to cut through the bottom of the bread, make 4 equally spaced slash marks down the length of the loaf. Make 4 additional slash marks on the other side—this will give the bread its characteristic "ear-like" design while it bakes.

8. Place the bread in the oven and immediately reduce the temperature to 375°F. Bake until golden, about 30–40 minutes. When the bread is finished baking, it should sound hollow when tapped on the bottom.

Italian Living Tradition

In Molise, this bread was traditionally stuffed—it was believed to be the perfect "little bag," or *m'bostarella* as it is called in dialect, for students to make school sandwiches out of.

This bread was traditionally made with a mix of bread flours, water, salt, mother yeast, and sometimes even potato starch. Nowadays many people have begun substituting commercial brewers' yeast for mother yeast, but the old-fashioned preparation is so easy that I have decided to include it here. Making this bread is a fun project to do with children; they will enjoy watching the yeast form and the bread come together with just a few simple ingredients.

WHOLE-WHEAT ROLLS
(PANINI DI SAN GIOVANNI)

Makes: 16 bun-size rolls | Serves: 16 | Serving Size: 1 roll
Prep Time: 15 minutes (plus 2 hours rising time) | Cooking Time: 25 minutes

Many regional Italian bread recipes have been around since antiquity. The more interesting ones may have originally been used as offerings to the gods. With the advent of Christianity, they were prepared for saints' days. This is St. Jonathan's—or San Giovanni's—bread. It is made with a mixture of grains known as crusca *(see Italian Living Tradition).*

1/2 cup mixed rye flour and spelt or oat flour

2 1/2 cups whole-wheat flour or additional rye flour

2 cups unbleached, all-purpose flour or corn flour, plus extra for work surface

1 1/4 cups lukewarm water (more if needed)

2 1/4 teaspoons active dry yeast

1 teaspoon unrefined sea salt

1 teaspoon extra virgin olive oil

Choices/Exchanges 2 Starch
Calories 140 | Calories from Fat 10
Total Fat 1g | Saturated Fat 0.0g | Trans Fat 0.0g
Cholesterol 0mg
Sodium 120mg

Potassium 110mg
Total Carbohydrate 28g | Dietary Fiber 3g | Sugars 0g
Protein 5g
Phosphorus 90mg

1. Mix and combine all flours, water, yeast, and salt in a large bowl. If necessary, add another 1/2 cup water, or enough to make a smooth dough that is not too hard to work.

2. Turn out onto a lightly floured work surface and knead for 10 minutes, until smooth and elastic. (Note that it is always better to work with a dough that seems slightly moist. If you resist the urge to add too much flour, the bread will have a lighter crumb.)

3. Place dough in a large bowl coated with the olive oil. Turn dough to coat. Cover and allow dough to rise for 1 hour.

4. Line a baking sheet with parchment paper and a dusting of flour. Dust a work surface with flour and place the dough on it. Shape the dough into 8 equal-size pieces and roll into smooth balls. Place balls on the baking sheet, cover with a clean kitchen towel, and allow to rise until doubled in size, at least 1 more hour.

5. Preheat oven to 350°F. Bake rolls until golden and cooked through, approximately 20–25 minutes.

❧ Italian Living Tradition ☙

Prior to the Industrial Revolution, the milling of wheat, and wheat itself, was often heavily taxed in Italy. Peasants could not afford finely milled grains, or to be choosy about which grains they ate. Instead, they made the best recipes they could out of the grains that were left over from milling. Barley, rye, oats, and other grains that were originally used to feed livestock would be combined and used in bread and pasta recipes; this mixture of grains was called *crusca*. Realizing that this practice made it easier for people to avoid taxes, medieval rulers often banned the milling of *crusca*.

WHOLE-WHEAT COUNTRY LOAVES
(PANE CASARECCIO INTEGRALE)

Makes: 2 (4 ×12-inch) loaves | Serves: 12 | Serving Size: 2 (1-inch) pieces
Prep Time: 15 minutes (plus 2 1/2 hours rising time) | Cooking Time: Approximately 40 minutes

This is simple, crusty bread from Calabria. It is perfect for soaking up the sauce from hearty, tomato-based stews, and it is best eaten on the day it is baked. Leftover, day-old pieces can be used for bruschetta, bread crumbs, or croutons. It can also be frozen, defrosted, and reheated in a 400°F oven for approximately 5 minutes, or until warm. To slice it, use a long, serrated knife, and cut 1-inch slices on the diagonal. For extra-crusty bread, place a baking pan with a shallow layer of boiling water on the bottom shelf in the oven while the bread is baking, or spray the walls of the oven with water after it is preheated.

1 package active dry yeast

1 1/4 cups warm water, divided

3 cups unbleached, all-purpose flour
   OR 1 1/2 cups rye flour and 1 1/2 cups corn flour, plus extra for work surface

1 teaspoon sugar

1 teaspoon unrefined sea salt or kosher salt

3 tablespoons extra virgin olive oil, divided

2 tablespoons semolina or rye flour

Choices/Exchanges 1 1/2 Starch, 1/2 Fat
Calories 150 | Calories from Fat 35
Total Fat 4g | Saturated Fat 0.5g | Trans Fat 0.0g
Cholesterol 0mg
Sodium 160mg

Potassium 40mg
Total Carbohydrate 25g | Dietary Fiber 1g | Sugars 0g
Protein 4g
Phosphorus 40mg

1. Dissolve yeast in 1/4 cup warm water in a small bowl. Let stand for 5 minutes until it bubbles.

2. Put flour, sugar, and salt into a large mixing bowl. Make a well in the center of the dry ingredients; add the dissolved yeast and another cup warm water. Mix well to form a dough. If the dough seems sticky, add more flour, 1 tablespoon at a time. (But be aware that adding too much flour will make the bread tough.) If the dough seems too dry and will not form a ball, add more water, 1 tablespoon at a time. Place the dough ball on a lightly floured work surface. Knead the dough by punching it down and pushing it, with both hands, away from you, then pulling it back towards you. Continue kneading the dough, using the back-and-forth motion, for approximately 5 minutes, or until you have a smooth, soft, and elastic dough.

3. Line a large bowl with 1 tablespoon olive oil. Place the dough into the bowl, and turn to coat with olive oil. Cover the bowl with plastic wrap and then clean kitchen towels. Place it in a draft-free area and allow it to rise until doubled in size. This will take 1–1 1/2 hours.

4. When dough has risen, preheat the oven to 425°F.

5. Punch down the dough. Dust a baking stone or baking sheet with the semolina or rye flour. Divide the dough into 2 equal-size pieces. Place the dough pieces on the baking stone or sheet and form them in to 2 (4 ×12-inch) loaves.

Make sure there is at least 4–5 inches between loaves so that when they rise, they will not stick together—or use separate baking sheets. Loosely cover with a clean kitchen towel and allow to rise for 1 more hour.

6. Uncover the bread; make 4 (1/8-inch) slits on the diagonal across each loaf. Brush each loaf with 1 tablespoon olive oil. Bake for 15 minutes.

7. Lower the temperature of the oven to 400°F and bake for 25 minutes, or until bread is golden brown. Allow to cool slightly. Serve warm.

Italian Living Tradition

Bread is taken very seriously in Italy. More than a mere culinary staple, bread is the cornerstone of the Italian culture, which takes deep pride in simply transforming the gifts of nature. Bread in Italy is even used metaphorically to express the pleasant mannerisms of people. Someone with a good character, for example, would be called "good...like bread." A big-hearted person would be "warm...like bread." If someone were flexible and easy to work with, they would be "soft...like bread." The list of Italian bread metaphors is endless.

WHOLE-WHEAT CRACKER RINGS WITH BLACK PEPPER AND FENNEL SEEDS (*TARALLI INTEGRALI CON PEPE E FINOCCHIO*)

Makes: 18–24 bread rings | Serves: 6–8 | Serving Size: 3 bread rings
Prep Time: 15 minutes (plus 2 1/2 hours rising time) | Cooking Time: 15–20 minutes

The southern Italian provinces of Lazio, Molise, Puglia, Basilicata, Campania, Abruzzo, and Calabria all share the tradition of serving taralli—*crunchy, cracker-like breads—with appetizers. In the old days, drying out these crackers was a way of preserving them. Today, they are a matter of taste and tradition. In Calabria, these crackers are prepared for the feast of St. Anthony. Traditional shapes for these crackers include rings, ropes, braids, sticks, and horseshoes. Wrapped in clear cellophane bags with a pretty tie,* taralli *make elegant gifts. I like to serve them with Sicilian Sweet-and-Sour Vegetable Medley (page 6), Southern Italian Fava Bean Purée (page 16), and almost any soup, along with olives and cheese.*

2 1/2 teaspoons active dry yeast

3/4 cup lukewarm water, divided

2 cups whole-wheat flour or gluten-free baking mix, plus extra for work surface

1 tablespoon freshly ground black pepper

2 teaspoons fennel seeds

1/4 teaspoon crushed red chile flakes

1/2 teaspoon unrefined sea salt

3 tablespoons plus 1/2 teaspoon extra virgin olive oil, divided

1 egg white, lightly beaten

Choices/Exchanges 1 1/2 Starch, 1 Fat
Calories 160 | Calories from Fat 50
Total Fat 6g | Saturated Fat 0.8g | Trans Fat 0.0g
Cholesterol 0mg
Sodium 160mg

Potassium 160mg
Total Carbohydrate 23g | Dietary Fiber 4g | Sugars 0g
Protein 5g
Phosphorus 115mg

1. In a small bowl, dissolve yeast with 1/4 cup lukewarm water.

2. Place the flour, pepper, fennel seeds, chile flakes, and salt in a large bowl. Add the yeast mixture, an additional 1/2 cup lukewarm water, and 3 tablespoons olive oil. Mix well to combine and form a dough.

3. Turn dough out onto a lightly floured surface. Knead energetically, adding a little more flour if needed, for about 8–10 minutes, until the dough is smooth and elastic.

4. Oil a large bowl with remaining 1/2 teaspoon olive oil and place the dough inside. Turn dough to coat with oil, and cover with plastic wrap and clean kitchen towels. Allow to rise until doubled in size, approximately 1 1/2 hours.

5. Preheat oven to 375°F.

6. Remove dough from bowl and break off a small chunk. Roll into a 6-inch rope that is approximately the width of a pencil, and form into a circle. Pinch the ends together tightly, and place ring on an ungreased baking sheet. Repeat with the rest of the dough. Cover rings with a clean kitchen towel and allow to rise until doubled in size, approximately 1 hour.

7. Brush tops of the rings with the egg white and bake until light golden, 15–20 minutes. Remove, cool on a rack, and store in a tightly covered container for up to a month.

Italian Living Tradition

Making bread dough from scratch can be labor-intensive, but it is worth the effort! In order to make this recipe more user-friendly, there are a few shortcuts you can take. First of all, the dough can be "kneaded" with a dough hook in a standing mixer. And instead of waiting for the dough to rise for 1 1/2 hours at room temperature, it can be covered well and left in the refrigerator for 12 hours or overnight. Then it can be rolled out and shaped into rings the following day. These crackers stay fresh for a month at room temperature, or they can be frozen for up to 6 months.

SAUCES AND CONDIMENTS
(SALSE E CONDIMENTI)

228   Fresh Tomato Sauce/*Salsa fresca di pomodoro*

230   Bread Crumbs and Hot Chile Peppers/*Mollica di pane e peperoncini*

231   Garlic and Oil/*Aglio e olio*

232   Emilia-Romagna–Style Green Herb Sauce/*Salsa verde all'Emiliana*

"Troppe salse vivande false."
"Too much sauce ruins the dish."
—Italian proverb

This chapter contains simple, straightforward sauces that are used to dress everything from grilled and sautéed vegetables to piping-hot pasta and gnocchi. Some of them, like the Emilia-Romagna–Style Green Herb Sauce (page 232), add an elegant, Italian touch to pan-fried chicken, veal, or fish fillets.

Historically, sauces have been used in Italy since before the Romans. The *garum* (fish sauce) that the Romans ate, however, had more in common with Asian fish sauces than with the ubiquitous tomato sauce that most people associate with Italy. It may be hard to believe, but prior to the 18th century, tomato sauce was not served in Italy; the tomato was native to the Americas and was not introduced to Italy until the 16th century. In the days before tomato sauce, pasta was dressed with sauces like Bread Crumbs and Hot Chile Peppers (page 230) and Garlic and Oil (page 231) in the south, and basil pesto and béchamel sauce in northern regions.

Spaghetti with tomato sauce is probably the most recognizable "Italian" food on the planet. But this relatively "new" invention didn't make it to northern Italy until after 1860, when Italy became uni-fied. It is said that when Italian general Giuseppe Garibaldi first ate this sauce at Melito di Porto Salvo in Calabria, he made his soldiers bring the recipe north. Since then, the classic recipe has held a special place in the culinary bloodline of all Italians, regardless of their provincial origins.

The quantity of sauce that you use is just as important as the type of sauce in the Italian kitchen. No one wants pasta that's drowning in a sauce. Sauces should be used to coat pasta and other ingredients. Their main function is to bind ingredients together and heighten flavor while introducing another texture to the dish and highlighting seasonal produce. The pairing of sauces with the correct pasta shapes and then pairing those pasta dishes with appropriate second courses is also important. Sauces such as Bread Crumbs and Hot Chile Peppers (page 230), Garlic and Oil (page 231), and pesto and béchamel sauces pair best with first courses when the second course will contain a tomato-based sauce. On the other hand, if you are serving Fresh Tomato Sauce (page 228) on pasta for a first course, the second course should not contain a tomato-based sauce. Roasted or grilled poultry, meat, or seafood would be a better match.

FRESH TOMATO SAUCE
(SALSA FRESCA DI POMODORO)

Serves: 4 | Serving Size: 1/2 cup
Prep Time: 10 minutes | Cooking Time: Approximately 25 minutes

The first recorded evidence of tomatoes in Italy dates back to 1548—they're definitely not one of the oldest traditional ingredients! Despite the fact that it is a relatively "new" addition to the Italian diet, the pomodoro (tomato) now holds one of the most prestigious places on the Italian table. Fresh tomato sauce is one of the pillars of the Italian kitchen. From this sauce, more elaborate sauces, soups, stews, pizzas, parmigianas, and more can be made.

Making a fresh tomato sauce is the best way to take advantage of the summer tomato harvest—and it's a healthier alternative to using store-bought sauces. Prepared tomato sauces are usually full of preservatives, sugar, and sodium. Try making large batches of this sauce and freezing or canning the excess so that you'll have fresh, homemade sauce on hand all year long. If good-quality fresh tomatoes are not available, substitute approximately 24 ounces of good-quality jarred or boxed strained Italian tomatoes.

10–12 fresh plum tomatoes (approximately 2–2 1/2 pounds)
2 tablespoons extra virgin olive oil
3 cloves garlic, finely chopped
Pinch crushed red chile flakes
1/8 teaspoon unrefined sea salt
1/4 teaspoon freshly ground black pepper
2 tablespoons finely chopped fresh basil or parsley, or a combination

Choices/Exchanges 2 Vegetable, 1 Fat
Calories 90 | Calories from Fat 45
Total Fat 5g | Saturated Fat 0.7g | Trans Fat 0.0g
Cholesterol 0mg
Sodium 60mg

Potassium 595mg
Total Carbohydrate 10g | Dietary Fiber 3g | Sugars 7g
Protein 2g
Phosphorus 60mg

1. Peel the tomatoes by scoring the skin of each one with a sharp knife from the top about 1/4 of the way down, in an "x" pattern. Then place scored tomatoes in a pot full of boiling water and boil until their skins begin to crack, approximately 2 minutes.

2. Remove tomatoes and plunge into ice-cold water. When tomatoes are cool enough to touch, peel them. If you want a chunky sauce, dice the tomatoes, and set them aside. If you want a smooth sauce, pass the tomatoes through a food mill to create a seedless purée.

3. Heat the olive oil in a large saucepan over medium heat. When it is hot, add the garlic and crushed red chile flakes. Cook just until the garlic begins to release its aroma.

4. Add the tomatoes, salt, pepper, and basil and/or parsley. Stir well to combine, cover, and reduce heat to low. Simmer for 20 minutes.

5. Serve sauce immediately or allow to cool to room temperature before storing. This sauce will keep in an airtight container in the refrigerator for 1 week, or in the freezer for 1 month.

❖ Italian Living Tradition ❖

Many people debate whether or not a little bit of sugar should be added to tomato sauce at the end of cooking. There are many factors that will influence the overall sweetness of your tomato sauce: the ripeness of the tomatoes, how long you cook the garlic, the sweetness of the basil, and how rapidly the sauce cooks. If you prefer a sweeter taste to your sauce, it is imperative to choose the tastiest tomatoes. Additional sweetness can be coaxed out of tomatoes by roasting them in a 425°F oven for approximately 20 minutes prior to using. It is also important not to let the garlic change color while cooking—the darker garlic gets, the more acrid the taste it imparts to a recipe. Look for the tiniest, dark-green basil leaves possible (homegrown basil is best). And allow the sauce to cook slowly and steadily for the desired amount of time to ensure the sweetest flavor and best taste possible.

BREAD CRUMBS AND HOT CHILE PEPPERS (MOLLICA DI PANE E PEPERONCINI)

Serves: 10 | Serving Size: Approximately 1 1/2 tablespoons
Prep Time: 5 minutes | Cooking Time: 3 minutes

Long before tomatoes flavored so many Italian recipes, toasted fresh bread crumbs were used as a condiment. As simple as they may be, the golden, oil-infused bits of bread do wonders to elevate even the most humble ingredients. Try serving this "sauce" over hot pasta or vegetables with grated pecorino Romano cheese over the top.

1/2 cup extra virgin olive oil
3/4 cup Fresh Bread Crumbs (page 291)
2 tablespoons crushed red chile flakes
1/4 cup sun-dried tomatoes, diced

1. In a large skillet, heat olive oil over medium-high heat. Add the bread crumbs, crushed red chilies, and sun-dried tomatoes. Sauté until they begin to change color and release their aroma, about 3 minutes.

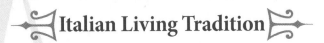

Italian Living Tradition

Many traditional Italian pasta dishes are dressed in a light condiment like this olive oil, bread crumb, and sun-dried tomato combination instead of heavy sauces. In addition to this recipe, sautéed bread crumbs are often combined with fresh anchovies and parsley. In Sicily, this dish is known as *Pasta con la mollica* (pasta with crumbs).

Choices/Exchanges 2 Fat
Calories 110 | Calories from Fat 100
Total Fat 11g | Saturated Fat 1.5g | Trans Fat 0.0g
Cholesterol 0mg
Sodium 55mg

Potassium 50mg
Total Carbohydrate 3g | Dietary Fiber 0g | Sugars 1g
Protein 1g
Phosphorus 5mg

GARLIC AND OIL
(AGLIO E OLIO)

Serves: 4 | Serving Size: 1 tablespoon
Prep Time: 1 minute | Cooking Time: 3 minutes

Preparing Garlic and Oil and serving it with spaghetti is the Italian equivalent of fixing a peanut butter and jelly sandwich in the U.S. It's made because it's quick and satisfying, not because of its creative appeal. While it's not flashy, the combination of olive oil, garlic, chile flakes, and parsley is one of the most nutrient-packed condiments you could ever treat your body to. In addition to pasta, try serving this sauce over vegetables and fish.

1/4 cup extra virgin olive oil
8 cloves garlic, minced
1/4 teaspoon crushed red chile flakes
1/4 cup finely chopped fresh flat-leaf parsley
1/8 teaspoon freshly ground black pepper

1. Heat olive oil in a large, wide skillet over medium heat. Add garlic and chile flakes, and cook just until they release their aroma. Add parsley and pepper, and stir. Serve by tossing into hot pasta or with fresh vegetables.

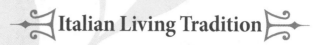
Italian Living Tradition

The ancient combination of garlic and oil is so ubiquitous to the Italian kitchen that it is often taken for granted. Having said that, the great flavor and nutritional benefits of this combination make it one of my favorites. I often choose garlic and oil over more expensive and intricate pairings. The secret to garlic recipes is to cook the garlic just until it releases its aroma—and not a moment longer. This ensures that the garlic is fragrant and sweet. If you allow the garlic to turn brown, it gives off a bitter flavor and completely overwhelms, rather than complements, the recipe.

Choices/Exchanges 1 1/2 Fat
Calories 70 | Calories from Fat 60
Total Fat 7g | Saturated Fat 1.0g | Trans Fat 0.0g
Cholesterol 0mg
Sodium 10mg

Potassium 105mg
Total Carbohydrate 2g | Dietary Fiber 1g | Sugars 0g
Protein 1g
Phosphorus 15mg

EMILIA-ROMAGNA–STYLE GREEN HERB SAUCE (SALSA VERDE ALL'EMILIANA)

Serves: 8 | Serving Size: 2 tablespoons
Prep Time: 5 minutes (plus overnight refrigeration) | Cooking Time: 0 minutes

The region of Emilia-Romagna is known as la grassa, *or "the fat one," because of its rich cuisine. In fact, Bolognese sauce, Prosciutto di Parma DOP (Denominazione di origine protetta/Protected Designation of Origin), and delicious griddle breads known as* piadine *all come from this region. Once you scratch beneath the surface, however, you will find many healthful recipes that the locals eat on a daily basis to stay in shape. This traditional condiment, used for boiled and grilled meats and leftover meatloaf, is one of them. Some versions of this sauce call for leftover stale bread instead of the hard-boiled egg yolks. Note that this sauce must be made a day in advance in order to allow the flavors to develop.*

2 hard-boiled egg yolks

1 clove garlic, minced

3 cups flat-leaf parsley leaves

2 oil-packed anchovy fillets, drained well

1 tablespoon capers, rinsed and drained

2 pickled green peperoncini, rinsed and finely chopped

2–3 tablespoons red wine vinegar

1/4 cup extra virgin olive oil (preferably first cold-pressed)

1/2 red or yellow bell pepper, cored, seeded, and diced finely

1/8 teaspoon unrefined sea salt

1/4 teaspoon freshly ground black pepper

⚜ Italian Living Tradition ⚜

Condiments like this one, which were originally made to dip leftover meats into, also make great marinades. Try marinating your favorite chicken or kabob recipe in this sauce (minus the bell peppers) for an hour before grilling.

1. Combine egg yolks, garlic, parsley, anchovy fillets, capers, peperoncini, and vinegar into a food processor, and pulse on and off until ingredients are finely chopped. Remove the center spout from food processor and slowly pour in the olive oil with the processor still running.

2. Remove mixture to a bowl. Stir in the bell pepper, taste, and season with salt and pepper. Cover and refrigerate overnight. Bring to room temperature before serving.

Choices/Exchanges 2 Fat
Calories 90 | Calories from Fat 70
Total Fat 8g | Saturated Fat 1.4g | Trans Fat 0.0g
Cholesterol 50mg
Sodium 105mg

Potassium 165mg
Total Carbohydrate 3g | Dietary Fiber 1g | Sugars 1g
Protein 2g
Phosphorus 35mg

DESSERTS
(DOLCI)

237   Fresh Fruit Kabobs/*Spiedini di frutta fresca*

238   Espresso Panna Cotta/*Panna cotta al caffè*

240   Strawberries in Balsamic Vinegar/*Fragole in aceto balsamico*

241   Fruit and Fresh Coconut Salad/*Macedonia di frutta con noce di cocco fresco*

242   Vanilla-Scented Roasted Figs/*Ficchi vanigliati al forno*

243   Poached Autumn Pears with Vanilla and Ginger Cream/*Pere al vaniglia con crema di zenzero*

244   Espresso and Spice–Poached Figs/*Ficchi al caffè e spezie*

246   Glazed Apples with Espresso Cream/*Mele glassate con crema di caffè*

247   Mixed-Berry Bruschetta/*Bruschetta ai frutti di bosco*

248   Peach and Apricot Mousse/*Spuma di pesca ed albicocche*

250   Crostini with Ricotta and Honey/*Crostini con ricotta al miele*

251   Whole-Wheat and Honey Cookies/*Biscotti integrale al miele*

252   Pomegranate-Orange Spice Pudding/*Budino alla melagrana con arance e canella*

253   Melon Sorbet/*Sorbetto di melone*

254   Chocolate, Espresso, and Cherry Biscotti/*Biscotti di cioccolato, caffè, e ciliege*

256   Coconut Ball Cookies/*Palline di noce di cocco*

257   Chocolate and Orange Sponge Cake/*Pan di Spagna di cioccolato ed arancia*

258   Pine Nut Cookies/*Biscotti di pinoli*

259   Yogurt Gelato/*Gelato allo yogurt*

260   Crunchy Almond and Pine Nut Cookies/*Fave dolci*

262   Piemontese "Ugly but Good" Cookies/*Brutti ma buoni*

264   Cinnamon-Infused Apple Cake/*Torta di mela e canella*

266   Ivrea's Polenta Cake/*Polentina di Ivrea*

268   Flourless Chocolate Cake/*Torta Caprese*

270   Tuscan Fig, Walnut, and Fennel Seed Torte/*Torta di ficchi, noci, e semi di finocchio*

272   Basilicata-Style Chestnut Cake/*Castagnaccio Lucano*

274   Pear, Ricotta, and Pine Nut Cake/*Torta soffice di pere con ricotta e pinoli*

276   Coconut and Chocolate Pudding/*Budino di noce di cocco e cioccolato*

"Il cibo gradito è meglio digerito."
"The food that is enjoyed is better digested."
—Italian proverb

During media interviews, journalists always ask me what "new" Italian dessert we should know about. Everyone wants to report a new trend in Italian sweet treats. My answer to the question is always the same: fruit! While it might not sound exciting, fruit really is the unsung hero of the Italian dessert tradition. Homecooked meals are always concluded with fresh, seasonal, local—many times it's from the trees out back—fruit. Sweet and packed with vitamins, minerals, and antioxidants, fruit-based desserts truly are the best of all. Heavier Italian desserts such as cannoli, panna cotta, and tiramisu are eaten on special occasions and holidays in Italy.

You may have heard that you should only eat fruit on an empty stomach or in between meals, but this is not necessarily so. Feel free to enjoy fruit with your meals or indulge in one of the fruit-based desserts in this chapter when your meal plan allows. It's important to note that not all sugars are created equal—and those found in fruit can be beneficial, when eaten in moderation. You won't find any artificial sweeteners in this chapter. I prefer to use ingredients that are naturally healthy and small amounts of natural sugar (see "natural sugar" in the Italian Culinary Glossary on page 295), organic honey, or agave nectar when needed.

As with vegetables, it's important to eat a wide variety of different colored fruits in order to get the largest spectrum of health benefits. Luckily, there are many fresh fruit–based desserts in this chapter that take advantage of summer's full bounty:

- Fresh Fruit Kabobs (page 237)
- Strawberries in Balsamic Vinegar (page 240)
- Fruit and Fresh Coconut Salad (page 241)
- Mixed-Berry Bruschetta (page 247)
- Pomegranate-Orange Spice Pudding (page 252)
- Melon Sorbet (page 253)
- Yogurt Gelato (page 259)
- Coconut and Chocolate Pudding (page 276)

When Italians can't use fresh fruits due to the cold weather, dried fruits become the go-to sweet treat. Drying fruits concentrates their sweetness and, in some cases, their nutrients. Dates, figs, peaches, and apricots are the most popular dried fruits in Italy. To dress them up a little, they are often macerated, poached, roasted, or tossed into a cookie, cake, or sweet bread recipe. The cooler weather desserts in the chapter are:

- Vanilla-Scented Roasted Figs (page 242)
- Espresso and Spice–Poached Figs (page 244)
- Poached Autumn Pears with Vanilla and Ginger Cream (page 243)
- Glazed Apples with Espresso Cream (page 246)
- Crostini with Ricotta and Honey (page 250)
- Espresso Panna Cotta (page 238)

Another popular, diabetes-friendly ingredient—which, although not traditional, is becoming more and more common in the kitchens of health-conscious Italian families—is yogurt. Yogurt contains protein, calcium, probiotics, and inulin, an ingredient that has been found to help stabilize glucose levels in some people with type 2 diabetes. In addition to being a great culinary match for fruit, yogurt also pairs well with a diabetes-friendly diet.

One other important and relatively healthful genre of Italian desserts is *casalinga,* or housewife-style baked goods. These rustic treats are often naturally low in sugar. Italians tend to eat them for breakfast, at teatime, or for a light dessert. Some of these recipes, such as Pine Nut Cookies (page 258), have important cultural significance. Others, such as Ivrea's Polenta Cake (page 266), Coconut Ball Cookies (page 256), Pear, Ricotta, and Pine Nut Cake (page 274), and Chocolate and Orange Sponge Cake (page 257), are impressive recipes that will test the limits of just how delicious diabetes-friendly desserts can be.

FRESH FRUIT KABOBS
(SPIEDINI DI FRUTTA FRESCA)

Serves: 5 | Serving Size: 2 kabobs
Prep Time: 15 minutes | Cooking Time: 0 minutes

Fruit salad on a stick is perfect for parties and outdoor gatherings. Even kids have been known to enjoy fruit more when it is presented this way. For an extra-special treat, serve these kabobs with Peach and Apricot Mousse (page 248) if desired. [Note: You will need ten bamboo or other disposable skewers to complete this dish.]

10 strawberries, hulled

10 (1-inch) cubes cantaloupe

10 (1-inch) cubes fresh pineapple

3 kiwi, peeled and cut into about 1-inch pieces

20 blueberries

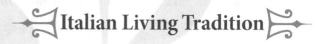
Italian Living Tradition

Spiedini, or skewers, are just as popular in Italy as they are in the U.S. An easy way to prepare kiwi is to slice it in half and scoop out the flesh with a spoon before slicing.

1. If using wooden or bamboo skewers, make sure all the splinters are removed by rolling two skewers together in your hands, or rubbing them over each other as if you are sharpening a knife.

2. Begin by threading a strawberry onto a skewer. Then thread the cantaloupe, pineapple, and kiwi, and finish the skewer with 2 blueberries on the pointed end. Make sure to push the blueberries up fairly high so they don't slip off the skewer. Repeat with the remaining skewers, and serve.

Choices/Exchanges 1 Fruit
Calories 60 | Calories from Fat 0
Total Fat 0g | Saturated Fat 0.0g | Trans Fat 0.0g
Cholesterol 0mg
Sodium 5mg

Potassium 300mg
Total Carbohydrate 15g | Dietary Fiber 3g | Sugars 11g
Protein 1g
Phosphorus 30mg

ESPRESSO PANNA COTTA (*PANNA COTTA AL CAFFÈ*)

Serves: 4 | Serving Size: 1/2 cup

Prep Time: 15 minutes (plus at least 4 hours refrigeration) | Cooking Time: 0 minutes

Panna cotta, Italian for "cooked cream," is a specialty of northern Italy's Piedmont region—an area known for its superior dairy products. Panna cotta, or some version of it, has long been popular throughout most of Europe and in other countries along the Mediterranean.

This creamy, espresso-laced panna cotta is light enough to eat every day but impressive enough to serve to guests. I use yogurt instead of the traditional cream to make the dish lighter.

[Note: You will need four (1/2-cup) ramekins to complete this dish.]

1/2 cup plus 2 tablespoons freshly made espresso coffee, divided
1 teaspoon unflavored gelatin
1/4 cup natural sugar
1 1/2 cups low-fat, low-sugar french vanilla yogurt, drained in a fine-mesh strainer
1/8 teaspoon unrefined sea salt
1/2 teaspoon cocoa powder

Choices/Exchanges 1/2 Low-Fat Milk, 1 Carbohydrate
Calories 120 | Calories from Fat 10
Total Fat 1g | Saturated Fat 0.7g | Trans Fat 0.0g
Cholesterol 5mg
Sodium 135mg
Potassium 225mg
Total Carbohydrate 24g | Dietary Fiber 0g | Sugars 17g
Protein 4g
Phosphorus 120mg

1. Pour 2 tablespoons espresso into a small bowl and sprinkle the gelatin on top. Whisk to combine, and let stand until thickened.

2. Pour the remaining 1/2 cup hot espresso into a small saucepan and whisk in the sugar until it has dissolved.

3. Stir in the yogurt and salt, and put the saucepan over medium heat.

4. When the mixture begins to bubble a little around the edges, take the pan off the heat.

5. With a fork, whisk the gelatin/espresso mixture and add it into the saucepan. Whisk until well combined, keeping the pan off heat. Allow the mixture to sit for a minute. Carefully divide the mixture into 4 ramekins and allow to come to room temperature. Cover and refrigerate for 4 hours or overnight.

6. To unmold easily, dip the bottom of each ramekin, one at a time, into some just-boiled water and hold there for about 8 seconds. Let each stand out of the water for another few seconds before wiping off the water and putting a small salad plate or saucer on top; then overturn the ramekin and let the panna cotta drop onto the plate. Sprinkle each with cocoa powder, and serve.

Italian Living Tradition

Panna cotta dates back to the 10th century, when it's believed that a woman of Hungarian origin first prepared it in Piedmont's Langhe area (also noted for its wine and white truffles). Original versions of panna cotta use heavy cream instead of yogurt. You can change the flavor of this recipe by replacing the espresso used in the gelatin mixture with 2 teaspoons of almond or vanilla extract, or by using a flavored yogurt.

STRAWBERRIES IN BALSAMIC VINEGAR (FRAGOLE IN ACETO BALSAMICO)

Serves: 8 | Serving Size: 1/2 cup
Prep Time: 5 minutes (plus at least 30 minutes macerating time) | Cooking Time: 0 minutes

This classic combination is so easy to prepare that it can hardly be considered a "recipe." It's a staple in my refrigerator all summer long. Use organic strawberries and good-quality balsamic vinegar, such as Aceto Balsamico di Modena (see Italian Living Tradition), in this recipe. Fruit and balsamic vinegar are a match made in heaven. Peaches, figs, and other berries could also be used in this recipe.

2 pints (4 cups) fresh strawberries, cleaned, trimmed, and thickly sliced

5 tablespoons good-quality balsamic vinegar

2 tablespoons pure honey

Freshly grated lemon zest or finely chopped fresh mint (for garnish)

1. Thirty minutes to 1 hour before serving, combine the strawberries, balsamic vinegar, and honey in a bowl. Stir to combine, and set aside at room temperature until ready to serve. (If you're making this dish the night before, cover with plastic wrap and store in the refrigerator overnight.)

2. Spoon into individual ramekins, garnish with lemon zest or mint, and serve.

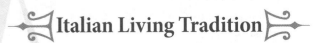

Italian Living Tradition

The origins of what we now call Aceto Balsamico di Modena can be traced all the way back to the 11th century. Authentic Aceto Balsamico di Modena is made from grape "must" (freshly pressed grape juice) that's partially fermented and boiled or concentrated from Italian grapes. It must be aged for at least 10 years in high-quality, natural wooden barrels. Be aware that words like *autentico, aceto balsamico bianco,* and *di Modena* may appear even on products that are *not* authentic Aceto Balsamico di Modena.

Choices/Exchanges 1 Fruit
Calories 50 | Calories from Fat 0
Total Fat 0g | Saturated Fat 0.0g | Trans Fat 0.0g
Cholesterol 0mg
Sodium 0mg

Potassium 150mg
Total Carbohydrate 13g | Dietary Fiber 2g | Sugars 9g
Protein 1g
Phosphorus 25 mg

FRUIT AND FRESH COCONUT SALAD (MACEDONIA DI FRUTTA CON NOCE DI COCCO FRESCO)

Serves: 10 | Serving Size: 1/2 cup
Prep Time: 5 minutes | Cooking Time: 0 minutes

You can use whatever fresh, seasonal fruit you prefer in this recipe. Coconuts can add variety and—best of all—healthy nutrients to your diet. In addition to adding flavor and texture to your recipes, they are rich in lauric acid, which can boost the immune system, and potassium. This recipe is a great way to include some coconut into your diet.

1 cup fresh coconut chunks
1 cup strawberries, cleaned, trimmed, and sliced
1 cup kiwi slices, peeled
1 cup fresh pineapple chunks
1 banana, sliced
Juice of 1 lemon
2 tablespoons pure honey

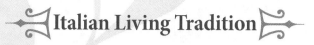

Italian Living Tradition

Fruit salad is known as a *Macedonia* in Italian, because it is an amalgamation of many ingredients, just as the modern-day Greek region of Macedonia is a mix of many cultural influences. Fruit salads are only served when fruit is in season. In the fall and winter, baked and roasted fruit would be served instead.

1. Add all the fruit (except the banana) to a medium bowl, and toss to combine.

2. Whisk the lemon juice and honey together in a small bowl.

3. Add the banana to the fruit mixture and pour lemon-honey dressing over top. Toss gently, and serve.

Choices/Exchanges 1 Fruit, 1/2 Fat
Calories 80 | Calories from Fat 30
Total Fat 3g | Saturated Fat 2.4g | Trans Fat 0.0g
Cholesterol 0mg
Sodium 0mg

Potassium 185mg
Total Carbohydrate 14g | Dietary Fiber 2g | Sugars 10g
Protein 1g
Phosphorus 25mg

VANILLA-SCENTED ROASTED FIGS
(FICCHI VANIGLIATI AL FORNO)

Serves: 6 | Serving Size: 2 figs
Prep Time: 5 minutes | Cooking Time: 10 minutes

Both fresh and dried figs can be used in this recipe. If you use fresh figs, note that they will only need half the time in the oven. If you use dried, keep in mind that roasting them will create a crunchy, candy-like texture on the outside and a chewy interior. I like to use fresh figs when they are in season and dried during other times of year.

12 dried figs, soaked in water for 1 hour, or 12 fresh figs

1/2 teaspoon extra virgin olive oil

12 walnut halves or other nut halves

1 teaspoon honey

1 teaspoon pure vanilla extract

2 tablespoons water

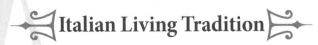

Italian Living Tradition

I've never encountered an Italian who doesn't love figs. Luckily, figs are fat-, sodium-, and cholesterol-free and make a great, portable snack.

1. Preheat oven to 350°F.

2. Cut the stems off the figs. Rub the olive oil over the figs and put them in an 8-inch baking pan, stem side up. Cut a cross in the top of each fig, cutting almost to the bottom, and push them slightly open with your finger. Press 1 walnut half into the center of each fig.

3. Combine the honey, vanilla, and water in a small bowl. Whisk well and pour over the figs.

4. Bake the figs until they open up like flowers, 8–10 minutes. Remove the pan from the oven. Serve hot.

Choices/Exchanges 1 1/2 Fruit, 1 Fat
Calories 120 | Calories from Fat 40
Total Fat 4g | Saturated Fat 0.5g | Trans Fat 0.0g
Cholesterol 0mg
Sodium 0mg

Potassium 0mg
Total Carbohydrate 21g | Dietary Fiber 3g | Sugars 17g
Protein 1g
Phosphorus 30mg

POACHED AUTUMN PEARS
WITH VANILLA AND GINGER CREAM
(PERE AL VANIGLIA CON CREMA DI ZENZERO)

Serves: 8 | Serving Size: 1/2 pear
Prep Time: 10 minutes | Cooking Time: 20 minutes

This dessert is so elegant and delicious that no one will even realize it's good for them. Pears are a great source of dietary fiber, which lowers cholesterol and may help prevent colon cancer. Ginger has been proven to reduce inflammation, an effect that can be particularly helpful to those suffering from disease.

4 bosc pears, peeled

2 tablespoons lemon juice

1 vanilla pod, split open OR 1 teaspoon vanilla paste

2 teaspoons grated fresh ginger, divided

2 tablespoons raw agave nectar

1/2 cup low-fat, low-sugar french vanilla yogurt

1 piece crystalized ginger, minced

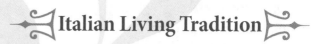

Italian Living Tradition

Poaching fruit is a classic Italian way of transforming nature's bounty into a sweet treat. With the all the overly sweet, processed cakes and desserts on the market, *dolci* like this one will be a welcome and refreshing change for your guests when entertaining.

1. Place pears in a medium saucepan and cover with water. Add lemon juice, vanilla pod, 1 teaspoon ginger, and agave nectar. Bring to boil over high heat. Then reduce heat to medium-low, and simmer for 20 minutes, or until pears are tender.

2. Turn off heat and drain pears, discarding liquid. Set aside to cool.

3. In the meantime, in a small bowl, mix yogurt with the remaining 1 teaspoon fresh ginger and the crystallized ginger, and set aside.

4. When pears are cool enough to handle, slice in half lengthwise. Place each half, cut side down, in the middle of a dessert plate. Spoon yogurt/ginger mixture around the sides of the pears. Allow to stand for 5 minutes at room temperature, then serve.

Choices/Exchanges 1 Fruit, 1/2 Carbohydrate
Calories 100 | Calories from Fat 0
Total Fat 0g | Saturated Fat 0.0g | Trans Fat 0.0g
Cholesterol 0mg
Sodium 10mg

Potassium 160mg
Total Carbohydrate 22g | Dietary Fiber 3g | Sugars 15g
Protein 1g
Phosphorus 35mg

ESPRESSO AND SPICE–POACHED FIGS
(FICCHI AL CAFFÈ E SPEZIE)

Serves: 4 | Serving Size: 3 figs and 2 tablespoons cream
Prep Time: 15 minutes | Cooking Time: 30 minutes (plus overnight refrigeration)

This is a fun, elegant recipe that can be made quickly but will still please even the most discerning palates. Figs are often poached in wine, but I love the deep, smoky flavor that espresso gives them.

1 1/2 cups brewed espresso
1/2 cup raw agave nectar
2 strips lemon peel
2 whole black peppercorns
1 (2-inch-long) cinnamon stick
12 dried white figs, stems peeled
2 tablespoons low-fat cream cheese
1/3 cup low-sugar vanilla yogurt
1 tablespoon pure honey
1 teaspoon pure vanilla extract

Choices/Exchanges 1 Fruit, 1 Carbohydrate
Calories 130 | Calories from Fat 10
Total Fat 1g | Saturated Fat 0.7g | Trans Fat 0.0g
Cholesterol 5mg
Sodium 50mg

Potassium 380mg
Total Carbohydrate 29g | Dietary Fiber 5g | Sugars 19g
Protein 3g
Phosphorus 60mg

1. Combine espresso, agave, lemon peel, pepper-corns, and the cinnamon stick in a small, deep saucepan. Place pan over medium-high heat and bring to a boil. Reduce heat to low, cover, and simmer 15 minutes.

2. Add whole figs to the syrup. Return to a simmer, cover, and poach gently until the figs are soft but not mushy, 15 minutes.

3. Transfer figs and syrup to a bowl, and let stand to cool until no more steam rises. When cool, cover the bowl with plastic wrap and refrigerate overnight.

4. Combine cream cheese, yogurt, honey, and vanilla in a medium mixing bowl. Stir together with a spoon or rubber spatula until well combined.

5. Remove chilled figs from the refrigerator and let stand until they reach room temperature. Transfer figs to another bowl, and strain the syrup, discarding the solids.

6. Place 3 figs, sliced in half, in the center of each plate. Top with vanilla cream cheese mixture. Spoon some of the poaching liquid over the plate, and serve.

Italian Living Tradition

In Italy, espresso is served at the end of meals. Since this dessert is poached in espresso, it satisfies the need for both coffee and sweets at the same time!

GLAZED APPLES WITH ESPRESSO CREAM
(MELE GLASSATE CON CREMA DI CAFFÈ)

Serves: 10 | Serving Size: 8 apple wedges and 2 tablespoons cream
Prep Time: 10 minutes | Cooking Time: 30 minutes

This fun, dippable dessert also makes a great snack or post-workout pick-me-up. You can omit the espresso in this recipe or replace it with your favorite flavored extract, if desired.

1/2 cup plus 1 tablespoon natural sugar

2 pounds golden delicious apples,
  peeled and each cut into 8 wedges

3 tablespoons (1 ounce) mascarpone cheese

1 cup low-fat vanilla yogurt, drained

1 tablespoon pure honey

1 tablespoon cold espresso

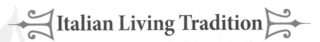
Italian Living Tradition

To an Italian, the next best thing to fresh fruit in the summer is baked or poached fruit in the winter. This recipe is no exception. It's simple enough to serve daily, but special enough for company.

1. Bring 1 cup water and 1/2 cup sugar to a boil in a 3-quart saucepan, stirring until sugar is dissolved. Reduce heat and simmer 5 minutes. Add apples and simmer, stirring occasionally, until just tender, about 15 minutes.

2. Transfer apples with a slotted spoon to a rack set over a baking pan, and let apples drain for 10 minutes. Reserve poaching liquid.

3. Preheat broiler to high.

4. Arrange apple wedges in a single layer in a flameproof, shallow baking pan and sprinkle with remaining 1 tablespoon sugar. Broil about 6 inches from heat, until apples are lightly browned on the edges, 3–5 minutes. Remove apples from oven and set aside to cool slightly.

5. In a small bowl, combine mascarpone, yogurt, honey, and espresso. Stir to mix well.

6. While apples are still warm, arrange them on plates and top with a dollop of cream mixture. Drizzle poaching liquid on top of apples. Serve immediately.

Choices/Exchanges 1 Fruit, 1 Carbohydrate
Calories 140 | Calories from Fat 20
Total Fat 2g | Saturated Fat 1.4g | Trans Fat 0.0g
Cholesterol 5mg
Sodium 25mg

Potassium 170mg
Total Carbohydrate 28g | Dietary Fiber 2g | Sugars 25g
Protein 2g
Phosphorus 50mg

MIXED-BERRY BRUSCHETTA
(BRUSCHETTA AI FRUTTI DI BOSCO)

Serves: 4 | Serving Size: 1 slice bread and 1/4 fruit mixture
Prep Time: 5 minutes | Cooking Time: About 7 minutes

Bruschetta is a popular Italian appetizer of toasted or grilled day-old artisan bread topped with an endless possibility of toppings. The term bruschetta *comes from the Italian word* bruciare, *which means "to burn." Originally, bruschetta were placed over open flames to toast.*

4 (1/4-inch) thin slices whole-wheat ciabatta,
 baguette, or gluten-free bread

1/4 cup trimmed strawberries

1/4 cup raspberries

1/4 cup blackberries

1/4 cup blueberries

3 teaspoons cornstarch, dissolved in 1/4 cup water

1 cinnamon stick

1/3 cup natural sugar

4 fresh mint leaves

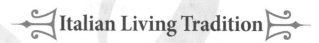

Italian Living Tradition

The fruit topping in this recipe is also used to make *crostate*, Italian pies, as well as toppings for yogurt and gelato.

1. Preheat broiler to high.

2. Toast bread slices on one side until golden, about 1–2 minutes. Remove from oven and set aside.

3. Prepare the filling by combining strawberries, raspberries, blackberries, and blueberries in a medium saucepan. Add cornstarch mixture, cinnamon stick, and sugar. Stir well to combine. Bring to a boil over high heat. Reduce heat to medium, stir slowly, and continue to cook 3–5 minutes, until mixture becomes thick like a pie filling.

4. Remove fruit mixture from heat and cool until almost room temperature. Discard cinnamon stick.

5. Place toasted bread on a serving platter. Top each slice with 1/4 of the fruit mixture, and garnish with mint. Serve immediately.

Choices/Exchanges 1 Starch, 1/2 Carbohydrate
Calories 130 | Calories from Fat 10
Total Fat 1g | Saturated Fat 0.1g | Trans Fat 0.0g
Cholesterol 0mg
Sodium 85mg

Potassium 105mg
Total Carbohydrate 29g | Dietary Fiber 2g | Sugars 19g
Protein 2g
Phosphorus 35mg

PEACH AND APRICOT MOUSSE
(*SPUMA DI PESCA ED ALBICOCCHE*)

Serves: 12 | Serving Size: 1/2 cup
Prep Time: 5 minutes (plus 30 minutes apricot-soaking time)
Cooking Time: 30 minutes (plus overnight refrigeration time)

Served cold, fruit mousses are popular summertime desserts in Italy. They are often served to children as a way to get them to eat more fruit. The addition of peach liqueur in this recipe, however, makes an easy and delicious but also sophisticated dessert for adults.

1 1/2 cups dried apricots (about 8 ounces), plus a few extra for garnish
1/2 cup Pêcher Mignon or other peach liqueur (do not use peach brandy)
1 tablespoon unflavored gelatin
1/4 cup raw agave nectar
2 cups low-fat, low-sugar french vanilla, apricot, or peach yogurt

---

Choices/Exchanges 1 Fruit, 1/2 Carbohydrate
Calories 120 | Calories from Fat 10
Total Fat 1g | Saturated Fat 0.3g | Trans Fat 0.0g
Cholesterol 0mg
Sodium 35mg

Potassium 320mg
Total Carbohydrate 23g | Dietary Fiber 2g | Sugars 17g
Protein 3g
Phosphorus 80mg

1. Combine dried apricots and 1 1/2 cups water in heavy, medium saucepan. Let stand 30 minutes. Place saucepan over high heat and bring to boil. Reduce heat and simmer gently until apricots are very soft, about 20 minutes. Allow to cool slightly.

2. Meanwhile, add 1/2 cup Pêcher Mignon to a small bowl and sprinkle gelatin over top. Set aside to soften. Once gelatin has dissolved, pour in agave nectar and mix well to combine.

3. Transfer apricots and the poaching liquid to a food processor, and purée until smooth.

4. Pour the purée into a large saucepan along with peach liqueur/gelatin mixture Bring to a boil, stirring gently in one direction. Boil for a few minutes until mixture thickens slightly. Reduce heat to simmer and stir until the mixure is thick like a paste. Transfer mixture to a large, heatproof bowl, and cool to room temperature.

5. Mix 1/3 of the yogurt into the apricot/peach mixture to lighten. Gently fold in the remaining yogurt in 2 batches. Cover bowl with plastic, and refrigerate mousse for 8 hours or overnight.

6. Spoon the mousse into pastry bag fitted with a large star tip. Pipe mousse into goblets or wine glasses. Dice a few additional dried apricots, sprinkle over mousse, and serve.

⊰ Italian Living Tradition ⊱

Spuma is the Italian word for mousse. There are many types of mousses, such as chocolate and fruit, in traditional Italian cuisine. Normally mousses are made with chocolate pieces and/or fruit purée that is blended with egg yolks for creaminess. Then freshly whipped cream and/or egg whites are folded in to lighten the consistency. In this recipe, I've substituted gelatin and yogurt for the eggs and cream to make a healthier mousse.

CROSTINI WITH RICOTTA AND HONEY (CROSTINI CON RICOTTA AL MIELE)

Serves: 4 | Serving Size: 1 slice
Prep Time: 1 minute | Cooking Time: 5 minutes

In Sicily, the locals eat fresh sheep and goat's milk ricotta for breakfast, as a topping and filling for pasta, and in desserts such as cannoli, cassata, and cheesecakes. This recipe can double as a rustic yet chic appetizer or a dessert.

3 ounces ricotta cheese

1 tablespoon pure honey

1/4 baguette, cut on the diagonal into 4 (1/4-inch) slices

1. Preheat broiler to high.

2. In a bowl, combine the ricotta and honey, and mix well.

3. Place the bread slices on a baking sheet and place under the broiler. Broil until golden, approximately 1–2 minutes. Remove from oven and carefully turn the bread slices over. Broil the other side for 1 more minute, or just until golden.

4. Remove bread from the oven and slather with the ricotta-honey mixture. Serve immediately.

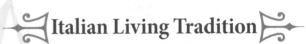

Italian Living Tradition

Crostini are thin slices of bread that are often grilled and can be topped with a myriad of savory toppings. They are common complements to alcoholic beverages served in the *apertivo* custom (see "apertivo" in Italian Culinary Glossary on page 295).

Choices/Exchanges 1 Starch, 1 Lean Protein
Calories 110 | Calories from Fat 30
Total Fat 3g | Saturated Fat 1.9g | Trans Fat 0.0g
Cholesterol 10mg
Sodium 150mg

Potassium 50mg
Total Carbohydrate 16g | Dietary Fiber 1g | Sugars 5g
Protein 5g
Phosphorus 55mg

WHOLE-WHEAT AND HONEY COOKIES (BISCOTTI INTEGRALE AL MIELE)

Serves: 18 | Serving Size: 1 cookie
Prep Time: 15 minutes | Cooking Time: 15 minutes

Hearty, nutritious cookies (called "biscotti," just like the famous twice-baked Italian cookies) are increasingly popular breakfast treats for all ages in Italy. This recipe incorporates the unique flavors of olive oil. Dried fruit, coconut, and citrus zest would make great additions to this recipe. You will need a pastry bag or a resealable plastic bag to pipe these cookies.

2 eggs

1/3 cup pure honey

3/4 cup whole-wheat flour, gluten-free baking mix, or almond flour

2 teaspoons pure vanilla

1 teaspoon yeast

1/2 cup extra virgin olive oil

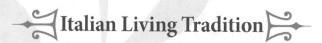
Italian Living Tradition

Simple but delicious, biscotti recipes like these have been enjoyed since Roman times in Italy.

1. Preheat oven to 400°F. Line a baking sheet with parchment paper.

2. Combine eggs and honey in a bowl with a wooden spoon. Add flour, vanilla, and yeast. Mix well to combine. Stir in the olive oil, mixing well to incorporate.

3. Spoon the dough into a pastry bag fitted with a 1-inch round tip, or a plastic sandwich bag with the tip cut off. Twist the ends to seal the bag, and press down, making cookies that are 2 1/2 inches long and 1 inch wide.

4. Bake until golden, approximately 15 minutes. Serve.

Choices/Exchanges 1/2 Starch, 1 1/2 Fat
Calories 90 | Calories from Fat 60
Total Fat 7g | Saturated Fat 1.0g | Trans Fat 0.0g
Cholesterol 20mg
Sodium 10mg

Potassium 25mg
Total Carbohydrate 7g | Dietary Fiber 0g | Sugars 5g
Protein 1g
Phosphorus 20mg

POMEGRANATE-ORANGE SPICE PUDDING
(BUDINO ALLA MELAGRANA CON ARANCE E CANELLA)

Serves: 8 | Serving Size: 1/2 cup

Prep Time: 5 minutes | Cooking Time: 20 minutes (plus a few hours refrigeration time)

This bright, festive dessert will be most appreciated during the holiday months. I love to smell the spices steeping in the pomegranate and orange juice while making this pudding. Because the pudding has a fruit juice base, its consistency will resemble that of jelly.

4 cups pomegranate juice

1/3 cup pure honey

1 cinnamon stick

4 tablespoons cornstarch

1/2 cup freshly squeezed orange juice

2 oranges, peeled, trimmed, and cut into supremes
  (see Italian Living Tradition on page 195)

Seeds of 1 pomegranate or zest of 1 orange (for garnish)

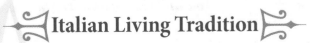

Italian Living Tradition

Once highly prized ingredients imported from North Africa and Central Asia, flavorful fruits such as pomegranates and oranges were often given as gifts during the holiday season in ancient times.

1. In a large saucepan, bring the pomegranate juice, honey, and cinnamon stick to a boil.

2. In a bowl, dissolve the cornstarch into the orange juice. Pour orange juice mixture into the saucepan, stirring vigorously. Increase heat under the saucepan to high and stir mixture, in one direction only, for 3 minutes. Reduce heat to medium-low and stir gently, always in one direction, until the mixture thickens and reduces to approximately 1/3 of its original volume, about 15 minutes.

3. Remove from heat. Let the mixture cool, and pour into a glass serving bowl, removing cinnamon stick.

4. Stir in the pieces of orange, cover with plastic wrap, and chill in the refrigerator for a few hours.

5. Sprinkle the pomegranate seeds or orange zest over the chilled pudding and serve.

Choices/Exchanges 1 Fruit, 1 Carbohydrate
Calories 130 | Calories from Fat 5
Total Fat 0.5g | Saturated Fat 0.0g | Trans Fat 0.0g
Cholesterol 0mg
Sodium 0mg

Potassium 340mg
Total Carbohydrate 30g | Dietary Fiber 1g | Sugars 22g
Protein 1g
Phosphorus 30mg

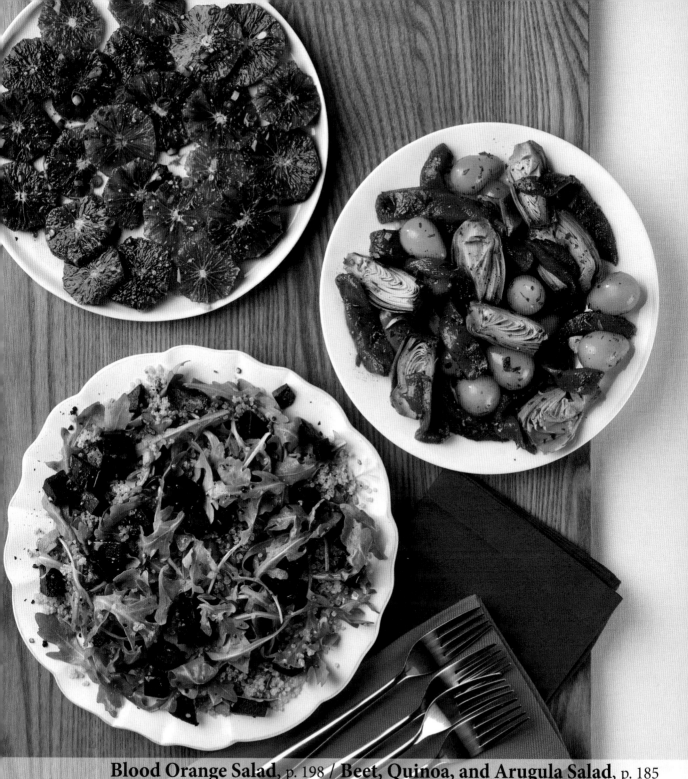

Blood Orange Salad, p. 198 / **Beet, Quinoa, and Arugula Salad**, p. 185
Red Pepper, Yellow Tomato, and Artichoke Salad, p. 187

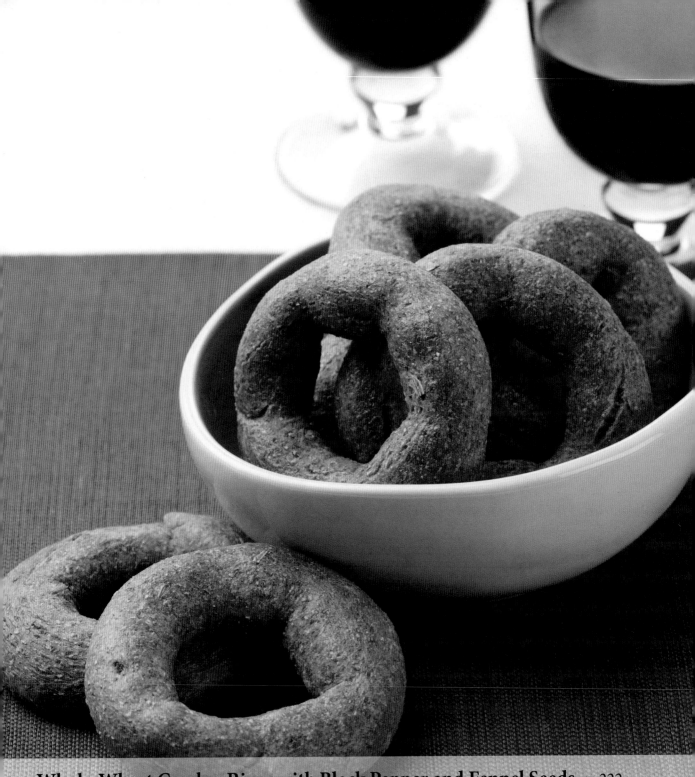

Whole-Wheat Cracker Rings with Black Pepper and Fennel Seeds, p. 222

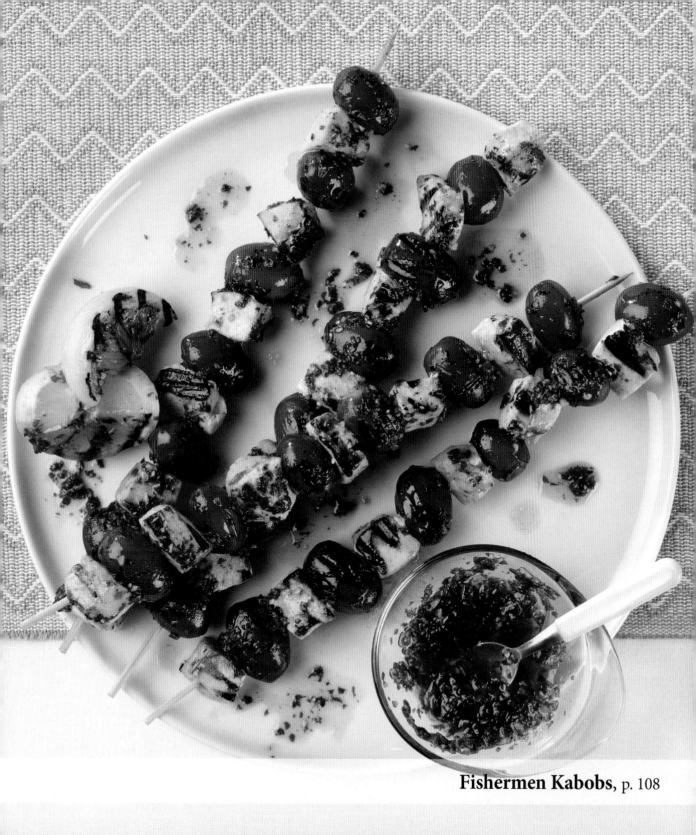

Fishermen Kabobs, p. 108

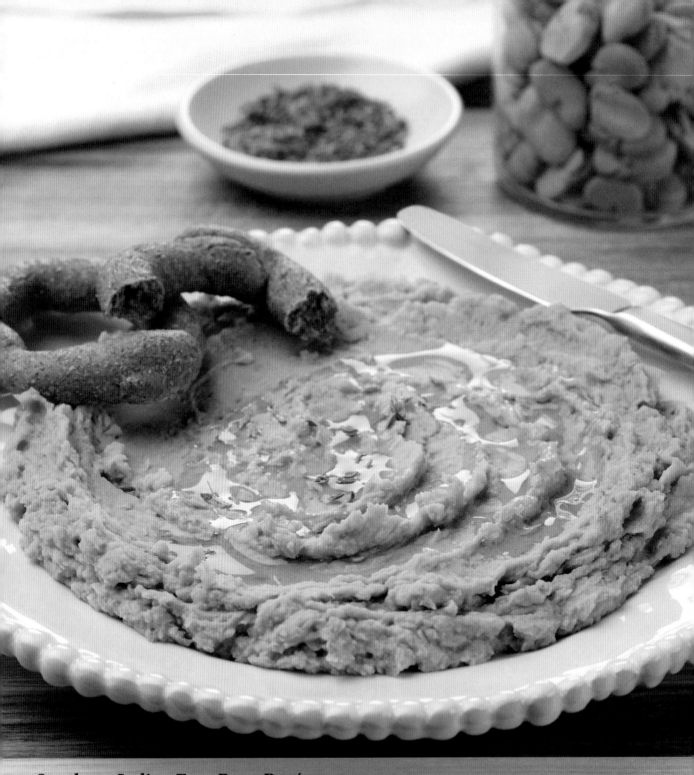

Southern Italian Fava Bean Purée, p. 16

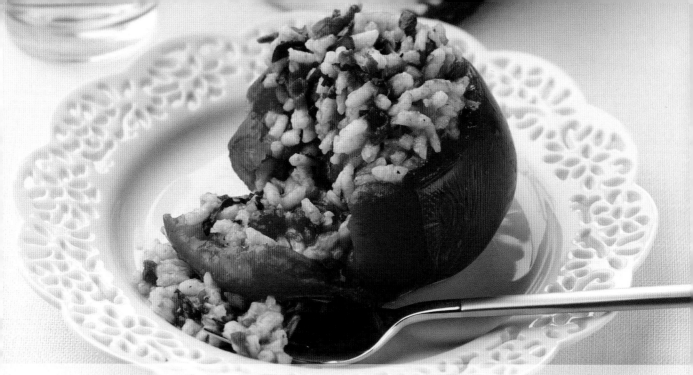

Roman-Style Rice and Herb–Stuffed Tomatoes, p. 20

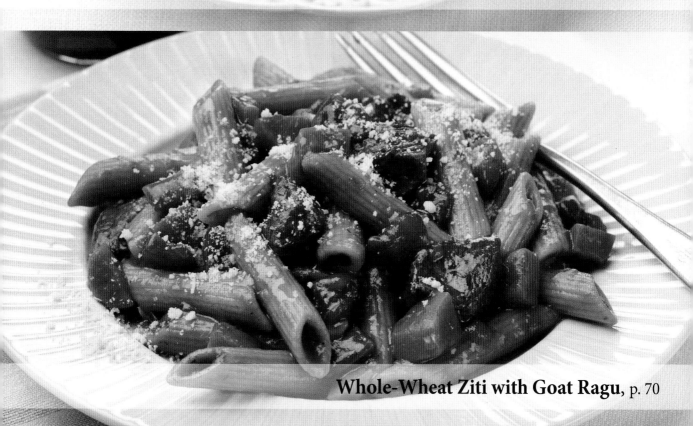

Whole-Wheat Ziti with Goat Ragu, p. 70

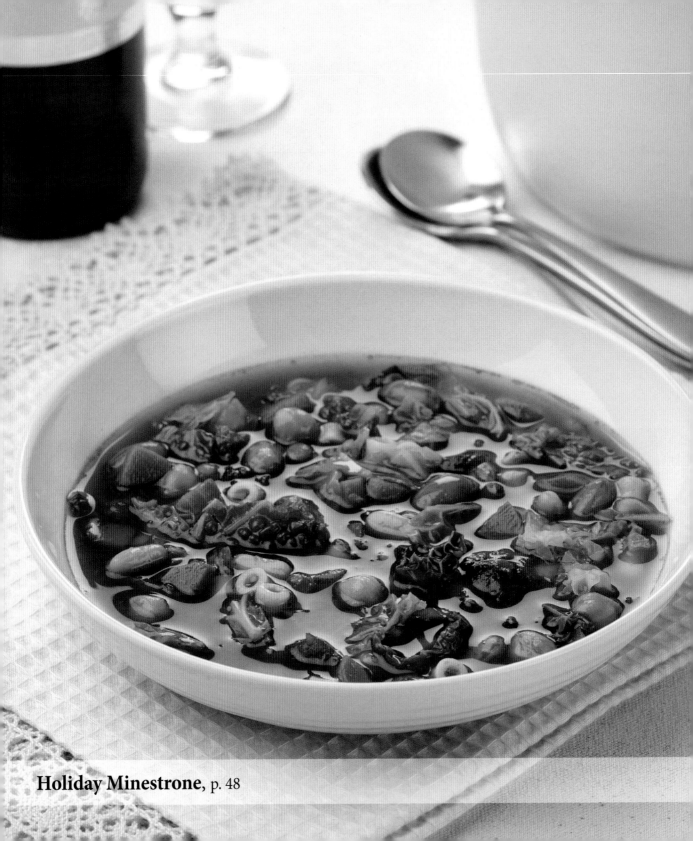

Holiday Minestrone, p. 48

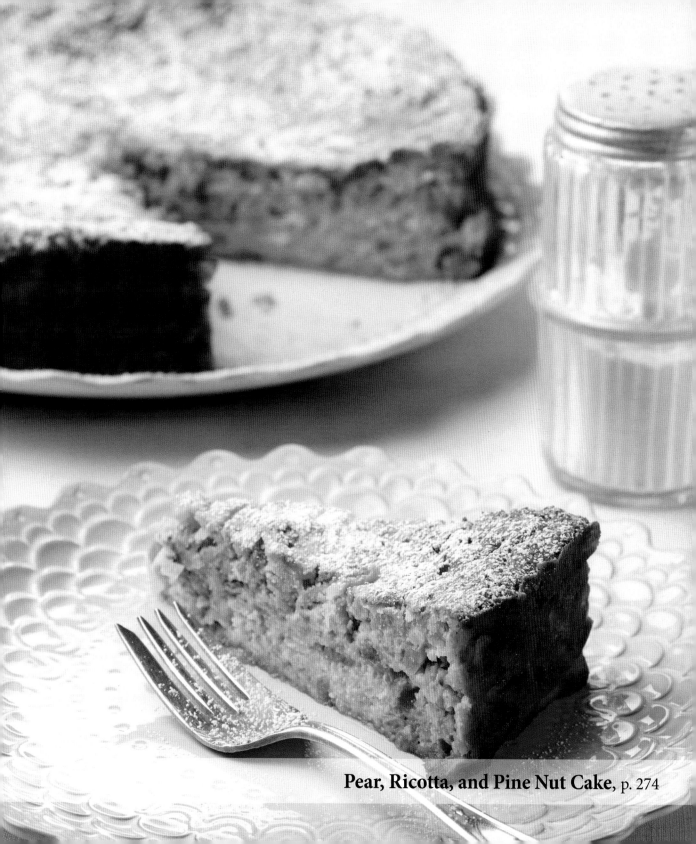

Pear, Ricotta, and Pine Nut Cake, p. 274

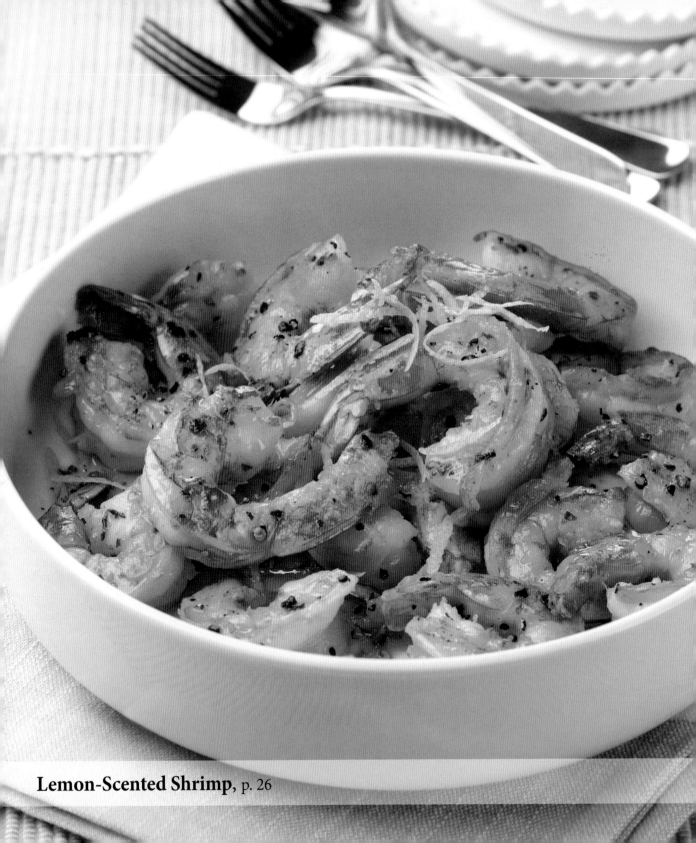

Lemon-Scented Shrimp, p. 26

MELON SORBET
(SORBETTO DI MELONE)

Serves: 6 | Serving Size: 3/4 cup
Prep Time: 5 minutes | Cooking Time: 5 minutes (plus at least 6 hours refrigeration time)

The word cantaloupe *may come from the name of the Italian town Cantalupo, which is said to be the first place in Europe where the cantaloupe was grown after being introduced from the Persian Empire. During the Roman Empire, cantaloupes were imported from North Africa and were revered as a symbol of fertility.*

It's best to make this dessert a day in advance. It should be refrigerated overnight before serving. Take advantage of summer's bounty with this recipe.

1 pound cantaloupe flesh, cubed

2 tablespoons lemon juice

1/4 cup pure honey

4 teaspoons powdered gelatin, diluted in 1/2 cup cold water

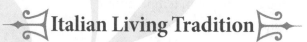

Italian Living Tradition

Roman naturalist Castore Durante discouraged those with diabetes from eating cantaloupes in his 16th-century book *Herbario Nuovo.* While cantaloupes do have a high glycemic index, they also contain a lot of fiber, which makes them safe for those with diabetes to consume in moderation.

1. Working in batches, if necessary, place the melon in a food processor, blender, or juicer. Add the lemon juice, and the honey. Pulse on and off until you have a liquid purée that is completely uniform in texture.

2. In a medium saucepan over medium heat add the gelatin mixture and 1 additional tablespoon water, and stir. Add the cantaloupe purée. Stir well from the bottom and sides to prevent the gelatin from crystallizing. Cook, stirring, for approximately 3–5 minutes, until mixture thickens.

3. Transfer the mixture to 6 (2-ounce) ramekins or cups, and cool to room temperature.

4. Cover and refrigerate for a minimum of 6 hours or overnight.

5. To unmold, run a butter knife around the borders of each ramekin. Place a serving dish on top of the ramekin, and turn it over to unmold the sorbet.

Choices/Exchanges 1 Carbohydrate
Calories 80 | Calories from Fat 0
Total Fat 0g | Saturated Fat 0.0g | Trans Fat 0.0g
Cholesterol 0mg
Sodium 30mg

Potassium 220mg
Total Carbohydrate 20g | Dietary Fiber 1g | Sugars 18g
Protein 1g
Phosphorus 40mg

CHOCOLATE, ESPRESSO, AND CHERRY BISCOTTI (*BISCOTTI DI CIOCCOLATO, CAFFÈ, E CILIEGE*)

Serves: 16 | Serving Size: 2 biscotti
Prep Time: 15 minutes | Cooking Time: About 55 minutes

If you've never made the ubiquitous Italian twice-baked cookie before, you'll be surprised at how easy it is. Biscotti were actually popular in North Africa and the Middle East prior to their presence in Europe. This unique version of biscotti combines chocolate, espresso, and cherries for a dramatic yet still rather light after-dinner treat.

4 large eggs, at room temperature

3/4 cup natural sugar

3 tablespoons pure honey

2 cups unbleached all-purpose flour or all-purpose gluten-free flour

1/4 cup unsweetened cocoa powder

2 tablespoons cold espresso or coffee

1 teaspoon vanilla

1/2 cup dried cherries

Choices/Exchanges 1 Starch, 1 Carbohydrate
Calories 140 | Calories from Fat 20
Total Fat 2g | Saturated Fat 0.5g | Trans Fat 0.0g
Cholesterol 45mg
Sodium 20mg

Potassium 80mg
Total Carbohydrate 29g | Dietary Fiber 1g | Sugars 16g
Protein 4g
Phosphorus 55mg

1. Preheat oven to 375°F. Grease and flour 2 (8 1/2 × 4 1/2 × 2 1/2-inch) loaf pans.

2. In a large bowl, add eggs and beat by hand or with an electric mixer on high speed until the mixture turns light yellow, about 3 minutes.

3. Slowly add the sugar and honey, and continue to beat until incorporated. With the mixer running on low speed (or while mixing by hand) add the flour, cocoa powder, espresso, and vanilla. Mix well to incorporate. Fold in the cherries.

4. Pour half of the batter into each pan. Smooth out the top of the batter. Bake in the middle of the oven for 25 minutes, or until dough turns golden.

5. Remove from the oven and reduce oven temperature to 350°F. Let biscotti cool for 10 minutes in the pan. Using oven mitts, turn over loaf pans to unmold cookies. Cool for an additional 10 minutes.

6. Cut each loaf crosswise into 1/4-inch sections. Lay each slice on its side on a baking sheet.

7. Bake for 8–10 minutes. Remove from oven, turn biscotti over, and bake for another 10–20 minutes. Cookies should be light brown and crisp when finished.

8. Cool thoroughly, and serve. Cookies will keep in an airtight container for up to a month.

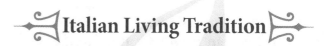

Italian Living Tradition

Biscotti are ever-present in cookie jars in Italian kitchens. They also make great edible gifts! Try placing a bunch in a cellophane bag and wrapping them with pretty ribbons to give as hostess gifts.

COCONUT BALL COOKIES
(PALLINE DI NOCE DI COCCO)

Serves: 21 | Serving Size: 2 cookies
Prep Time: 5 minutes (plus 30 minutes resting time) | Cooking Time: 12–14 minutes

These delicate cookies contain only three ingredients! The delicious little bites take only minutes to make. Since they are naturally gluten-free, they're perfect for Passover. I recommend using air-insulated baking sheets or stacking two baking sheets one on top of the other, and baking these cookies in the upper third of the oven to prevent the bottoms from overbrowning.

3/4 cup natural sugar

2 eggs

1 cup organic dehydrated coconut (see Where to Buy Guide on page 299)

1. Combine sugar and eggs in a bowl and whisk for 3–5 minutes, until the mixture is white and foamy. Add the coconut and whisk well to combine. Cover with plastic wrap and allow to rest for 30 minutes at room temperature, without touching.

2. Preheat oven to 325°F degrees. Line 2 baking sheets with parchment paper.

3. With slightly wet hands (I keep a little ramekin of water next to me while I work), roll dough into 1-inch balls and place them 1 inch apart on baking sheets.

4. Bake for 12–14 minutes, or until they begin to turn color slightly and are cooked through. Cool slightly and serve at room temperature.

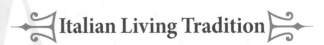

Italian Living Tradition

These types of little cookies are called *biscottini per il te* (tea cookies) in Italy, and Italians would not consider them a dessert. They can be made ahead and frozen and will last up to a week in an airtight container. I recommend serving them with various other cookies on a decorative tray.

Choices/Exchanges 1/2 Carbohydrate, 1/2 Fat
Calories 60 | Calories from Fat 30
Total Fat 3g | Saturated Fat 2.2g | Trans Fat 0.0g
Cholesterol 20mg
Sodium 10mg

Potassium 25mg
Total Carbohydrate 8g | Dietary Fiber 1g | Sugars 7g
Protein 1g
Phosphorus 15mg

CHOCOLATE AND ORANGE SPONGE CAKE (PAN DI SPAGNA DI CIOCCOLATO ED ARANCIA)

Serves: 10 | Serving Size: 1 (1-inch) slice
Prep Time: 15 minutes | Cooking Time: 40 minutes

This classic Italian cake is eaten for breakfast or as a snack, or it can be used as a base for more elaborate holiday desserts. It's also a delicious base for shortcakes and sundaes. You can double the recipe and freeze one cake, wrapped in plastic wrap, for another time. Use almond flour instead of all-purpose flour for a gluten-free alternative—this is a popular substitution during Passover.

Nonstick cooking spray
6 large eggs, separated, divided
3/4 cup raw agave nectar
1 teaspoon vanilla extract
Zest of 1 orange
2 teaspoons baking powder (gluten-free, if needed)
1/3 cup unsweetened cocoa powder
1 teaspoon espresso
1 1/8 cups unbleached all-purpose flour or almond flour

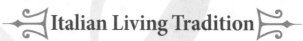

Italian Living Tradition

Sponge cakes are used as a base in Italian cooking schools, where pastry chefs learn to use them in layered cakes, trifles, Florentine *zuccoto*, Sicilian *cassata*, and much more. In Italy, a plain slice is often eaten with *caffè latte* for breakfast in the morning.

1. Preheat oven to 350°F. Grease a 1 1/2-quart loaf pan (8 1/4 × 9 × 2 3/4 inches) with nonstick cooking spray.

2. Beat egg whites in a large bowl until stiff peaks form, and set aside.

3. Cream agave nectar and egg yolks together, and continue beating until they are very light yellow in color. Stir in the vanilla, orange zest, baking powder, cocoa, and espresso. Gently fold the egg whites into the batter.

4. Sprinkle the flour on top of the batter and carefully incorporate until just combined. Pour batter into prepared baking pan and bake for 40 minutes, or until cake is golden and sides begin to pull away from the pan.

5. Remove from the oven and allow to cool completely. Serve.

Choices/Exchanges 1/2 Starch, 1 Carbohydrate, 1 Lean Protein
Calories 160 | Calories from Fat 35
Total Fat 4g | Saturated Fat 1.3g | Trans Fat 0.0g
Cholesterol 110mg

Sodium 140mg
Potassium 110mg
Total Carbohydrate 26g | Dietary Fiber 2g | Sugars 12g
Protein 6g
Phosphorus 100mg

PINE NUT COOKIES
(BISCOTTI DI PINOLI)

Serves: 18 | Serving Size: 2 cookies
Prep Time: 15 minutes | Cooking Time: 12–14 minutes

Bakeries specializing in sweets, known as pasticcerie *throughout the region of Calabria, prominently display this rustic yet delicious and satisfying cookie. When I was growing up, these cookies were integral to wedding and holiday cookie trays, and they were prepared not only by Calabrians, but also Italian-Americans hailing from other southern Italian regions.*

This recipe uses fewer eggs than the traditional version, which gives these cookies a lighter but equally delicious taste.

1 cup natural sugar

1/4 cup pure honey

1/4 teaspoon salt

3 large eggs

2 1/4 cups flour

1/2 teaspoon baking powder (gluten-free, if needed)

2 teaspoons almond extract

6 tablespoons pine nuts

⊰ Italian Living Tradition ⊱

Many people like to make large batches of these cookies and keep them on hand for unexpected guests. They taste great as part of breakfast, during teatime, or as a snack. Don't be surprised if your guests eat a handful at a time!

1. Preheat oven to 375°F.

2. Place sugar, honey, salt, and eggs in a bowl. Beat mixture with an electric mixer until eggs are foamy. Fold in flour, baking powder, and almond extract. The batter should be the consistency of chocolate chip cookie dough. If it is too thin, add a little more flour, 1 tablespoon at a time, until it reaches the right consistency.

3. Line 2 baking sheets with parchment paper. Drop rounded teaspoons full of dough about 2 inches apart on the baking sheets. Sprinkle each cookie with 6–8 pine nuts and bake for 12–14 minutes, until light golden brown.

4. Remove cookies from oven and serve.

Choices/Exchanges 1/2 Starch, 1 Carbohydrate
Calories 120 | Calories from Fat 20
Total Fat 2g | Saturated Fat 0.4g | Trans Fat 0.0g
Cholesterol 25mg
Sodium 20mg

Potassium 40mg
Total Carbohydrate 22g | Dietary Fiber 0g | Sugars 12g
Protein 3g
Phosphorus 45mg

YOGURT GELATO
(GELATO ALLO YOGURT)

Serves: 6 | Serving Size: 1/3 cup

Prep Time: 5 minutes (plus approximately 3 hours freezing time) | Cooking Time: 0 minutes

Italy's glorious gelaterie *now serve yogurt-flavored gelato—which is quite different from the frozen yogurt available elsewhere. It is usually made with whole milk, whole milk yogurt, sugar, and glucose in the artisanal fashion. This recipe has been adapted to make it diabetes-friendly.*

2 cups low-fat, low-sugar french vanilla
   or plain yogurt

1 teaspoon pure vanilla extract

1/4 cup pure honey

1 cup fresh raspberries or other berries (optional)

1. Combine yogurt, vanilla, and honey. Mix well to combine.

2. Transfer to ice cream or gelato maker, if using, until mixture reaches the desired consistency. If you're not using an ice cream or gelato maker, proceed to step 3.

3. Transfer mixture to a deep, 9-inch, freezer-safe container and place in the freezer. After 45 minutes, open the door and check the mixture. As it starts to freeze around the edges, remove it from the freezer and stir it vigorously with a spatula or whisk in order to break up any frozen sections. This action helps to ensure a creamier product. (You can use a hand-held mixer, if you have one, for best results.) Return mixture to the freezer.

4. Continue to check the mixture every 30 minutes, stirring vigorously (by hand or with the hand-held mixer) as it's freezing. Repeat this process until the gelato is frozen through. It will likely take around 3 hours to freeze completely. Serve with berries on the side, if using.

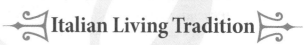

Italian Living Tradition

According to Italian historians, gelato became famous in mainland Italy in the 16th century. There was a famous Sicilian chef named Francesco Procopio Cutò who made flavored ices and gelato in the traditional Sicilian fashion. He opened a café and ice cream shop in Paris called Café Procope; the longest continuously operating café in Paris, it is still open today.

Choices/Exchanges 1 1/2 Carbohydrate
Calories 130 | Calories from Fat 10
Total Fat 1g | Saturated Fat 0.5g | Trans Fat 0.0g
Cholesterol 5mg
Sodium 55mg

Potassium 220mg
Total Carbohydrate 25g | Dietary Fiber 1g | Sugars 17g
Protein 4g
Phosphorus 115mg

CRUNCHY ALMOND AND PINE NUT COOKIES
(FAVE DOLCI)

Serves: 25 | Serving Size: 2 cookies
Prep Time: 15 minutes | Cooking Time: 15–20 minutes

Many people are surprised to learn that Italy, just like Mexico, has the tradition of celebrating the Day of the Dead. Between November 1 (All Saints' Day) and November 2 (All Souls' Day), Italians serve traditional baked goods (usually rustic breads or cookies), go to Mass, and gather with friends and loved ones. As you eat these special treats, it is customary to remember the lives of departed loved ones; this is a way to show respect and connect to them.

First-timers to these cookies will find them very hard in texture—similar to the cookies that Americans call biscotti. They are meant to be dunked into coffee, tea, or sweet wine. The good news is that their tough texture helps them to travel well. For a variation on this recipe, you can swap the almond flour for hazelnut flour and replace the pine nuts with chopped, peeled hazelnuts.

4 cups almond flour, plus extra for work surface

1/2 cup pine nuts

1 cup confectioners' sugar

1 large egg and 2 egg yolks, whisked together in a small bowl

1 teaspoon baking powder (use gluten-free, if needed)

Grated zest of 1 lemon

1 tablespoon grappa or orange or lemon juice

1 teaspoon pure cinnamon

Choices/Exchanges 1/2 Carbohydrate, 2 Fat
Calories 130 | Calories from Fat 90
Total Fat 10g | Saturated Fat 1.0g | Trans Fat 0.0g
Cholesterol 20mg
Sodium 25mg

Potassium 135mg
Total Carbohydrate 9g | Dietary Fiber 2g | Sugars 6g
Protein 4g
Phosphorus 100mg

1. Preheat oven to 350°F. Line a large (18 × 26-inch) baking sheet with parchment paper, and place it on top of another equal-size baking sheet. (The double pans help prevent the bottoms of the cookies from turning dark.)

2. In a food processor, combine the almond flour, pine nuts, and confectioners' sugar, and pulse on and off until you obtain a fine powder.

3. Transfer the mixture to a large bowl, and stir in the eggs, baking powder, lemon zest, grappa or juice, and cinnamon. Mix well with a wooden spoon to combine.

4. Dust a work surface with almond flour and turn the mixture out onto it. Knead lightly until a smooth, compact dough forms. (If dough is too sticky to work with, add additional flour, a few tablespoons at a time, until it resembles the consistency of play dough. If the dough is too dry and a ball will not form, add water or orange or lemon juice, a few tablespoons at a time, until it becomes more malleable.)

5. Break off small pieces of dough and roll into 1/2-inch balls. Place the balls 1/2 inch apart on the baking sheet.

6. Bake until lightly golden and cooked through, approximately 15–20 minutes. Cookies will last for 4 days in an airtight container.

⚜ Italian Living Tradition ⚜

Many Italian towns and regions have their own culinary traditions for honoring the departed. *Pan dei morti* (bread of the dead) as well as *ossa dei morti* (bones of the dead) cookies are also prepared in many places. Today, some of these ancient customs are being left behind for the much more commercial and seemingly "modern" appeal of Halloween, but some areas still uphold them.

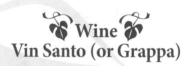

🍇 Wine 🍇
Vin Santo (or Grappa)

PIEMONTESE "UGLY BUT GOOD" COOKIES
(BRUTTI MA BUONI)

Serves: 10 | Serving Size: 2 cookies
Prep Time: 15 minutes | Cooking Time: Approximately 25 minutes

While these cookies originally come from the northern Italian province of Piedmont, they are popular in other Italian provinces as well. Antico Forno Molinari, a traditional bakery in Frascati, outside of Rome, has been making them since the 19th century. In Piedmont, bakers have their own variations on these cookies; they often use the same ingredients but change the amount of nuts that is chopped. For example, some people like to use half chopped hazelnuts and half whole hazelnuts.

1 1/2 cups whole hazelnuts plus 10 halved nuts, divided
3/4 cup confectioners' sugar
1/8 teaspoon unrefined sea salt
1 large egg white, lightly beaten
2 teaspoons pure vanilla extract
1 teaspoon pure honey

Choices/Exchanges 1 Carbohydrate, 3 Fat
Calories 190 | Calories from Fat 140
Total Fat 15g | Saturated Fat 1.1g | Trans Fat 0.0g
Cholesterol 0mg
Sodium 35mg

Potassium 165mg
Total Carbohydrate 14g | Dietary Fiber 3g | Sugars 10g
Protein 4g
Phosphorus 75mg

1. Preheat oven to 350°F.

2. Spread the hazelnuts on a large-rimmed baking sheet and toast for about 12 minutes, until the nuts are fragrant and the skins blister. Transfer the hazelnuts to a kitchen towel and let cool, then rub them together to remove their skins.

3. In a food processor, pulse the hazelnuts with the confectioners' sugar and salt until finely chopped. Scrape the hazelnut mixture into a medium bowl. Stir in the egg white, vanilla, and honey.

4. Line a baking sheet with parchment paper. Roll teaspoon-size mounds of the hazelnut dough into rough circles (they needn't be perfectly round). Place onto the prepared baking sheet 1 inch apart and place a halved hazelnut into the center. Press down slightly.

5. Bake the cookies in the center of the oven for about 14 minutes, or until browned in a few spots. (You can change the cooking time to about 13 minutes for chewy cookies or 15 minutes for slightly crisp cookies.)

6. Let the cookies cool on the baking sheet before serving.

⟨Italian Living Tradition⟩

These cookies can be stored in an airtight container for up to 4 days. Traditionally, this type of cookie would have been made during the hazelnut harvest. But any kind of nut can be used. Walnuts, almonds, or pistachios can be swapped for the hazelnuts in these scrumptious, gluten-free treats.

CINNAMON-INFUSED APPLE CAKE
(*TORTA DI MELA E CANELLA*)

Serves: 16 | Serving Size: 1 (3/4-inch) slice
Prep Time: 15 minutes | Cooking Time: 45 minutes

If you are looking to create a new breakfast, brunch, snack, teatime, or dessert favorite, this cake is for you. I think this cake is even better the day after it's made; the flavors continue to strengthen. This cake will stay fresh for a few days in a sealed container at room temperature. You can also wrap it in plastic wrap and aluminum foil and freeze it for up to a month.

Nonstick cooking spray

3/4 cup raw agave nectar

1/3 cup canola oil

3 large eggs

3 cups almond flour

3/4 cup powdered stevia

2 teaspoons pure cinnamon

1 teaspoon vanilla

4 large golden delicious apples, cored, peeled, and diced

1 tablespoon confectioners' sugar, for dusting

Choices/Exchanges 1 Fruit, 1/2 Carbohydrate, 2 Fat
Calories 190 | Calories from Fat 130
Total Fat 14g | Saturated Fat 1.2g | Trans Fat 0.0g
Cholesterol 25mg
Sodium 15mg

Potassium 185mg
Total Carbohydrate 28g | Dietary Fiber 3g | Sugars 5g
Protein 5g
Phosphorus 105mg

1. Preheat oven to 350°F. Grease a 10-inch spring-form cake pan with nonstick cooking spray.

2. Place the agave nectar, oil, and eggs in a medium bowl, and mix to combine. Stir in the almond flour, mixing well to combine. Add the stevia, cinnamon, and vanilla, and mix well to combine. Stir in apples.

3. Spoon the batter into the greased cake pan, spread the mixture evenly, and smooth the top. Shake the pan to ensure that there are no gaps in the batter.

4. Bake on the center rack of the oven for 40–45 minutes, or until a knife or toothpick inserted in the center of the cake comes out clean.

5. Remove cake from the oven and allow to cool to room temperature.

6. Remove cake from the pan, dust with confectioners' sugar, and serve.

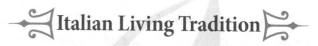

Italian Living Tradition

Rustic, farmhouse-style desserts like this one are best enjoyed in the fall. I like to serve this cake after a meal consisting of a bean soup such as Barley, Chestnut, and White Bean Minestrone (page 54), Cannellini Bean, Tomato, and Orzo Soup (page 56), or Farmhouse Vegetable and Farro Soup (page 58), and a salad such as Belgian Endive, Radicchio, and Grapefruit Salad (page 191), or Arugula Salad with Pears, Parmesan, and Cocoa Nibs (page 192).

IVREA'S POLENTA CAKE
(POLENTINA DI IVREA)

Serves: 12 | Serving Size: 1 (3/4-inch) slice
Prep Time: 15 minutes | Cooking Time: 30 minutes

There is a town in the province of Torin (in Piedmont) named Ivrea, which is the home of a famous polenta cake created in 1922 called "La polenta di Ivrea." This cake is traditionally covered with a drizzle of honey and orange juice. I created this recipe as a diabetes-friendly alternative to the original. Fortunately, everyone who tries it loves it and is surprised to learn that it is diabetes friendly—and naturally gluten-free. You can turn to this easy, straightforward cake for a delicious addition to brunch, teatime, or dessert.

2/3 cup expeller-pressed canola or vegetable oil, plus extra for greasing pan

1 cup natural sugar

1/2 cup almond flour

1 cup fine polenta (or cornmeal)

1 1/2 teaspoons baking powder (use gluten-free, if needed)

3 large eggs

Zest of 2 lemons

1 teaspoon vanilla

Juice of 1 orange, for drizzling (optional)

Choices/Exchanges 1 1/2 Carbohydrate, 2 Fat
Calories 200 | Calories from Fat 90
Total Fat 10g | Saturated Fat 1.0g | Trans Fat 0.0g
Cholesterol 45mg
Sodium 80mg

Potassium 100mg
Total Carbohydrate 26g | Dietary Fiber 2g | Sugars 18g
Protein 4g
Phosphorus 80mg

1. Preheat oven to 350°F. Line the base of a 9-inch springform cake pan with baking parchment and grease bottom and sides lightly with canola oil.

2. Combine 2/3 cup canola oil and sugar, either by hand in a bowl with a wooden spoon or using a freestanding mixer, until pale and fully combined.

3. Mix together the almond flour, polenta, and baking powder, and beat part of this dry mixture into the oil/sugar mixture, followed by 1 egg. Then alternate adding the dry ingredients and eggs, beating all the while, until all of the dry mixture and eggs are incorporated. Finally, beat in the lemon zest and vanilla, and pour, spoon, or scrape the mixture into your prepared cake pan.

4. Bake for about 30 minutes, or until lightly golden and a cake tester or toothpick inserted into the center comes out clean. The edges of the cake should have begun to shrink away from sides of the pan.

5. Remove from the oven and allow to cool completely. Release the sides of the pan and invert cake onto a cake platter. Drizzle with orange juice, if desired. Serve immediately, or store at room temperature overnight or in the refrigerator for up to 3 days.

Italian Living Tradition

This cake is the northern Italian answer to popular Mediterranean semolina cakes, which are doused with simple syrup and served as very sweet desserts. Made with just a few pantry ingredients, this is the type of cake that Italian housewives would whip up upon the arrival of unexpected guests or to serve with the Sunday meal.

FLOURLESS CHOCOLATE CAKE
(TORTA CAPRESE)

Serves: 12 | Serving Size: 1/12 cake
Prep Time: 15 minutes | Cooking Time: 35–40 minutes

Torta Caprese means "Capri-style cake" in Italian. Because it contains no flour, this cake works well for people who are gluten-intolerant, and it makes a perfect Passover dessert. The original version of this cake contains no almond flour, additional chocolate, and butter. I have lightened up the recipe and added the berry accompaniment to make this rich dessert diabetes-friendly.

1 cup mixed berries

1 tablespoon good-quality balsamic vinegar

1 tablespoon (21 grams) stevia powder

Nonstick cooking spray

1/3 cup dark chocolate chips

1/4 cup hot espresso or strong coffee

2 teaspoons vanilla extract

1 egg white

1 egg, yolk and white separated, divided

2/3 cup canola oil

2/3 cup raw agave nectar

1/2 cup unsweetened cocoa powder

1/2 cup almond flour

Choices/Exchanges 1 Carbohydrate, 3 Fat
Calories 190 | Calories from Fat 150
Total Fat 17g | Saturated Fat 2.3g | Trans Fat 0.0g
Cholesterol 15mg
Sodium 15mg

Potassium 160mg
Total Carbohydrate 12g | Dietary Fiber 3g | Sugars 4g
Protein 3g
Phosphorus 65mg

1. Combine the berries with balsamic vinegar and stevia in a medium bowl. Stir to combine, cover, and set aside at room temperature until serving cake. (If you are serving the cake the next day, you can store the berries in the refrigerator.)

2. Preheat oven to 350°F. With nonstick cooking spray, grease a springform pan that is 9 inches in diameter with 2 3/4-inch-high sides. Line bottom of the pan with parchment paper.

3. In a large glass or metal bowl, stir chocolate chips, hot espresso, and vanilla together until chocolate is melted and mixture is smooth. Allow mixture to cool until lukewarm.

4. Using clean beaters and a standing electric mixer, beat 2 egg whites until stiff peaks form.

5. In a separate bowl, whisk egg yolk, canola oil, and agave nectar until batter is smooth and resembles maple syrup in consistency. Stir in cocoa powder and almond flour, mixing well until incorporated.

6. Fold egg yolk mixture into lukewarm chocolate mixture. Fold in egg whites 1/3 at a time.

7. Place prepared cake pan on a baking sheet. Transfer batter to pan. Bake until a cake tester or toothpick inserted into center comes out with moist crumbs attached, about 35–40 minutes.

8. Cool cake for 5 minutes, then gently press down the edges. Let cake cool completely in pan.

(Cake can be prepared up to 1 day ahead. If preparing ahead of time, cover with plastic wrap and refrigerate. Let stand at room temperature 1 hour before continuing.) Run knife around pan sides to loosen cake. Remove sides of pan; transfer cake to platter. Remove parchment paper, and serve.

Italian Living Tradition

You can make this into a lemon-flavored *Torta Caprese* by omitting the chocolate chips and instead adding the grated zest of 3 lemons and the juice of 1 lemon.

TUSCAN FIG, WALNUT, AND FENNEL SEED TORTE
(TORTA DI FICCHI, NOCI, E SEMI DI FINOCCHIO)

Serves: 14 | Serving Size: 1 (1/2-inch) slice
Prep Time: 15 minutes | Cooking Time: 25–30 minutes

This traditional, dense torte is a family favorite that I often make for my father. When I used to teach cake-baking workshops for beginners, I was often pleasantly surprised that people preferred this cake over the super-sugary cakes often served at birthday parties. You can make this recipe ahead of time and freeze it. It also travels well and makes a great host/hostess gift. The original version of this dish uses regular flour and sugar instead of the combination of corn and rice flour and the agave nectar in this gluten-free recipe. Try serving thin slices with breakfast, brunch, or afternoon tea or coffee.

1/4 cup plus 1 teaspoon canola oil, divided
1/3 cup corn flour, plus extra for pan
1/3 cup rice flour
2 teaspoons baking powder (use gluten-free, if needed)
1 teaspoon fennel seeds, crushed in a mortar
1/4 teaspoon salt
4 large eggs, separated, divided
1/2 cup powdered stevia
1 teaspoon vanilla
5 ounces chopped dried white figs
1 cup walnuts, toasted and chopped, divided
1/2 cup low-fat, low-sugar vanilla yogurt (for garnish)
3 medium fresh figs (for garnish)
Handful of fresh mint leaves (for garnish)

Choices/Exchanges 1 Fruit, 1/2 Carbohydrate, 2 Fat
Calories 190 | Calories from Fat 110
Total Fat 12g | Saturated Fat 1.4g | Trans Fat 0.0g
Cholesterol 55mg
Sodium 140mg

Potassium 190mg
Total Carbohydrate 24g | Dietary Fiber 2g | Sugars 7g
Protein 4g
Phosphorus 110mg

1. Preheat oven to 350°F. Grease (with 1 teaspoon canola oil) and flour a 9-inch springform pan.

2. Mix corn flour, rice flour, baking powder, fennel seeds, and salt in a small bowl.

3. Beat egg yolks and stevia together in another bowl until thick and pale yellow, about 3 minutes. Slowly beat in 1/4 cup canola oil and vanilla. Stir in the flour mixture, then the figs and 1/2 cup walnuts.

4. Using clean beaters, beat egg whites in a separate bowl until stiff peaks form. Stir 1/3 of the egg whites into batter, then carefully fold in the remaining egg whites.

5. Transfer batter to the prepared pan. Bake cake in the center of the oven until a cake tester or toothpick inserted into center comes out clean, about 25–30 minutes.

6. Cool cake in the pan on a rack. Place cake on a platter and garnish with yogurt, fresh figs, and mint. Serve.

❖Italian Living Tradition❖

While they may seem rustic compared to the more elevated pastry creations of today's bakers, fruit-and-nut–studded cakes like this one were served as offerings to the gods in antiquity. Homestyle or *casareccio*-style cakes like these are usually served at breakfast and snack time.

BASILICATA-STYLE CHESTNUT CAKE (*CASTAGNACCIO LUCANO*)

Serves: 24 | Serving Size: 1 (3/4-inch) slice
Prep Time: 15 minutes | Cooking Time: 30 minutes

The Italian word castagnaccio *refers to a sweet or savory cake or bread made from chestnuts or chestnut flour. Dense chestnut groves are prominent throughout Italy, and the southern Italian region of Basilicata is no exception. In this magical region, I am aware of three varieties of this cake—all of which are traditional Christmastime treats. One version is made like a pie (or* crostata, *in Italian) with a chocolate-chestnut filling between a layer of crust and lattice dough on the top. A second version is a mini pastry-dough calzone with the same filling. This recipe makes a very dense, intensely chestnut-flavored cake, which is probably better served as a snack or for breakfast, because it is less sweet than many other desserts. The honey from the mountains in Basilicata is very special and adds a lot of flavor to traditional versions of this cake; try to use organic, local, wildflower honey in this recipe for that great honey flavor.*

Nonstick cooking spray

3 eggs, separated, divided

1/4 cup raw agave nectar

1/2 cup organic local wildflower honey

1 tablespoon vanilla

1 3/4 cups skim milk

1/2 cup expeller-pressed canola or vegetable oil

4 cups chestnut flour (see Where to Buy Guide)

1 tablespoon active dry yeast

1/3 cup good-quality cocoa powder

1/8 teaspoon unrefined sea salt

1 teaspoon ground cloves

Zest of 1 orange

1/2 cup chopped, peeled, roasted chestnuts, walnuts, or raisins

---

Choices/Exchanges 1 Carbohydrate, 3 Fat
Calories 200 | Calories from Fat 140
Total Fat 15g | Saturated Fat 1.4g | Trans Fat 0.0g
Cholesterol 25mg
Sodium 30mg

Potassium 195mg
Total Carbohydrate 13g | Dietary Fiber 3g | Sugars 9g
Protein 6g
Phosphorus 130mg

1. Preheat oven to 350°F. Grease 2 (9-inch) baking pans with nonstick cooking spray, line with parchment paper, and spray the top of the parchment and sides of pans again.

2. In the bowl of a standing mixer fitted with the whisk attachment, or in a large metal bowl using electric beaters, whisk the egg whites on high speed until stiff peaks form. Transfer to another bowl.

3. Add egg yolks, agave nectar, and honey to mixer bowl and switch to a paddle attachment. Mix on medium speed until combined, approximately 1 minute. Reduce speed to low, and add in vanilla, milk, and oil. Mix until combined. Next add in chestnut flour, yeast, cocoa, salt, cloves, and orange zest.

4. When combined, remove bowl from mixer, and stir in chestnuts (or walnuts or raisins). Fold in egg whites, 1/3 at a time, being careful not to deflate them.

5. Divide mixture evenly into both pans. Smooth out the top with a spatula, and tap the bottoms of pans lightly on the counter.

6. Place onto the center rack of the oven and bake until a toothpick inserted in the center comes out clean and the cake begins to pull away from the edges of the pan, approximately 30 minutes.

❧Italian Living Tradition ❧

Chestnut flour is low in fat and calories, and many people consider it to be a good alternative to almond flour in recipes. It is most often used in the fall and winter for making breads, fritters, and pastas to pair with rich sauces.

PEAR, RICOTTA, AND PINE NUT CAKE
(TORTA SOFFICE DI PERE CON RICOTTA E PINOLI)

Serves: 18 | Serving Size: 1 (1/2-inch) slice
Prep Time: 15 minutes (plus raisin-soaking time) | Cooking Time: 40–50 minutes

Sicily's famed ricotta cheese plays a leading role in the region's most prized desserts. Everything from cannoli alla Siciliana to cassata cakes highlights this smooth, creamy cheese by-product, which is made from the whey of cow's milk cheese. Luckily, many organic, gourmet, and Italian grocers now sell high-quality ricotta. Sometimes, you can even find artisan-made, hand-dipped ricotta. If you go to an Italian deli that makes cannolis, ask them for some of their ricotta to use in this cake—they usually keep it in the back.

3/4 pound skim milk ricotta

2/3 cup raw agave nectar

4 large egg whites

1/4 cup natural sugar

1 cup golden raisins, soaked in 3/4 cup orange juice for 20 minutes

6 ounces pine nuts

Grated zest of 2 oranges

6 large egg yolks, whisked until foamy

4 large pears, peeled, diced or grated in a food processor, and drained of excess liquid

2 tablespoons confectioners' sugar (for garnish)

Choices/Exchanges 1 Fruit, 1/2 Carbohydrate, 2 Fat
Calories 200 | Calories from Fat 90
Total Fat 10g | Saturated Fat 2.0g | Trans Fat 0.0g
Cholesterol 65mg
Sodium 35mg

Potassium 230mg
Total Carbohydrate 27g | Dietary Fiber 3g | Sugars 19g
Protein 6g
Phosphorus 130mg

1. Preheat oven to 350°F. Grease and flour a 10-inch springform pan.

2. Place the ricotta and agave nectar in a large bowl and mix until ricotta is smooth.

3. Beat the egg whites on high speed with sugar until stiff peaks form.

4. Drain the raisins, pat them dry, and dice them. Add the pine nuts, orange zest, raisins, egg yolks, and pears to the ricotta mixture, and mix with a wooden spoon until incorporated.

5. Fold egg whites into ricotta mixture with a spatula, stirring counterclockwise. (Start at the "3 o'clock" position and turn your wrist counter-clockwise until you reach the same point.) Continue folding in the egg whites just until they are incorporated and mixture is smooth.

6. Pour the mixture into the prepared pan and hit pan on the counter a few times to release air bubbles. Position a rack in the center of the oven, and bake cake until a knife inserted in the top comes out clean, 40–50 minutes.

7. Cool to room temperature, sprinkle with confectioners' sugar, and cut into thin wedges to serve.

Italian Living Tradition

The combination of golden raisins, pine nuts, and orange zest gives this cake a uniquely Sicilian flair. Keep in mind that those same flavors make a great addition to savory rice pilafs and cookies as well.

COCONUT AND CHOCOLATE PUDDING
(BUDINO DI NOCE DI COCCO E CIOCCOLATO)

Serves: 8 | Serving Size: 1/2 cup

Prep Time: 5 minutes (plus approximately 2 1/2 hours cooling time) | Cooking Time: 5 minutes

The decadent combination of creamy coconut milk and rich chocolate in this recipe will make it hard for anyone to believe that it is diabetes-friendly. Cool and comforting, this chocolaty dessert is a welcome treat for all age groups. This can be frozen in an ice cream maker, if desired.

1/2 cup unsweetened cocoa powder (preferably natural)

4 cups skim milk, divided

1 teaspoon pure vanilla extract

1/2 cup raw agave nectar

2 tablespoons cornstarch

1/4 cup organic dried coconut flakes or fresh coconut flakes (for garnish)

Choices/Exchanges 1 Carbohydrate, 1/2 Fat
Calories 100 | Calories from Fat 30
Total Fat 3g | Saturated Fat 2.5g | Trans Fat 0.0g
Cholesterol 0mg
Sodium 70mg

Potassium 325mg
Total Carbohydrate 14g | Dietary Fiber 3g | Sugars 7g
Protein 6g
Phosphorus 175mg

1. Add cocoa to a medium bowl and whisk in just enough milk (about 2/3 cup) to make a smooth paste. Stir in vanilla. Set aside.

2. Mix agave and cornstarch in a medium sauce-pan. Gradually whisk in the remaining milk. Heat over medium heat, stirring frequently with a wooden spoon or heatproof spatula, until the mixture begins to barely simmer around the edges. Then, stirring constantly and scraping the sides and corners of the pan to prevent scorch-ing, let the mixture simmer for 2 1/2–3 minutes to fully cook the cornstarch.

3. Scrape the hot mixture into the bowl with the cocoa mixture. Whisk until well blended.

4. Cool by placing the bowl in an ice bath for about 45 minutes.

5. Transfer mixture to a deep, 9-inch, freezer-safe container or baking dish and cover with plastic wrap. Put into the freezer.

6. After 1 1/2 hours, open the freezer and check the mixture. As it starts to freeze near the edges, remove it from the freezer and stir it vigorously with a spatula or whisk. Serve immediately or transfer to the refrigerator to store. Garnish with coconut flakes before serving.

⊰ Italian Living Tradition ⊱

Budini, or puddings, are a part of the classic *cucina casalinga,* or housewives' (or home cooks') repertoire, in Italy. They're simple desserts that can be whipped up with only a few cupboard ingredients and then shared enthusiastically with family. On Sundays, holidays, and special occasions, puddings are used as fillings for cakes or served with cake or cookies and fruit for a more elaborate dessert.

HOW TO COOK LIKE AN ITALIAN

282 Roasted Peppers/*Peperoni arrostiti*

283 Dried Beans/*Fagioli secchi*

284 Braised Cannellini Beans/*Fagioli cannellini*

285 Lentils/*Lenticchie*

286 Polenta/*Polenta*

287 Homemade Vegetable Stock/*Brodo di verdura*

288 Homemade Seafood Stock/*Brodo di pesce*

289 Homemade Chicken Stock/*Brodo di pollo*

290 Homemade Meat Stock/*Brodo di carne*

291 Fresh Bread Crumbs/*Molliche di pane*

292 Homemade Croutons/*Crostini*

"Tutto fa brodo."
"Every little bit counts."
—Italian proverb

These simple recipes are the backbone of the Italian kitchen. Replacing store-bought ingredients with these homemade staple ingredients will improve the overall taste of your dishes, and save you time and money, while cutting excess sodium, calories, and preservatives from your meals. Whenever I prepare these recipes, I make them in large quantities and store them; every recipe in this chapter can be prepared and then frozen for later use. With roasted peppers, stocks, beans, lentils, and fresh bread crumbs in your freezer, you'll always be prepared to whip up healthful, inexpensive soups, pastas, salads, and purées in no time.

ROASTED PEPPERS
(PEPERONI ARROSTITI)

Serving Size: 1/2 large pepper
Prep Time: 5 minutes (plus 30 minutes cooling time)
Cooking Time: Approximately 30–40 minutes

Bell peppers (any color)
Olive oil

1. Preheat oven to 500°F. Place whole bell peppers on a baking sheet and place in the oven for 30–40 minutes, or until the skins are wrinkled and peppers are charred, turning them each time a side is charred (approximately twice during cooking).

2. Remove peppers from oven and cover tightly with aluminum foil to create steam. Set aside.

3. When peppers are cool enough to handle, after approximately 30 minutes, cut into quarters, peel off skin, and remove seeds. Place pepper pieces in a jar, cover with olive oil, and seal with a lid. (Drain oil from peppers before using.) Refrigerate for up to 2 weeks. Alternatively, place pepper pieces in a sealable plastic bag and freeze until using.

Choices/Exchanges 1 Vegetable
Calories 25 | Calories from Fat 0
Total Fat 0g | Saturated Fat 0.0g | Trans Fat 0.0g
Cholesterol 0mg
Sodium 0mg

Potassium 175mg
Total Carbohydrate 5g | Dietary Fiber 2g | Sugars 3g
Protein 1g
Phosphorus 20mg

DRIED BEANS
(FAGIOLI SECCHI)

Serving Size: 1/2 cup cooked beans
Prep Time: 1 hour (or overnight) bean-soaking time
Cooking Time: Approximately 25–50 minutes

Purchasing dried beans and cooking them yourself is more economical and healthful than purchasing the canned variety. Popular bean types used in Italian recipes include cannellini beans, borlotti (cranberry) beans, fava beans, chickpeas, and broad beans. All of these can be prepared in advance using this recipe and then stored in the refrigerator for up to a week for later use in various other recipes.

Dried beans (any variety)
1/4 teaspoon unrefined sea salt

1. All beans must be soaked overnight in cold water, or covered in boiling water for 1 hour prior to cooking.

2. To prepare, drain the soaked beans and place them in a saucepan. Add salt, cover beans with water, and bring to a boil over high heat.

3. Reduce heat to medium-low, cover, and let cook until beans are tender, about 25–50 minutes. (This may take longer depending on the size of the beans.)

4. Drain and cool. If not using right away, store beans in an airtight container in the refrigerator for up to 1 week.

Choices/Exchanges 1 1/2 Starch
Calories 110 | Calories from Fat 0
Total Fat 0g | Saturated Fat 0.0g | Trans Fat 0.0g
Cholesterol 0mg
Sodium 120mg

Potassium 370mg
Total Carbohydrate 20g | Dietary Fiber 8g | Sugars 0g
Protein 8g
Phosphorus 120mg

BRAISED CANNELLINI BEANS
(FAGIOLI CANNELLINI)

Serves: 4 | Serving Size: 1/2 cup
Prep Time: 8 hours (or overnight) bean-soaking time
Cooking Time: 30–40 minutes

1 cup dried cannellini beans
4 rosemary sprigs, divided
1 tablespoon extra virgin olive oil
1/4 teaspoon unrefined sea salt

1. In a large bowl, add cannellini beans and enough cold water to cover them by 4 inches. Let soak in a cool place or in the refrigerator for at least 8 hours or overnight.

2. Drain the beans and transfer them to a 2-quart saucepan. Pour in enough water to cover by 2 fingers, and drop in 2 rosemary sprigs. Bring the water to a boil, and then lower the heat so the water is barely at a simmer. Cook until the beans are tender but not mushy, with just enough liquid to cover them, about 30–40 minutes. (If necessary, add more water, 1 tablespoon at a time, to keep the beans covered as they simmer.)

3. Remove the beans from the heat and gently stir in olive oil, sea salt, and 2 more rosemary sprigs. Let the beans stand to cool and absorb the cooking liquid. The end result should be tender beans with a creamy consistency in just enough liquid to coat them. If not using right away, store beans in an air-tight container in the refrigerator for up to 1 week.

Choices/Exchanges 1 1/2 Starch, 1/2 Fat
Calories 140 | Calories from Fat 35
Total Fat 4g | Saturated Fat 0.6g | Trans Fat 0.0g
Cholesterol 0mg
Sodium 120mg

Potassium 345mg
Total Carbohydrate 19g | Dietary Fiber 6g | Sugars 0g
Protein 7g
Phosphorus 145mg

LENTILS
(LENTICCHIE)

Serving Size: 1/2 cup
Prep Time: 1 minute | Cooking Time: 5–30 minutes

Unlike beans, lentils do not need to be soaked overnight. Instead, simply pour the lentils into a shallow bowl and sort through them with your fingers, making sure that there are no stones or unwanted particles.

Dried lentils (any variety)
1/4 teaspoon unrefined sea salt
1/4 teaspoon freshly ground black pepper
1 bay leaf

1. Rinse the lentils in a colander.

2. Place lentils in a saucepan and add enough water to cover the lentils twice. Add sea salt, pepper, and the bay leaf. Bring to boil over high heat. Then reduce heat to low and simmer, uncovered, until lentils are tender, about 5–30 minutes depending on the variety. (Red lentils are the quickest-cooking variety, followed by green and brown, and then black.)

3. If not using right away, store cooked lentils in an airtight container in the refrigerator for up to 1 week.

Choices/Exchanges 1 1/2 Starch
Calories 120 | Calories from Fat 5
Total Fat 0.5g | Saturated Fat 0.0g | Trans Fat 0.0g
Cholesterol 0mg
Sodium 120mg

Potassium 365mg
Total Carbohydrate 20g | Dietary Fiber 8g | Sugars 2g
Protein 9g
Phosphorus 180mg

POLENTA
(POLENTA)

Serves: 8 | Serving Size: 1/2 cup
Prep Time: 2 minutes | Cooking Time: Approximately 30 minutes

Cornmeal is a staple ingredient throughout Italy today. Polenta is an easy and delicious side dish.

4 cups water (or more, if needed)
1 cup dried polenta
1/4 teaspoon unrefined sea salt
1/4 teaspoon freshly ground black pepper

1. Add 4 cups water to a medium saucepan and bring to a boil over high heat. Slowly pour in the polenta by the handful in a gentle stream, stirring and whisking simultaneously with a whisk or wooden spoon to avoid lumps. Continue stirring until mixture starts to thicken, about 3 minutes.

2. Lower heat to medium-low (or a temperature that allows a very low simmer) and cook for at least 20–25 minutes, stirring about every 5 minutes. Be sure to crush any lumps that may form against the side of the pan. If the polenta is too thick, add 1/2 cup water to soften it. Polenta is done when it easily comes away from the sides of the pan. Add sea salt and pepper.

3. Remove saucepan from heat and cool, allowing polenta to solidify. If not using right away, store polenta in an airtight container in the refrigerator for up to 1 week.

Choices/Exchanges 1 1/2 Starch
Calories 110 | Calories from Fat 5
Total Fat 0.5g | Saturated Fat 0.0g | Trans Fat 0.0g
Cholesterol 0mg
Sodium 270mg

Potassium 50mg
Total Carbohydrate 24g | Dietary Fiber 1g | Sugars 1g
Protein 2g
Phosphorus 30mg

STOCKS
(BRODO)

I highly recommend making your own stocks because they taste better, are more economical, and contain far less sodium than commercial varieties. Try making stock in large quantities and freezing it, preportioned, so that you'll always have it on hand to add to your favorite recipes. Each of these recipes yields about 3 1/2 quarts (14 cups) of stock.

Homemade Vegetable Stock
(Brodo di verdura)

Serves: 14 | Serving Size: 1 cup
Prep Time: 5 minutes | Cooking Time: 30 minutes

1 onion, peeled and halved

1 carrot, peeled, trimmed, and halved

1 stalk celery, trimmed and halved (can include leaves, if desired)

1/4 pound (4 ounces) cherry tomatoes

4 sprigs fresh basil, with stems

1 small bunch fresh flat-leaf parsley, with stems

1/2 teaspoon salt

1. In a large stock pot, place the onion, carrot, celery, cherry tomatoes, basil, and parsley. Cover with 4 quarts (16 cups) water. Bring to a boil over high heat, then reduce heat to medium-low. Add salt and simmer, uncovered, for 30 minutes.

2. Drain stock, reserving liquid. Discard the rest.

Choices/Exchanges Free Food
Calories 5 | Calories from Fat 0
Total Fat 0g | Saturated Fat 0.0g | Trans Fat 0.0g
Cholesterol 0mg
Sodium 75mg

Potassium 30mg
Total Carbohydrate 1g | Dietary Fiber 0g | Sugars 0g
Protein 0g
Phosphorus 5mg

Homemade Seafood Stock
(*Brodo di pesce*)

Serves: 14 | Serving Size: 1 cup
Prep Time: 5 minutes | Cooking Time: 30 minutes

1 onion, peeled and halved
1 carrot, peeled, trimmed, and halved
1 stalk celery, trimmed and halved
Shells from 2 pounds shrimp
1/2 teaspoon salt
1 dried bay leaf
1 tablespoon whole black peppercorns

1. In a large stock pot, place onion, carrot, celery, and shrimp shells. Cover with 4 quarts (16 cups) water. Bring to a boil over high heat, then reduce heat to medium-low.

2. Skim off the residue that forms on top of the stock and discard. Add salt, bay leaf, and peppercorns. Simmer, uncovered, for about 30 minutes.

3. Drain stock, reserving liquid. Discard the rest.

Choices/Exchanges Free Food
Calories 5 | Calories from Fat 0
Total Fat 0g | Saturated Fat 0.0g | Trans Fat 0.0g
Cholesterol 0mg
Sodium 75mg

Potassium 25mg
Total Carbohydrate 1g | Dietary Fiber 0g | Sugars 0g
Protein 0g
Phosphorus 5mg

Homemade Chicken Stock
(*Brodo di pollo*)

Serves: 14 | Serving Size: 1 cup
Prep Time: 5 minutes | Cooking Time: 40 minutes

1 medium onion, peeled and cut in half
1 medium carrot, peeled, trimmed, and cut in half
1 medium stalk celery, trimmed and cut in half
1 1/4 pounds chicken bones or carcasses
1 teaspoon whole black peppercorns
1 dried bay leaf
1/2 teaspoon salt

1. In a large stock pot, place onion, carrot, celery, chicken bones, peppercorns, and bay leaf. Cover with 4 quarts (16 cups) water. Bring to a boil over high heat, then reduce heat to medium-low.

2. Skim off the residue that forms on top of the stock and discard. Add salt and simmer, uncovered, for 40 minutes.

3. Drain stock, reserving liquid. Discard the rest.

Choices/Exchanges Free Food
Calories 10 | Calories from Fat 0
Total Fat 0g | Saturated Fat 0.0g | Trans Fat 0.0g
Cholesterol 0mg
Sodium 75mg

Potassium 35mg
Total Carbohydrate 1g | Dietary Fiber 0g | Sugars 0g
Protein 1g
Phosphorus 10mg

Homemade Meat Stock
(Brodo di carne)

Serves: 14 | Serving Size: 1 cup
Prep Time: 5 minutes | Cooking Time: 1 hour

1 medium onion, peeled and cut in half

1 medium carrot, peeled, trimmed, and cut in half

1 medium stalk celery, trimmed and cut in half

3 pounds beef, veal, lamb, or goat bones (shin, leg, rib, or collar), cut into 4-inch pieces

1 dried bay leaf

1 teaspoon peppercorns

1/2 teaspoon salt

1. In a large stock pot, place onion (can be grilled first, if desired), carrot, celery, bones, bay leaf, and peppercorns. Cover with 4 quarts (16 cups) water. Bring to a boil over high heat, then reduce heat to medium-low.

2. Skim off the residue that forms on top of the stock and discard. Add salt and simmer, uncovered, for 40 minutes.

3. Drain stock, reserving liquid. Discard the rest.

Choices/Exchanges Free Food
Calories 5 | Calories from Fat 0
Total Fat 0g | Saturated Fat 0.0g | Trans Fat 0.0g
Cholesterol 0mg
Sodium 75mg

Potassium 35mg
Total Carbohydrate 1g | Dietary Fiber 0g | Sugars 0g
Protein 1g
Phosphorus 5mg

FRESH BREAD CRUMBS
(MOLLICHE DI PANE)

Serves: 16 | Serving Size: 1/4 cup
Prep Time: 5 minutes | Cooking Time: 0 minutes

You'll be amazed at the difference switching from store-bought to fresh bread crumbs will make in your recipes. Try using one of the bread recipes from this book.

1 (8-ounce) loaf dense, day-old country-style bread

1. Cut the loaf of bread into 1-inch cubes and, working in batches if necessary, place them in a food processor, being careful not to fill it more than halfway. Pulse on and off until the crumbs are as fine as possible.

2. If not using immediately, freeze bread crumbs in a plastic freezer bag for up to a month.

Choices/Exchanges 1/2 Starch
Calories 30 | Calories from Fat 5
Total Fat 0.5g | Saturated Fat 0.0g | Trans Fat 0.0g
Cholesterol 0mg
Sodium 55mg

Potassium 15mg
Total Carbohydrate 6g | Dietary Fiber 0g | Sugars 0g
Protein 1g
Phosphorus 10mg

HOMEMADE CROUTONS
(CROSTINI)

Serves: 4 | Serving Size: 1 cup
Prep Time: 5 minutes | Cooking Time: 2–5 minutes

2 (1/4-inch) slices Italian bread or any gluten-free bread
1 tablespoon extra virgin olive oil

1. Preheat the broiler to high.

2. Cut slices of Italian or gluten-free bread into 1-inch cubes and place on a baking sheet. Drizzle olive oil onto the bread cubes and toss to combine.

3. Place under the broiler and toast until golden, 1–2 minutes on each side.

Choices/Exchanges 1 Fat
Calories 45 | Calories from Fat 35
Total Fat 4g | Saturated Fat 0.5g | Trans Fat 0.0g
Cholesterol 0mg
Sodium 30mg

Potassium 5mg
Total Carbohydrate 3g | Dietary Fiber 0g | Sugars 0g
Protein 0g
Phosphorus 5 mg

THE ITALIAN PANTRY

The foundation of any good *cucina* is its pantry. Italian cooks have always relied upon well-stocked pantries to create traditional foods. *La dispensa*, the pantry, was traditionally a place where summer produce could be preserved for the winter months and spices, olive oil, and aged cheeses could be stored. While we now have modern refrigerators and freezers, it is still important to develop your pantry.

Keeping a well-stocked pantry helps modern cooks save time and money. When time is of the essence, it's great to be able to open up your cupboard and create a delicious meal in minutes—often in less time than it takes to wait at a restaurant or order delivery. By keeping healthful, good-quality products around, you'll have less need to eat out. Your pantry can transform snow days and bad weather into an opportunity to enjoy delicious meals in your own home. With a little planning and effort, a well-stocked pantry can also save you money; try stocking up on your favorite items the next time they are on sale. Buy in bulk and store what you don't need. Below, you'll find a list of common Italian pantry items. Use this list as a guide to help you fill your pantry and make the most out of your Italian cooking experience.

Due to the healthful nature of most Italian ingredients and the popularity of Italian cuisine, many of the ingredients in this book can be found in supermarkets, health food stores, or organic markets as well as Italian markets. These ingredients are increasingly available in most major supermarkets.

The Italian Culinary Glossary on page 295 gives definitions for some of the more unusual ingredients and explains where they can be purchased. And the Where to Buy Guide (page 299) lists current Internet resources that can help you get your hands on hard-to-find ingredients. If you need to substitute or omit an ingredient, don't feel bad! That's the way many delicious recipes have evolved over the centuries.

Common Pantry Items

Baking
Active dry yeast
Agave nectar
Almond extract
Almond flour
Baking powder
Baking soda
Cornstarch
Dehydrated coconut flakes (organic)
Kosher salt
Natural sugar
Pumpkin purée
Pure vanilla extract
Rice flour
Rye flour
Semolina
Unbleached all-purpose flour
Unrefined sea salt
Unsweetened cocoa powder (good quality)
Whole-wheat flour

Beans and Legumes
Brown lentils
Cannellini beans (dried and/or low-sodium canned)
Chickpeas (dried and/or no-salt-added canned)
Cranberry beans (dried and/or low-sodium canned)
Peeled fava beans (dried)

Herbs (Dried)
Oregano
Rosemary
Sage
Thyme

Italian Specialty
Anchovy fillets (packed in olive oil)
Artichoke hearts (canned)
Bread crumbs (plain)
Canned diced tomatoes (low sodium and fire roasted)
Canned tuna (packed in water)
Capers (packed in water)
Dried porcini mushrooms
Espresso coffee
Olives (oil cured, green and black, kalamata and gaeta)
Roasted red peppers (jarred)
Sun-dried tomatoes
Tomato paste (reduced sodium)
Tomato purée (reduced sodium)

Nuts and Dried Fruit
Almonds (blanched and raw)
Chestnuts (jarred or packaged, whole roasted or steamed)
Hazelnuts
Pine nuts
Pistachios (shelled)
Walnuts

Oils and Vinegars
Balsamic vinegar (preferably Aceto Balsamico di Modena)
Canola oil or vegetable oil (expeller-pressed)
Distilled white vinegar
Extra virgin olive oil (preferably first cold-pressed)
Nonstick cooking spray (organic)
Red wine vinegar
White wine vinegar

Pasta (Whole wheat or gluten-free)
Couscous
Ditalini
Fusilli
Orecchiette
Orzo
Pastina
Penne rigate
Spaghetti
Ziti

Rice and Grains
Arborio rice
Cornmeal/polenta
Farro
Spelt berries

Spices
Anise seeds
Bay leaves (dried)
Cloves (ground and whole)
Crushed red chile flakes (preferably from Calabria and Basilicata)
Cumin seeds
Fennel seeds
Kosher salt
Nutmeg
Pure cinnamon (ground and sticks)
Saffron
Unrefined sea salt
Whole black peppercorns

Cooking Wine
Dry white wine
Marsala

ITALIAN CULINARY GLOSSARY

⊙=Organic Market, **❶**=Italian Market, **❸**=Supermarket

Apertivo

This word comes from the French term *apér-itif*, derived from the Latin *aperire,* meaning "to open." The *apertivo* is to many Italians what happy hour is to Americans. You can meet friends in a bar after work and prior to dinner for an *apertivo*—drinks—and appetizers. During these occasions, a wide array of appetizers is served with the drinks.

Baby squid—⊙, ❶, ❸

Call your local market to make sure they have the smaller, tender variety of squid in stock before making a trip.

Baccalà—⊙, ❶, ❸

Salt-dried cod, reconstituted by soaking in water. It is typically served cold in a salad, boiled as a stew, or fried, and it's commonly served on Christmas Eve in Italy. Call stores first to check availability.

Besciamella

White sauce made with flour, butter, and milk. It is typically used in lasagna, as a pasta sauce, or as a dressing. This sauce is called *béchamel* in French.

Borlotti (cranberry) beans—⊙, ❶, ❸

Known as cranberry beans in the U.S., this type of bean is very popular in the Mediterranean region.

Branzino

Mediterranean sea bass. This firm-fleshed fish is usually grilled, roasted, or baked and is often served cold.

Bruschetta

Toasted bread rubbed with garlic and often topped with olive oil and fresh vegetables.

Cannellini beans—⊙, ❶, ❸

Also known as white kidney beans, cannellini beans are popular in the Mediterranean region.

Carpaccio

Raw beef thinly sliced and served with olive oil and capers. This dish was created as an antipasto at Harry's Bar in Venice in the 1950s; it was named after Venetian artist Vittore Carpaccio.

Casalinga, alla

This phrase means "housewife style." It is used to refer to homemade dishes or dishes cooked in a down-home style.

Castagne—⊙, ❶, ❸

Chestnuts, traditionally roasted over coals or boiled. Preroasted or steamed and peeled chestnuts can be purchased in vacuum-sealed jars or packages.

Cavatelli—⊙, ❶, ❸

Little "cave-shaped" pasta popular in the southern Italian regions of Basilicata, Calabria, and Puglia, where they are still made by hand. *Cavatelli* are appreciated for their ability to absorb liquid.

Cena

Dinner.

Chickpeas—⊙, ❶, ❸

Also known as garbanzo beans, chickpeas and their flour are common ingredients throughout the Mediterranean.

Colazione
Breakfast.

Contorno
Side dish that complements a main course.

Couscous—Ⓞ, Ⓘ, Ⓢ
Eaten predominately in North Africa, Sicily, and the eastern Mediterranean, couscous is a tiny, round pasta made of semolina and coarsely ground durum wheat flour. The name originates from the Berber word *k'seksu*. Traditionally hand rolled, manufactured couscous is available in instant varieties in supermarkets. Israeli couscous, known as *moghrabieh* in Arabic, consists of larger, pearl-like pasta beads and is a popular base for stews in the eastern Mediterranean.

Crostini
Toasted bread with a savory topping.

Digestivo—Ⓘ
An after-dinner drink that "aids digestion," such as amaro, grappa, or other liqueurs.

Dolce
Literally means "sweet." This is the Italian term for desserts.

DOP
An acronym that stands for *Denominazione di origine protetta* (Protected Designation of Origin, or PDO, in English). DOP is a designation used on the label of high-quality Italian foods to indicate that the product was locally made and packaged.

Dried apricots—Ⓞ, Ⓘ, Ⓢ
There were once more than 21 varieties of apricots in the Mediterranean. Choose the juiciest, plumpest fruit possible.

Dried figs—Ⓞ, Ⓘ, Ⓢ
Greece, the Italian region of Calabria, and Turkey export high-quality figs around the globe. Figs are available in white and black varieties, but it is the white fig that works best in the recipes in this book. If the only figs you can find are extremely dry, soak them in citrus juice or water for a few hours until they plump up.

Expeller-pressed canola and vegetable oils—Ⓞ, Ⓘ, Ⓢ
When cooking with oils other than olive oil, look for the words "expeller pressed" on the label; that means the oil was extracted without chemicals.

Fagioli—Ⓞ, Ⓘ, Ⓢ
The Italian word for beans. They are generally cooked freshly shelled or dried.

Fava beans, peeled—Ⓞ, Ⓢ
Used extensively in southern Italy, North Africa, and the Middle East, fava beans are one of the world's oldest crops. The peeled variety are white and require soaking before using.

First cold-pressed extra virgin olive oil—Ⓞ, Ⓘ, Ⓢ
This oil is extracted from the first pressing of the olives, which means better quality and flavor. True extra virgin olive oils are all first cold-pressed. Since many international consumers are not aware of this, many extra virgin olive oils sold outside of the Mediterranean region will say both "extra virgin" and "first cold pressed" on the label.

Fresh mozzarella (preferably buffalo milk)—Ⓞ, Ⓘ, Ⓢ

Because mozzarella is a fresh cheese, its quality is extremely important. Varieties made with buffalo milk have the richest flavor, and even though buffalo mozzarella is expensive, a little bit goes a long way. If buffalo-milk mozzarella is not available in your area, look for the freshest mozzarella possible.

Frutti di bosco

Berries such as raspberries, blueberries, blackberries, and strawberries.

Frutti di mare

The general term for seafood. This term mainly refers to mollusks and crustaceans, either raw or cooked.

Gnocchi

Potato, flour, or semolina dumplings generally served as a first course.

Goat cheese—Ⓞ, Ⓘ, Ⓢ

Goat cheese and other goat dairy products may be easier for people with lactose intolerance to digest. Look for the freshest variety possible.

Goat meat—Ⓞ, Ⓘ

Goat meat is growing in popularity in the U.S. because it's extremely low in fat and easy to digest. It can be a challenge to find, however. Call your local ethnic butchers to special-order, if possible, or see the Where to Buy Guide (page 299).

Grappa—Ⓘ

A clear brandy distilled from the pulp of crushed grapes.

Maccheroni—Ⓞ, Ⓘ

A type of pasta ranging in shape from the rigatoni-like to the slightly more elongated *casareccio*-style (homemade) shapes. *Maccheroni*

is often served with hearty tomato and meat sauces. The word *maccheroni* used to refer to a type of homemade pasta found throughout Italy and was used instead of the word *pasta*. This term is the origin for the English word *macaroni*.

Mascarpone—Ⓞ, Ⓘ, Ⓢ

Fresh, soft cream cheese. The unsweetened variety is used in pasta or risotto, while sweetened mascarpone is used with fruit or desserts like tiramisu.

Natural sugar—Ⓞ, Ⓢ

Also called "turbinado," natural sugar is a partially refined light brown cane sugar. For the recipes in this book, regular sugar or organic sugar can be substituted.

Parmigiano-reggiano cheese—Ⓞ, Ⓘ, Ⓢ

This is an aged cow's milk cheese from the Emilia-Romagna region of Italy. Italian law mandates that only parmigiano-reggiano cheese made in specific areas can be called by this name. Look for DOP (*Denominazione di origine protetta*/Protected Designation of Origin) varieties for the best quality.

Pearl barley—Ⓞ, Ⓢ

A variety of barley in which the hull and bran layers are removed. It is polished to give it the "pearl" name.

Pecorino Romano cheese—Ⓞ, Ⓘ, Ⓢ

An aged sheep's milk cheese from the Lazio region of Italy around Rome. The word *pecorino* denotes "coming from sheep," and many Italian areas have their own version of pecorino cheese. Pecorino varieties such as pecorino Crotonese, pecorino Sardo, pecorino di Moliterno, and many others have their own distinct flavors and are worth sampling if you can find them.

Peperoncini—◐, ❶

Hot chile peppers that are used mainly in southern Italy.

Peperoni di Senise—❶

Sweet red peppers from Senise that are sun-dried and sometimes finely ground. They are used as a seasoning in Basilicata.

Pesto—◐, ❶, ❺

A sauce originally mashed with a mortar and pestle. This term usually refers to the Genovese sauce made with basil leaves, olive oil, pine nuts, and grated cheese.

Polenta —◐, ❶, ❺

Cornmeal cooked slowly in water, milk, or broth. It can be served as a porridge, a side dish, or cooled and cut into squares, which are sometimes grilled, fried, or sauced with tomato.

Pranzo

Lunch.

Primo

A first course such as a pasta or rice dish.

Pure cinnamon—◐

In the Mediterranean region, "pure" cinnamon is used. It has a more mellow flavor than the American variety, which (by law) can be mixed with 20% cassia. In the store, look for "true cinnamon," sometimes also called Sri Lankan cinnamon or Ceylon cinnamon.

Ragù

A stewed or braised meat sauce.

Ricotta—◐, ❶, ❺

A soft cheese traditionally made from sheep or goat's milk. It can be eaten fresh or used as a filling for ravioli or pastries. Ricotta can also be salted (called *ricotta salata)*, dried, and used for grating.

Risotto—◐, ❶, ❺

A dish of creamy stubby rice—such as arborio or *carnaroli* rice—that is cooked slowly in broth to make it flavorful.

Saffron—◐, ❶, ❺

The world's most expensive spice, saffron is cultivated from the stigmas of the crocus flower in the autumn. Its English name is derived from the plural feminine form of the Arabic word for yellow—*saffra*. Saffron provides a bright yellow pigment and unique flavor to drinks, savory dishes, and sweets. Medicinally, saffron is said to have diuretic properties, increase energy, suppress coughs, rejuvenate the heart, and ease labor pains.

Saor, in

This term refers to the Venetian method of marinating fish in a sweet-and-sour mixture usually made of raisins, onions, pine nuts, and vinegar.

Secondo

The second course of a meal, usually the meat or fish course.

Semola—❶

The Italian term for semolina, the fine, yellow flour made from the heart of wheat. Semolina is used for pasta, gnocchi, breads, and desserts.

Sformato

A mold of cooked and minced vegetables. This term also refers to a dessert similar to custard or flan.

Spiedini

Skewers or kabobs.

Spuma

Literally means "foam"; the term for mousse.

Spuntino

Snack or light lunch, which can be either sweet or savory.

Stuzzichini

Appetizers or finger foods.

Unfiltered extra virgin olive oil—Ⓞ, Ⓘ

Unfiltered olive oil contains small particles of olive flesh, which reduce the shelf life of the oil. Many people, myself included, feel that unfiltered olive oil has a better taste because the olive particles continue to flavor the oil. It can sometimes be found in chain supermarkets during the holidays.

Unrefined sea salt—Ⓞ, Ⓢ

This is my go-to salt. It is relatively inexpensive and has not been processed or exposed to harsh chemicals. It contains a wide variety of the minerals and elements necessary for optimal health that are native to the area it comes from. It does not have added iodine, as most commercial brands of table salt do. There is no noticeable difference in flavor between unrefined sea salt and other salts, so kosher salt, table salt, and other sea salts can be used in its place in the recipes in this book.

Veal roast, boneless breast of—Ⓞ, Ⓘ, Ⓢ

Check the availability with your local butcher or supermarket before making a trip; veal often needs to be special-ordered.

White sesame—Ⓞ, Ⓘ, Ⓢ

The attractive flowers of the tropical sesame plant produce sesame seeds as they dry up. They yield approximately one tablespoon of seeds per pod. The seeds contain protein, phosphorus, niacin, sulfur, and carbohydrates. They are also used to make culinary oils and pastes.

WHERE TO BUY GUIDE

Note that source information is accurate as of the time of this book's publication.

CHEFSHOP.COM
chefshop.com

Great for: *bigoli* pasta, 00 flour, cannellini and other beans, and rice.

CYBERCUCINA
cybercucina.com
800-796-0116

Great for: borlotti (cranberry) beans, fava beans, Aceto Balsamico di Modena. They also have a great selection of gluten-free pasta and artisan pasta, risotto, farro, grains, legumes, and polenta.

FORMAGGIO KITCHEN
formaggiokitchen.com
888-212-3224

Great for: 00 flour, chestnut flour, arborio rice, and capers in sea salt.

GUSTIAMO
gustiamo.com
718-860-2949

Great for: *fior di sale* (salt from Sicily), borlotti (cranberry) beans, dry porcini mushrooms, *carnaroli* rice, and Caffè Sant'Eustachio espresso.

IL MERCATO ITALIANO
ilmercatoitaliano.net
920-884-6010

Great for: *fior di sale* (salt from Sicily), semolina flour, whole anchovies, and Italian tuna.

ITALIAN HARVEST
italianharvest.com

Great for: sweet paprika from Calabria, borlotti (cranberry) beans, and Aceto Balsamico di Modena.

MELISSA'S PRODUCE
melissas.com
800-588-1281
roberts@melissas.com

Great for: High-quality produce such as figs, pomegranates, artichokes, peppers, fresh and dried beans and legumes, and more.

PO VALLEY FOODS
povalleyfoods.com

Great for: *pizzoccheri alla valtellina* (buckwheat pasta), buckwheat penne, arborio and *carnaroli* rice, and polenta.

SALUMERIA ITALIANA
salumeriaitaliana.com
800-400-5916

Great for: pecorino Sardo cheese, pecorino Romano cheese, parmigiano-reggiano cheese (DOP), 00 flour, and *semola* (semolina) flour.

SUPERMARKET ITALY
supermarketitaly.com
201-729-0739

Great for: Tutto Calabria brand roasted red peppers, olives, and hot chile peppers.

THE TASTE OF CALABRIA
calabriataste.com

Great for: pecorino Crotonese cheese, grana padano cheese, dried chile flakes, dried porcini mushrooms, and wild oregano.

WHOLE FOODS MARKETS
wholefoodsmarkets.com (for locations)

Great for: olives, olive oils, vinegars, gluten-free pastas, flours, baking products, pecorino Romano cheese, mascarpone, parmigiano-reggiano cheese, Pomi brand boxed tomato purée and chopped tomatoes, agave nectar, pure honey, natural sugar, and unrefined sea salt.

ZINGERMAN'S
zingermans.com
888-636-8162

Great for: *cruschi* peppers from Basilicata and roasted figs from Calabria.

RESOURCES

Books

Bianchi A. *Italian Festival Food: Recipes and Traditions from Italy's Regional Country Food Fairs.* New York, Wiley, 1999

Caggiano B. *From Biba's Italian Kitchen.* New York, Hearst Books, 1995

Caggiano B. *Trattoria Cooking: More then 200 Authentic Recipes from Italy's Family-Style Restaurants.* New York, Macmillan, 1992

Concu G. *Itinerario del Gusto in Sardegna.* Nuoro, Imago Multimedia, 2012

Curti, L, Fraioli JO. *Food Festivals of Italy: Celebrated Recipes from 50 Food Fairs.* Layton, UT, Gibbs Smith, 2008

Davidson A. *The Oxford Companion to Food.* New York, Oxford University Press, 1999

Diotaiuti L. *The Al Tiramisu Restaurant Cookbook: An Elevated Approach to Authentic Italian Cuisine.* Washington, DC, Create Space, 2013

Field C. *Celebrating Italy: The Tastes and Traditions of Italy as Revealed through Its Feasts, Festivals, and Sumptuous Foods.* New York, Harper Perennial, 1997

Kostioukovitch E. *Why Italians Love to Talk About Food.* New York, Farrar, Straus, and Giroux, 2006

Lazari L. *1000 Ricette di Puglia.* Milano, Congedo Publishing, 2011

Marchesi G. *Buon appetito Maestro: A tavola con Giuseppe Verdi.* Parma, Battei, 2001

Marchesi G. *La Cucina di Verdi: Armonie di note, profumi e sapori sulla tavola del Maestro.* Valesi RR, Ed. Milano, Editoriale Giorgio Mondadori, 2003

Palmer MA. *Cucina di Calabria: Treasured Recipes and Family Traditions from Southern Italy.* London, Hippocrene Books, 1997

Riolo A. *Arabian Delights: Recipes and Princely Entertaining Ideas from the Arabian Peninsula.* Washington, DC, Capital Books, 2007

Riolo A. *The Mediterranean Diabetes Cookbook.* Alexandria, VA, American Diabetes Association, 2011

Riolo A. *Nile Style: Egyptian Cuisine and Culture.* New York, Hippocrene Books, 2013

Riolo A. *The Ultimate Mediterranean Diet Cookbook.* Boston, Fair Winds Press, 2015

Tomalini M. *Il Meglio Della Cucina Italiana.* Milano, De Vecchi Editore, 2001

Valli CG, Meneghelli E. *La cucina dell'Alto Lago di Garda.* Verona, Cierre Edizioni, 2000

Online Articles

Mediterranean Diet's Anti-Diabetes Benefits Revealed [article online], 7 Jan 2014. Reuters. Available from http://www.cbsnews.com/news/mediterranean-diets-anti-diabetes-benefits-revealed/. Accessed 4 March 2014

Nauert R. Mediterranean Diet May Benefit Mind as Well as Body [article online], 2014. Available from http://psychcentral.com/news/2013/09/04/mediterranean-diet-may-benefit-mind-as-well-as-body/59177.html. Accessed 19 May 2014

Preidt R. Chocolate, Tea, Berries May Cut Diabetes Risk [article online], 2014. Available from http://consumer.healthday.com/diabetes-information-10/misc-diabetes-news-181/choco-tea-berries-diabetes-j-of-nutrition-u-east-anglia-release-batch-1107-684032.html. Accessed 4 March 2014

Terranova G. La qualità dell'olio per curare i tumori scoperti all'Unical i benefici dell'extravergine [article online], 24 Jan 2014. *Il Quotidiano della Calabria.* Available from http://www.ilquotidianodellacalabria.it/news/idee-societa/721861/La-qualita-dell-olio-per-curare.html. Accessed 19 May 2014

Websites

Benefits of Vegetables [Internet], c2015. Organic Information Services Pvt Ltd. Available from http://www.organicfacts.net/health-benefits/vegetable/vegetables.html. Accessed 3 February 2014

Enjoying Olive Oil [Internet], c1998-2014. The Olive Oil Source Editors. Available from http://www.oliveoilsource.com/page/enjoying-olive-oil. Accessed 25 January 2014

Harlan TS. Why are Fruits and Nuts Good for You? Fruit and Nuts in the Medittteranean Diet [Internet], c2015. Harlan Bros Production LLC. Available from http://www.drgourmet.com/eatinghealthy/meddietfruitnuts.shtml. Accessed 3 February 2014

Mediterranean Diet Pyramid [Internet], c2015. International Olive Council. Available from http://www.internationaloliveoil.org/estaticos/view/87-mediterranean-diet-pyramid._Accessed 2 April 2014

Olio di Oliva di Calabria [Internet], c2010. Portale Calabria Editors. Available from http://www.portalecalabria.com/site/enogastronomia/olio/olio.asp. Accessed 25 January 2014

Olivo del Mediterraneo [Internet]. Raffaella Petruccelli, Pierluigi Mariotti, and Stefano Cerreti. Available from http://pomologia.ivalsa.cnr.it/olivo/olivo.htm. Accessed 3 February 2014

Research: Fruits and Vegetables [Internet], c2008–2015. Produce for Better Health Foundation. Available from http://www.fruitsandveggiesmorematters.org/research. Accessed 3 February 2014

Seafood and Nutrition: Seafood & Current Dietary Recommendations [Internet], c2015. Seafood Health Facts. Available from http://seafoodhealthfacts.org/seafood_nutrition/practitioners/seafood_dietary.php. Accessed 10 April 2014

INDEX

A

Abruzzese-Style Roasted Baby Goat with Peppers/*Capretto alla Neretese*, 152–153

Aceto Balsamico di Modena, 240

agricultural festival, 31

al cartoccio, 115

alcohol, x, 248–249. *See also* wine

all'onda, 32

almond, 52–53, 86–87

almond flour, 260–261, 264–269

Alto Crotonese olive oil, 9

American Diabetes Association (ADA), vi, viii

anchovy, 24–25, 76–77, 116–117, 128–129, 168–169, 193, 199, 232

antioxidant, viii

apertivo, 4, 295

Apicius, 50, 94

appetizer (*antipasti*)

  Crostini with Chickpea Cream/*Crostini con ceci*, 10–11

  defined, 3

  Lemon-Scented Shrimp/*Gamberi al limone*, 26–27

  Puglian Fava Bean Purée with Sautéed Chicory/*Fave e cicoria Pugliese*, 18–19

  Ricotta, Grilled Eggplant, and Fresh Mint Bruschetta/*Bruschetta Calabrese*, 8–9

  Roman-Style Rice and Herb–Stuffed Tomatoes/*Pomodori ripieni di riso alla Romana*, 20–21

  Sicilian Sweet-and-Sour Vegetable Medley/*Caponata*, 6–7

  Southern Italian Fava Bean Purée/*Maccu*, 16–17

  Stuffed Eggplant/*Melanzane ripiene*, 22–23

  Stuffed Peppers/*Peperoni ripieni*, 24–25

  Tuscan Crudités with Olive Oil Dip/*Pinzimonio*, 5

  Umbrian Frittata Skewers with Chickpea Dipping Sauce/*Spiedini di frittata con crema di ceci d'Umbria*, 14–15

  Vegetable and Parmesan Carpaccio/*Carpaccio di verdure e parmigiano*, 12–13

  Zucchini Carpaccio with Green Peppercorns/*Carpaccio di zucchine al pepe verde*, 28

apple, 246, 264–265

apricot, 248–249, 296

artichoke, 12–13, 96–97, 116–117, 164–165, 187

Artichoke, Mushroom, and Caramelized Onion Frittata/*Frittata di carciofi, funghi, e cipolle caramellate*, 96–97

Artichokes with Garlic and Oil/*Carciofi all'aglio e olio*, 164–165

artigiano, 209–210

arugula, 185, 192

Arugula Salad with Pears, Parmesan, and Cocoa Nibs/*Insalata di rucola con pere, parmigiano, e pennini di cacao*, 192

asparagus, 178–179, 188–189

Asparagus, Orange, and Fennel Salad/*Insalata di asparagi, arance, e finocchi*, 188–189

B

baby squid, 112–113, 200–201, 295

Baccalà, 295

baking, 293

balsamic vinegar, 138–139, 171, 178–179, 190, 240

banana, 241

Barley, Chestnut, and White Bean Minestrone/*Minestra d'orzo, castagne, e cannellini*, 54–55

basil, 62–63, 66–67, 86–87, 98–99, 204–205, 228–229

Basilicata-Style Chestnut Cake/*Castagnaccio Lucano*, 272–273

bean

  Barley, Chestnut, and White Bean Minestrone/*Minestra d'orzo, castagne, e cannellini*, 54–55

  borlotti, 48–49, 168–169, 295

  Braised Cannellini Beans/*Fagioli cannellini*, 284

  cannellini, 40–41, 48–49, 56–59, 186, 196–197, 284, 295

  Cannellini Bean, Tomato, and Orzo Soup/*Zuppa di cannellini e pomodoro con pasta di riso*, 56–57

  Cannellini Bean, Tuna, and Red Onion Salad/*Insalata di cannellini, tonno, e cipolle rosse*, 186

  Cannellini Bean Soup with Seafood/*Zuppa di fagioli con frutti di mare*, 40–41

  chickpea, 10–11, 14–15, 38–39, 48–49, 100–101, 203, 295

  Chickpea Salad/*Insalata di ceci*, 203

Dried Beans/*Fagioli secchi*, 283

fava, 16–19, 52–53, 296

green, 204–205

haricots verts, 175

pantry, 294

pasta and, 32

Puglian Fava Bean Purée with Sautéed Chicory/*Fave e cicoria Pugliese*, 18–19

Sardinian Fava Bean Soup/*Zuppa di fave Sarda*, 52–53

Southern Italian Fava Bean Purée/*Maccu*, 16–17

Venetian-Style Beans with Swiss Chard/*Fagioli alla Veneziana con bietole*, 168–169

white, 54–55

beef, 50–51, 154–155

Beet, Quinoa, and Arugula Salad/*Insalata di barbabietole, quinoa, e rucola*, 185

Belgian Endive, Radicchio, and Grapefruit Salad/*Insalata d'indivia, radicchio, e pompelmo*, 191

berry, 268–269. *See also under specific type*

Besciamella, 295

biscotti, 254–255. *See also* cookie

blackberry, 247

Blood Orange Salad/*Insalata d'arance sanguose*, 198

blueberry, 237, 247

Bongusto, Fred, 145

Braised, Stuffed Calamari with Tomato Sauce/*Calamari ripieni in salsa di pomodoro*, 112–113

Braised Cannellini Beans/*Fagioli cannellini*, 284

branzino, 295

bread (*pane*)

baguette, 44–45, 214–215, 250

Bread Crumbs and Hot Chili Peppers/*Mollica di pane e peperoncini*, 230

bruschetta, 8–9, 247, 295

crostini, 250, 296

Crostini with Ricotta and Honey/*Crostini con ricotta al miele*, 250

crouton, 60–61, 196–197, 292

crumbs, 22–25, 102–103, 154–155, 176–177, 230, 291

culture, 209, 221

Fresh Bread Crumbs/*Molliche di pane*, 291

Homemade Bread with Mother Yeast from Molise/*Pane spiga*, 216–217

Mixed-Berry Bruschetta/*Bruschetta ai frutti di bosco*, 247

No-Knead Italian "Baguettes"/*Filoni (senza impanare)*, 214–215

sesame-semolina, 10–11

Tyrolean Rye Bread with Fennel and Cumin/*Ur-Paarl della Val Venosta*, 212–213

Whole-Wheat Country Loaves/*Pane casareccio integrale*, 220–221

Whole-Wheat Cracker Rings with Black Pepper and Fennel Seeds/*Taralli integrali con pepe e finocchio*, 222–223

Whole-Wheat Rolls/*Panini di San Giovanni*, 218–219

broccoli, 60–61, 68–69

Bruzio olive oil, 9

C

cabbage, 48–49, 100–101, 163

Cacciatore-Style Chicken/*Pollo alla cacciatora*, 140–141

cake, 257, 264–269, 272–275

Calabria, vii, 9

Calabrian New Year's Celebration, xi

Calabrian-Style Roasted Potatoes/*Patate Calabrese al forno*, 176–177

Calabrian Wedding Soup/*Minestra maritata*, 50–51

calamari, 34–35, 40–41, 112–113

Campania-Style Rustic Vegetable Stew/*Cianfotta*, 98–99

Cannellini Bean, Tomato, and Orzo Soup/*Zuppa di cannellini e pomodoro con pasta di riso*, 56–57

Cannellini Bean, Tuna, and Red Onion Salad/*Insalata di cannellini, tonno, e cipolle rosse*, 186

Cannellini Bean Soup with Seafood/*Zuppa di fagioli con frutti di mare*, 40–41

cantaloupe, 237, 253

caper, 24–25, 120–123, 136–137, 232

carbohydrate, viii

carpaccio, 107, 295

carrot, 142–143, 161

Carrot and Zucchini Ribbons/*Nastri di carote e zucchine*, 161

Cartia, Rocco, 18, 22

casalinga, 236, 295

castagne, 295

Catholic Church, viii, 17

Cauliflower and Herb Salad from Le Marche/*Insalata di cavolfiore alla Marchigiana*, 199

cavatelli, 295

cena, 295

chard, 80–81

Chargrilled Asparagus with Balsamic and Parmesan/*Asparagi grigliati con balsamico e parmigiano*, 178–179

cheese

Arugula Salad with Pears, Parmesan, and Cocoa Nibs/*Insalata di rucola con pere, parmigiano, e pennini di cacao*, 192

Chargrilled Asparagus with Balsamic and Parmesan/*Asparagi grigliati con balsamico e parmigiano*, 178–179

fontina, 80–81

mascarpone, 246, 297

mozzarella, 196–197, 297

Pan-Fried Fennel with Parmesan/*Finocchi con parmigiano*, 162

parmesan, 12–13, 162, 178–179, 192

parmigiano-reggiano, 22–23, 76–77, 80–81, 297

pecorino, 16–17, 44–45, 50–51, 102–103, 176–177, 297

ricotta, 8–9, 64–65, 82–83, 250, 274–275, 298

rind, 54–55, 57

Vegetable and Parmesan Carpaccio/*Carpaccio di verdure e parmigiano*, 12–13

cherry, 254–255

chestnut, 42–43, 54–55, 144–145, 272–273

chestnut flour, 272–273

chicken

Cacciatore-Style Chicken/*Pollo alla cacciatora*, 140–141

Chicken Breasts with Citrus, Capers, and Pine Nuts/*Petti di pollo al limone, caperi, e pinoli*, 136–137

Chicken Stew with Mushrooms and Onions/*Stufato di pollo con funghi e cipolle*, 134–135

Classic Roasted Chicken/*Pollo al forno*, 142–143

Herb-Marinated Chicken Breasts/*Petti di pollo marinate con erbe*, 132–133

Homemade Chicken Stock/*Brodo di pollo*, 289

Marinated Chicken with Rosemary and Balsamic Vinegar/*Pollo marinato con rosmarino ed aceto balsamico*, 138–139

Monday Salad/*Insalata del lunedi*, 196–197

Roasted Chicken with Grapes and Chestnuts/*Pollo con le uve e castagne*, 144–145

Roman Chicken, Pepper, and Tomato Stew/*Pollo in umido alla Romana*, 94–95

chickpea, 10–11, 14–15, 38–39, 48–49, 100–101, 203, 295

Chickpea Salad/*Insalata di ceci*, 203

Chickpea Soup with Rosemary-Infused Shrimp/*Crema di ceci con gamberi*, 38–39

chicory, 18–19

chocolate, 6–7, 192, 254–255, 257, 268–269, 276–277

Chocolate, Espresso, and Cherry Biscotti/*Biscotti di cioccolato, caffè, e ciliege*, 254–255

Chocolate and Orange Sponge Cake/*Pan di Spagna di cioccolato ed arancia*, 257

Christian Era, vii, 159, 218

Christmas, 43

Christmas Eve Feast of the Seven Fishes, x, 91

Cicchetti, 4

Cicero, 10

cinnamon, 244–245, 252, 264–265, 298

Cinnamon-Infused Apple Cake/*Torta di mela e canella*, 264–265

Cipriani, Giuseppe, 12–13

citrus, 130–131, 136–137, 198

Citrus and Herb–Infused Scallop Stew/*Capesante in umido con erbe ed agrumi*, 130–131

Classic Meatballs/*Polpette*, 154–155

Classic Roasted Chicken/*Pollo al forno*, 142–143

Classic Roman fare, xii

clove, 152–153, 272–273

cocoa, 192, 238–239, 254–255, 257, 268–269, 276–277

coconut, 241, 256, 276–277

Coconut and Chocolate Pudding/*Budino di noce di cocco e cioccolato*, 276–277

Coconut Ball Cookies/*Palline di noce di cocco*, 256

coffee, 238–239, 244–246. *See also* espresso

colazione, 296

condiment. *See* sauces and condiments (*salse e condimenti*)

contorno, 296

cookie, 251, 254–256, 258, 260–263. *See also* biscotti

cooking

Braised Cannellini Beans/*Fagioli cannellini*, 284

Dried Beans/*Fagioli secchi*, 283

Fresh Bread Crumbs/*Molliche di pane*, 291

Homemade Chicken Stock/*Brodo di pollo*, 289

Homemade Croutons/*Crostini*, 292

Homemade Meat Stock/*Brodo di carne*, 290

Homemade Seafood Stock/*Brodo di pesce*, 288

Homemade Vegetable Stock/*Brodo di verdura*, 287

Lentils/*Lenticchie*, 285

Polenta/*Polenta*, 286

Roasted Peppers/*Peperoni arrostiti*, 282

cornmeal, 128–129, 214–215, 298

couscous, 86–87, 296

cracker, 222–223

Cream of Chestnut Soup/*Crema di castagna*, 42–43

creme, 33

Crostini with Chickpea Cream/*Crostini con ceci*, 10–11

Crostini with Ricotta and Honey/*Crostini con ricotta al miele*, 250

Crunchy Almond and Pine Nut Cookies/*Fave dolci*, 260–261

crusca, 218–219

cucina casalinga, 33

cucina povera, 32

cumin, 212–213

D

dandelion green, 193

D'Annunzio, Gabriele, 8

Day of the Dead, 260–261

desserts (*dolci*)

Basilicata-Style Chestnut Cake/*Castagnaccio Lucano*, 272–273

Chocolate, Espresso, and Cherry Biscotti/*Biscotti di cioccolato, caffè, e ciliege*, 254–255

Chocolate and Orange Sponge Cake/*Pan di Spagna di cioccolato ed arancia*, 257

Cinnamon-Infused Apple Cake/*Torta di mela e canella*, 264–265

Coconut and Chocolate Pudding/*Budino di noce di cocco e cioccolato*, 276–277

Coconut Ball Cookies/*Palline di noce di cocco*, 256

Crostini with Ricotta and Honey/*Crostini con ricotta al miele*, 250

Crunchy Almond and Pine Nut Cookies/*Fave dolci*, 260–261

Espresso and Spice–Poached Figs/*Ficchi al caffè e spezie*, 244–245

Espresso Panna Cotta/*Panna cotta al caffè*, 238–239

Flourless Chocolate Cake/*Torta Caprese*, 268–269

Fresh Fruit Kabobs/*Spiedini di frutta fresca*, 237

Fruit and Fresh Coconut Salad/*Macedonia di frutta con noce di cocco fresco*, 241

Glazed Apples with Espresso Cream/*Mele glassate con crema di caffè*, 246

Ivrea's Polenta Cake/*Polentina di Ivrea*, 266–267

Melon Sorbet/*Sorbetto di melone*, 253

Mixed-Berry Bruschetta/*Bruschetta ai frutti di bosco*, 247

Peach and Apricot Mousse/*Spuma di pesca ed albicocche*, 248–249

Pear, Ricotta, and Pine Nut Cake/*Torta soffice di pere con ricotta e pinoli*, 274–275

Piemontese "Ugly but Good" Cookies/*Brutti ma buoni*, 262–263

Pine Nut Cookies/*Biscotti di pinoli*, 258

Poached Autumn Pears with Vanilla and Ginger Cream/*Pere al vaniglia con crema di zenzero*, 243

Pomegranate-Orange Spice Pudding/*Budino alla melagrana con arance e canella*, 252

Strawberries in Balsamic Vinegar/*Fragole in aceto balsamico*, 240

Tuscan Fig, Walnut, and Fennel Seed Torte/*Torta di ficchi, noci, e semi di finocchio*, 270–271

Vanilla-Scented Roasted Figs/*Ficchi vanigliati al forno*, 242

Whole-Wheat and Honey Cookies/*Biscotti integrale al miele*, 251

Yogurt Gelato/*Gelato allo yogurt*, 259

digestivo, 296

dining out, 3–4. *See also* restaurant

dinner, ix, 31

Diotaiuti, Luigi, vii, 70

dip, 5, 14–15

DOC (*Denominazione di origine controllata*), viii

DOCG (*Denominazione di origine controllata e garantita*), viii

dolce, 296

dried apricot, 296

Dried Beans/*Fagioli secchi*, 283

dried fig, 296

Duchess-Style dish, 125

Durante, Castore, 253

E

eating out, 4. *See also* restaurant

eggplant, 6–9, 22–23, 98–99, 166–167, 171, 174, 202

Eggplant Croquettes/*Polpette di melanzane*, 102–103

Emilia-Romagna–Style Green Herb Sauce/*Salsa verde all'Emiliana*, 232

endive, 191

entertaining, 3, 160

Epiphany, 43

escarole, 50–51

espresso, 238–239, 244–246, 254–255, 268–269

Espresso and Spice–Poached Figs/ *Ficchi al caffè e spezie*, 244–245

Espresso Panna Cotta/ *Panna cotta al caffè*, 238–239

expeller, 296

F

fagioli, 296

fall menu, x, 184

Farmhouse Vegetable and Farro Soup/ *Zuppa di verdure e farro*, 58–59

farro, 58–59, 204–205

farrotto, 205

fennel bulb, 5, 12–13, 72–73, 114–115, 162, 166–167, 188–189

fennel seed, 212–213, 222–223, 270–271

fig, 242, 244–245, 270–271, 296

first cold-pressed extra virgin olive oil, 296

first courses/*primi*

Barley, Chestnut, and White Bean Minestrone/ *Minestra d'orzo, castagne, e cannellini*, 54–55

Calabrian Wedding Soup/ *Minestra maritata*, 50–51

Cannellini Bean, Tomato, and Orzo Soup/ *Zuppa di cannellini e pomodoro con pasta di riso*, 56–57

Cannellini Bean Soup with Seafood/ *Zuppa di fagioli con frutti di mare*, 40–41

Chickpea Soup with Rosemary-Infused Shrimp/ *Crema di ceci con gamberi*, 38–39

Cream of Chestnut Soup/ *Crema di castagna*, 42–43

Farmhouse Vegetable and Farro Soup/ *Zuppa di verdure e farro*), 58–59

Holiday Minestrone/ *Millecosedde*, 48–49

Potato Gnocchi/ *Gnocchi di patate*, 78–79

Pumpkin Risotto/ *Risotto di zucca*, 74–75

Pumpkin Soup/ *Crema di zucca*, 36–37

Red Pepper and Sweet Potato Gnocchi/ *Gnocchi di peperoni rossi e patate dolce*, 82–83

Roman-Style Broccoli and Pecorino Soup/ *Zuppa di broccoletti*, 60–61

Rustic Lentil Soup/ *Zuppa di lenticchie*, 46–47

Sardinian Fava Bean Soup/ *Zuppa di fave Sarda*, 52–53

Spaghetti Squash "Pasta" with Shrimp, Tomatoes, and Basil/ *"Pasta" di zucca con gamberi, pomodori, e basilico*, 62–63

Spaghetti with Fresh Tuna and Fennel/ *Pasta con tonno e finocchio*, 72–73

Spinach Fettuccine with Walnut-ricotta Pesto/ *Fettuccine di spinaci con pesto di noci e ricotta*, 64–65

Trapani-Style Almond Couscous/ *Cuscus alla mandorla Trapanese*, 86–87

Turnip Gnocchi with Herb Sauce/ *Gnocchi di rapa con salsa d'erbe*, 84–85

Tuscan Buckwheat Pasta with Cheese, potatoes, and Greens/ *Pizzoccheri della Valtellina*, 80–81

Tuscan Seafood Stew/ *Cacciucco Livornese*, 34–35

Venetian-Style Whole-Wheat Spaghetti with Sauce/ *Bigoli in salsa*, 76–77

Whole-Wheat Fusilli with Pesto and Cherry Tomatoes/ *Fusilli con pesto e pomodori*, 66–67

Whole-Wheat Orecchiette Pasta with Broccoli and Garlic/ *Orecchiette integrale con broccoli*, 68–69

Whole-Wheat Ziti with Goat Ragu/ *Ziti integrale con ragu di capra*, 70–71

Zucchini Soup with Crostini/ *Zuppa di zucchini con crostini*, 44–45

fish. *See also* seafood

Cannellini Bean, Tuna, and Red Onion Salad/ *Insalata di cannellini, tonno, e cipolle rosse*, 186

Cannellini Bean Soup with Seafood/ *Zuppa di fagioli con frutti di mare*, 40–41

Christmas Eve Feast of the Seven Fishes, 91

Fish Stew over Polenta/ *Pesce in umido con la polenta*, 128–129

Fishermen Kabobs/ *Spiedini alla marinara*, 108–109

Fresh Tuna Steaks with Sautéed Artichokes/ *Tonno con carciofi*, 116–117

monkfish, 34–35

sauce, 227

Sea Bass with Fennel Baked in Parchment/ *Branzino con finocchio al cartoccio*, 114–115

Sea Bream with Duchess-Style Sweet Potatoes/ *Orata con patate dolce alla ducchessa*, 124–125

Seafood Salad/ *Insalata di pesce*, 200–201

Sicilian-Style Fish with Vegetables/*Dentice alla Siciliana con verdure al forno*, 122–123

Smoked Fish, Orange, and Radicchio Salad with Olives/*Insalata di pesce affumicato, arance, e radicchio*, 194–195

sole, 126–127

Spaghetti with Fresh Tuna and Fennel/*Pasta con tonno e finocchio*, 72–73

swordfish, 108–109, 120–121

Swordfish with Olives, Capers, Herbs, and Tomatoes/*Pesce spade alla ghiotta*, 120–121

Trout Fillets with Sun-Dried Tomato and Cured-Olive Crust/*Filetti di trota impanati con pomodori secchi ed olive curate*, 118–119

tuna, 72–73, 116–117, 186

Tuscan Seafood Stew/*Cacciucco Livornese*, 34–35

Venetian-Style Sole in a Sweet-and-Sour Sauce/*Sfogi in saor*, 126–127

Fish Stew over Polenta/*Pesce in umido con la polenta*, 128–129

Fishermen Kabobs/*Spiedini alla marinara*, 108–109

flavonoid, viii

Flourless Chocolate Cake/*Torta Caprese*, 268–269

Fresh Bread Crumbs/*Molliche di pane*, 291

Fresh Fruit Kabobs/*Spiedini di frutta fresca*, 237

Fresh Tomato Sauce/*Salsa fresca di pomodoro*, 228–229

Fresh Tuna Steaks with Sautéed Artichokes/*Tonno con carciofi*, 116–117

frittata, 14–15, 96–97, 173

fruit. *See also under specific type*

citrus, 136–137, 198

dessert, as, 235

dried, 235

Fresh Fruit Kabobs/*Spiedini di frutta fresca*, 237

Fruit and Fresh Coconut Salad/*Macedonia di frutta con noce di cocco fresco*, 241

pantry, 294

frutti di bosco, 297

frutti di mare, 297

G

Garibaldi, Giuseppe, 227

garlic, 68–69, 164–165, 170, 180, 228–229, 231

Garlic and Oil/*Aglio e olio*, 231

gelato, 259

ghiotta cooking style, 121

ginger, 243

Glazed Apples with Espresso Cream/*Mele glassate con crema di caffè*, 246

gluten-free, vi, 31

gnocchi, ix, 32, 78–79, 82–85, 297

goat, 70–71, 152–153, 297

goat cheese, 297

grain, 294. *See also under specific type*

grape, 144–145

grapefruit/grapefruit juice, 191

grappa, 297

Greek, ancient, vii, 31–32

green onion, 198

green peppercorn, 28

greens, 19

H

Haricots Verts with Hazelnuts/*Fagiolini alle nocciole*, 175

hazelnut, 175, 262–263

herb

Cauliflower and Herb Salad from Le Marche/*Insalata di cavolfiore alla Marchigiana*, 199

Citrus and Herb–Infused Scallop Stew/*Capesante in umido con erbe ed agrumi*, 130–131

Emilia-Romagna–Style Green Herb Sauce/*Salsa verde all'Emiliana*, 232

fresh, 139

Herb-Marinated Chicken Breasts/*Petti di pollo marinate con erbe*, 132–133

Herb-Roasted Turkey/*Tacchino al forno*, 148–149

Mixed Mushroom and Herb Medley/*Funghi in padella con erbe*, 172

pantry, 294

Roman-Style Rice and Herb–Stuffed Tomatoes/*Pomodori ripieni di riso alla Romana*, 20–21

Swordfish with Olives, Capers, Herbs, and Tomatoes/*Pesce spade alla ghiotta*, 120–121

Turnip Gnocchi with Herb Sauce/*Gnocchi di rapa con salsa d'erbe*, 84–85

Zucchini and Herb Croquettes/*Polpette di zucchine*, 104–105

Herbario Nuovo (Durante), 253

holiday, x, 3, 43, 91

Holiday Minestrone/*Millecosedde*, 48–49

Homemade Bread with Mother Yeast from Molise/*Pane spiga*, 216–217

Homemade Chicken Stock/*Brodo di pollo*, 289

Homemade Croutons/*Crostini*, 292

Homemade Meat Stock/*Brodo di carne*, 290

Homemade Seafood Stock/*Brodo di pesce*, 288

Homemade Vegetable Stock/*Brodo di verdura*, 287

honey, 250–251, 253, 258–259, 272–273

I

IGT (*Indicazione geografica tipica*), viii

il saor, 127

ingredient, 92, 281

insalata mista, 183

insalata verde, 183

Itali, vii

Italian
culture, 71
food, vi–vii
proverb, vi–vii, 3, 31–32, 91, 159, 183, 209, 227, 235, 281

Italian *Sagra* (Festival) menu, xi

Italian Witch, 43

Ivrea's Polenta Cake/*Polentina di Ivrea*, 266–267

J

Johnson, Alba, 98

K

Kale Sautéed in Garlic, Oil, and Hot Chili Peppers/*Ravizzone con aglio, olio, e peperoncino*, 170

kiwi, 237, 241

L

La Befana festival, 43

label, viii

laganon, 31–32

Lamezia olive oil, 9

lemon/lemon juice, 26–27, 116–117, 130–133, 136–137, 269

Lemon-Scented Shrimp/*Gamberi al limone*, 26–27

lentil, 46–47, 285

Lentils/*Lenticchie*, 285

liqueur, 248–249

locavore eating, 105

lunch, ix, 31

M

maccheroni, 297

Macedonia, 241

Magna Grecia, 31–32

marinara, 109

Marinated Chicken with Rosemary and Balsamic Vinegar/*Pollo marinato con rosmarino ed aceto balsamico*, 138–139

Marinated Eggplant/*Melanzane al funghetto*, 171

Marinated Eggplant Salad/*Melanzane in insalata alla Calabrese*, 202

mattanza, 73

meal planning, ix–xii, 3–4, 31, 91

meat, 91, 290. *See also under specific type*

Mediterranean diet, viii, 53, 168

Melon Sorbet/*Sorbetto di melone*, 253

menu, xi–xiv, 159, 183–184

Mesopotamia, vii

minestre, 33

mint, 8–9, 20–21, 173

Mixed-Berry Bruschetta/*Bruschetta ai frutti di bosco*, 247

Mixed Grilled Vegetables/*Verdure miste alla griglia*, 166–167

Mixed Mushroom and Herb Medley/*Funghi in padella con erbe*, 172

Modica, 6, 192

Molise, 216–217

Monday Salad/*Insalata del lunedi*, 196–197

mother yeast, 216–217

mousse, 248–249

mushroom, 14–15, 96–97, 134–135, 140–141, 172

mussels, 34–35, 40–41, 110–111

Mussels in Saffron-Tomato Broth/*Cozze in brodo di zafferano*, 110–111

N

natural sugar, 297

No-Knead Italian "Baguettes"/*Filoni (senza impanare)*, 214–215

nut
almond, 52–53, 86–87, 260–261
Basilicata-Style Chestnut Cake/*Castagnaccio Lucano*, 272–273
chestnut, 42–43, 54–55, 144–145, 272–273
Crunchy Almond and Pine Nut Cookies/*Fave dolci*, 260–261
Haricots Verts with Hazelnuts/*Fagiolini alle nocciole*, 175
hazelnut, 175, 262–263
pantry, 294
Pear, Ricotta, and Pine Nut Cake/*Torta soffice di pere con ricotta e pinoli*, 274–275
pine, 66–69, 122–123, 126–127, 136–137, 204–205, 260–261, 274–275
Pine Nut Cookies/*Biscotti di pinoli*, 258
Trapani-Style Almond Couscous/*Cuscus alla mandorla Trapanese*, 86–87
Tuscan Fig, Walnut, and Fennel Seed Torte/*Torta di ficchi, noci, e semi di finocchio*, 270–271
walnut, 64–65, 193, 242, 270–271

O

octopus, 34–35

Oenotria, vii

oil, 294

olive, 118–121, 194–195

olive oil, 5, 9, 164–165, 170, 180, 193, 231, 296, 299

onion, 96–97, 134–135, 186

orange/orange juice, 116–117, 130–131, 188–189, 194–195, 198, 252, 257, 274–275

Our Lady of the Rosary feast, 77

P

Pan-Fried Fennel with Parmesan/*Finocchi con parmigiano*, 162

panifici, 209, 215

panna cotta, 238–239

Pan-Seared Sea Scallops/*Capesante in padella*, 106–107

pantry, 293–294

parchment, 114–115

parsley, 203, 231–232

pasta, ix

    bean and, 32

    bigoli, 76–77

    buckwheat, 81

    Cannellini Bean, Tomato, and Orzo Soup/*Zuppa di cannellini e pomodoro con pasta di riso*, 56–57

    ditalini, 48–49

    history of, 31–32

    lagane, 32

    pantry, 294

    pastina, 50–51

    pizzoccheri, 80–81

    Spaghetti Squash "Pasta" with Shrimp, Tomatoes, and Basil/*"Pasta" di zucca con gamberi, pomodori, e basilico*, 62–63

Spaghetti with Fresh Tuna and Fennel/*Pasta con tonno e finocchio*, 72–73

Spinach Fettuccine with Walnut-Ricotta Pesto/*Fettuccine di spinaci con pesto di noci e ricotta*, 64–65

Tuscan Buckwheat Pasta with Cheese, Potatoes, and Greens/*Pizzoccheri della Valtellina*, 80–81

Venetian-Style Whole-Wheat Spaghetti with Sauce/*Bigoli in salsa*, 76–77

Whole-Wheat Fusilli with Pesto and Cherry Tomatoes/*Fusilli con pesto e pomodori*, 66–67

Whole-Wheat Orecchiette Pasta with Broccoli and Garlic/*Orecchiette integrale con broccoli*, 68–69

Whole-Wheat Ziti with Goat Ragu/*Ziti integrale con ragu di capra*, 70–71

Peach and Apricot Mousse/*Spuma di pesca ed albicocche*, 248–249

pear, 98–99, 192, 243, 274–275

Pear, Ricotta, and Pine Nut Cake/*Torta soffice di pere con ricotta e pinoli*, 274–275

pearl barley, 297

pepper

    Abruzzese-Style Roasted Baby Goat with Peppers/*Capretto alla Neretese*, 152–153

    black, 222–223

    Bread Crumbs and Hot Chili Peppers/*Mollica di pane e peperoncini*, 230

    chili, 82–83, 170, 230

    green bell, 150–151

    Kale Sautéed in Garlic, Oil, and Hot Chili Peppers/*Ravizzone con aglio, olio, e peperoncino*, 170

peperoncini, 232, 298

peperoni di Senise, 82–83, 298

Pepper, Potato, and Eggplant Medley/*Peperoni, patate, e melanzane al forno*, 174

red bell, 5

Red Pepper, Yellow Tomato, and Artichoke Salad/*Insalata di peperoni rossi, pomodori gialli, e carciofi*, 187

red roasted, 82–83, 106–107, 187, 282

Roasted Peppers/*Peperoni arrostiti*, 282

Roman Chicken, Pepper, and Tomato Stew/*Pollo in umido alla Romana*, 94–95

Stuffed Peppers/*Peperoni ripieni*, 24–25

Veal, Potato, and Pepper Stew/*Spezzatino di vitello*, 150–151

pesto, 64–67, 86–87, 204–205, 298

Piemontese "Ugly but Good" Cookies/*Brutti ma buoni*, 262–263

pignata, 51

pineapple, 237, 241

pine nut, 66–69, 122–123, 126–127, 136–137, 204–205, 260–261, 274–275

Pine Nut Cookies/*Biscotti di pinoli*, 258

Poached Autumn Pears with Vanilla and Ginger Cream/*Pere al vaniglia con crema di zenzero*, 243

polenta, 128–129, 266–267, 286, 298

Polenta/*Polenta*, 286

polyphenol, viii

Pomegranate-Orange Spice Pudding/*Budino alla melagrana con arance e canella*, 252 potato, 32, 78–81, 142–143, 150–151, 174, 176–177

Potato Gnocchi/*Gnocchi di patate*, 78–79

poultry, 91. *See also under specific type*

pranzo, 298

presentation, 4, 161

primo, 298

Procopio Cutò, Francesco, 259

Protected Designation of Origin (PDO), 296

pudding, 276–277

Puglian Fava Bean Purée with Sautéed Chicory/*Fave e cicoria Pugliese*, 18–19

Pumpkin Risotto/*Risotto di zucca*, 74–75

Pumpkin Soup/*Crema di zucca*, 36–37

puntarelle, 18

pure cinnamon, 298

Q

quinoa, 104–105, 185

R

radicchio, 5, 191, 194–195

ragu, 70–71, 298

raisin, 6–7, 98–99, 122–123, 126–127, 136–137, 274–275

raspberry, 247, 259

Red Pepper, Yellow Tomato, and Artichoke Salad/*Insalata di peperoni rossi, pomodori gialli, e carciofi*, 187

Red Pepper and Sweet Potato Gnocchi/*Gnocchi di peperoni rossi e patate dolce*, 82–83

Reggio Calabria, 8

resources, 301–302

restaurant, 3–4, 31–32

rice, 20–21, 32, 74–75, 294

Ricotta, Grilled Eggplant, and Fresh Mint Bruschetta/*Bruschetta Calabrese*, 8–9

risotto, ix, 32–33, 74–75, 298

Roasted Chicken with Grapes and Chestnuts/*Pollo con le uve e castagne*, 144–145

Roasted Peppers/*Peperoni arrostiti*, 282

romaine lettuce, 196–197, 202

Roman, vii

Roman Chicken, Pepper, and Tomato Stew/*Pollo in umido alla Romana*, 94–95

Roman-Style Broccoli and Pecorino Soup/*Zuppa di broccoletti*, 60–61

Roman-Style Rice and Herb–Stuffed Tomatoes/*Pomodori ripieni di riso alla Romana*, 20–21

rosemary, 38–39, 138–141

Rustic Lentil Soup/*Zuppa di lenticchie*, 46–47

rye flour, 212–213, 218–219

S

saffron, 40–41, 100–101, 110–111, 298

sagre, 31, 159, 209

salads (*insalate*)

Arugula Salad with Pears, Parmesan, and Cocoa Nibs/*Insalata di rucola con pere, parmigiano, e pennini di cacao*, 192

Asparagus, Orange, and Fennel Salad/*Insalata di asparagi, arance, e finocchi*, 188–189

Beet, Quinoa, and Arugula Salad/*Insalata di barbabietole, quinoa, e rucola*, 185

Belgian Endive, Radicchio, and Grapefruit Salad/*Insalata d'indivia, radicchio, e pompelmo*, 191

Blood Orange Salad/*Insalata d'arance sanguose*, 198

Cannellini Bean, Tuna, and Red Onion Salad/*Insalata di cannellini, tonno, e cipolle rosse*, 186

Cauliflower and Herb Salad from Le Marche/*Insalata di cavolfiore alla Marchigiana*, 199

Chickpea Salad/*Insalata di ceci*, 203

Marinated Eggplant Salad/*Melanzane in insalata alla Calabrese*, 202

Monday Salad/*Insalata del lunedi*, 196–197

nutrition, 183

Red Pepper, Yellow Tomato, and Artichoke Salad/*Insalata di peperoni rossi, pomodori gialli, e carciofi*, 187

Seafood Salad/*Insalata di pesce*, 200–201

seasonal menu, 183–184

Smoked Fish, Orange, and Radicchio Salad with Olives/*Insalata di pesce affumicato, arance, e radicchio*, 194–195

Tomatoes with Balsamic Vinegar/*Insalata di pomodori all'aceto balsamico*, 190

Tuscan Farro Salad/*Insalata di farro alla Toscana*, 204–205

Val d'Aosta–Style Dandelion Salad/*Insalata di dente di leone Valdostana*, 193

salt, 299

saor, in, 298

Sardinian Fava Bean Soup/*Zuppa di fave Sarda*, 52–53

Saturn, 159

sauces and condiments (*salse e condimenti*), 227–232

Sautéed Zucchini with Vinegar and Mint/*Zucchine in padella con aceto e menta*, 173

scallop, 40–41, 106–107, 130–131, 200–201

scaloppine, 136–137

Scappi, Bartolomeo, 74

Sea Bass with Fennel Baked in Parchment/*Branzino con finocchio al cartoccio*, 114–115

Sea Bream with Duchess-Style Sweet Potatoes/*Orata con patate dolce alla ducchessa*, 124–125

seafood. *See also* fish; *under specific type*

    Braised, Stuffed Calamari with Tomato Sauce/*Calamari ripieni in salsa di pomodoro*, 112–113

    Cannellini Bean Soup with Seafood/*Zuppa di fagioli con frutti di mare*, 40–41

    Citrus and Herb–Infused Scallop Stew/*Capesante in umido con erbe ed agrumi*, 130–131

    Homemade Seafood Stock/*Brodo di pesce*, 288

    Lemon-Scented Shrimp/*Gamberi al limone*, 26–27

    Mussels in Saffron-Tomato Broth/*Cozze in brodo di zafferano*, 110–111

    Pan-Seared Sea Scallops/*Capesante in padella*, 106–107

    Seafood Salad/*Insalata di pesce*, 200–201

    Tuscan Seafood Stew/*Cacciucco Livornese*, 34–35

sea salt, 299

seasonal menu, ix–xii

second courses (*secondi*), 91–92

    Abruzzese-Style Roasted Baby Goat with Peppers/*Capretto alla Neretese*, 152–153

    Artichoke, Mushroom, and Caramelized Onion Frittata/*Frittata di carciofi, funghi, e cipolle caramellate*, 96–97

    Braised, Stuffed Calamari with Tomato Sauce/*Calamari ripieni in salsa di pomodoro*, 112–113

    Cacciatore-Style Chicken/*Pollo alla cacciatora*, 140–141

    Campania-Style Rustic Vegetable Stew/*Cianfotta*, 98–99

    Chicken Breasts with Citrus, Capers, and Pine Nuts/*Petti di pollo al limone, caperi, e pinoli*, 136–137

    Chicken Stew with Mushrooms and Onions/*Stufato di pollo con funghi e cipolle*, 134–135

    Citrus and Herb–Infused Scallop Stew/*Capesante in umido con erbe ed agrumi*, 130–131

    Classic Meatballs/*Polpette*, 154–155

    Classic Roasted Chicken/*Pollo al forno*, 142–143

    Eggplant Croquettes/*Polpette di melanzane*, 102–103

    Fish Stew over Polenta/*Pesce in umido con la polenta*, 128–129

    Fishermen Kabobs/*Spiedini alla marinara*, 108–109

    Fresh Tuna Steaks with Sautéed Artichokes/*Tonno con carciofi*, 116–117

    Herb-Marinated Chicken Breasts/*Petti di pollo marinate con erbe*, 132–133

    Herb-Roasted Turkey/*Tacchino al forno*, 148–149

    Marinated Chicken with Rosemary and Balsamic Vinegar/*Pollo marinato con rosmarino ed aceto balsamico*, 138–139

    Mussels in Saffron-Tomato Broth/*Cozze in brodo di zafferano*, 110–111

    Pan-Seared Sea Scallops/*Capesante in padella*, 106–107

    Roasted Chicken with Grapes and Chestnuts/*Pollo con le uve e castagne*, 144–145

    Roman Chicken, Pepper, and Tomato Stew/*Pollo in umido alla Romana*, 94–95

    Sea Bass with Fennel Baked in Parchment/*Branzino con finocchio al cartoccio*, 114–115

    Sea Bream with Duchess-Style Sweet Potatoes/*Orata con patate dolce alla ducchessa*, 124–125

    Sicilian-Style Fish with Vegetables/*Dentice alla Siciliana con verdure al forno*, 122–123

    Spiced Chickpea Stew/*Stufato di ceci alle spezie*, 100–101

    Swordfish with Olives, Capers, Herbs, and Tomatoes/*Pesce spade alla ghiotta*, 120–121

    Trout Fillets with Sun-Dried Tomato and Cured-Olive Crust/*Filetti di trota impanati con pomodori secchi ed olive curate*, 118–119

    Veal, Potato, and Pepper Stew/*Spezzatino di vitello*, 150–151

    Vegetable-Stuffed Turkey Breast/*Petto di tacchino ripieno di verdure*, 146–147

    Venetian-Style Sole in a Sweet-and-Sour Sauce/*Sfogi in saor*, 126–127

    Zucchini and Herb Croquettes/*Polpette di zucchine*, 104–105

secondo, 298

semola, 298

semolina, 220–221

sformato, 3, 298

shopping, 92, 293, 299–300

shrimp, 26–27, 34–35, 38–41, 62–63, 200–201

Sicilian-Style Fish with Vegetables/*Dentice alla Siciliana con verdure al forno*, 122–123

Sicilian Sweet-and-Sour Vegetable Medley/*Caponata*, 6–7

side dishes (*contorni*), 159–160

Artichokes with Garlic and Oil/*Carciofi all'aglio e olio*, 164–165

Calabrian-Style Roasted Potatoes/*Patate Calabrese al forno*, 176–177

Carrot and Zucchini Ribbons/*Nastri di carote e zucchine*, 161

Chargrilled Asparagus with Balsamic and Parmesan/*Asparagi grigliati con balsamico e parmigiano*, 178–179

Haricots Verts with Hazelnuts/*Fagiolini alle nocciole*, 175

Kale Sautéed in Garlic, Oil, and Hot Chili Peppers/*Ravizzone con aglio, olio, e peperoncino*, 170

Marinated Eggplant/*Melanzane al funghetto*, 171

Mixed Grilled Vegetables/*Verdure miste alla griglia*, 166–167

Mixed Mushroom and Herb Medley/*Funghi in padella con erbe*, 172

Pan-Fried Fennel with Parmesan/*Finocchi con parmigiano*, 162

Pepper, Potato, and Eggplant Medley/*Peperoni, patate, e melanzane al forno*, 174

Sautéed Zucchini with Vinegar and Mint/*Zucchine in padella con aceto e menta*, 173

Spinach Sautéed in Garlic and Oil/*Spinaci all'aglio e olio*, 180

Sweet-and-Sour Cabbage/*Cavoli acidi*, 163

Venetian-Style Beans with Swiss Chard/*Fagioli alla Veneziana con bietole*, 168–169

skewer, 14–15, 108, 237

Slow Food, 209, 212–213

Smoked Fish, Orange, and Radicchio Salad with Olives/*Insalata di pesce affumicato, arance, e radicchio*, 194–195

soup, 31, 33

Barley, Chestnut, and White Bean Minestrone/*Minestra d'orzo, castagne, e cannellini*, 54–55

Calabrian Wedding Soup/*Minestra maritata*, 50–51

Cannellini Bean, Tomato, and Orzo Soup/*Zuppa di cannellini e pomodoro con pasta di riso*, 56–57

Cannellini Bean Soup with Seafood/*Zuppa di fagioli con frutti di mare*, 40–41

chicken stock, 36–37, 44–47, 50–51

Chickpea Soup with Rosemary-Infused Shrimp/*Crema di ceci con gamberi*, 38–39

Cream of Chestnut Soup/*Crema di castagna*, 42–43

Farmhouse Vegetable and Farro Soup/*Zuppa di verdure e farro*, 58–59

Holiday Minestrone/*Millecosedde*, 48–49

Homemade Chicken Stock/*Brodo di pollo*, 289

Homemade Meat Stock/*Brodo di carne*, 290

Homemade Seafood Stock/*Brodo di pesce*, 288

Homemade Vegetable Stock/*Brodo di verdura*, 287

Pumpkin Soup/*Crema di zucca*, 36–37

Roman-Style Broccoli and Pecorino Soup/*Zuppa di broccoletti*, 60–61

Rustic Lentil Soup/*Zuppa di lenticchie*, 46–47

Sardinian Fava Bean Soup/*Zuppa di fave Sarda*, 52–53

seafood stock, 38–39

Tuscan Seafood Stew/*Cacciucco Livornese*, 34–35

vegetable stock, 42–43, 74–75

Zucchini Soup with Crostini/*Zuppa di zucchini con crostini*, 44–45

Southern Italian Fava Bean Purée/*Maccu*, 16–17

Southern Italian picnic, xii

Spaghetti Squash "Pasta" with Shrimp, Tomatoes, and Basil/*"Pasta" di zucca con gamberi, pomodori, e basilico*, 62–63

Spaghetti with Fresh Tuna and Fennel/*Pasta con tonno e finocchio*, 72–73

spice, 244–245, 252, 294

Spiced Chickpea Stew/*Stufato di ceci alle spezie*, 100–101

spiedini, 298

spinach, 58–59, 112–113, 146–147, 180

Spinach Fettuccine with Walnut-ricotta Pesto/*Fettuccine di spinaci con pesto di noci e ricotta*, 64–65

Spinach Sautéed in Garlic and Oil/*Spinaci all'aglio e olio*, 180 sponge cake, 257

spring menu, 159, 183

spuma, 248–249, 298

spuntino, 299

squid, 200–201, 295

stew

    Campania-Style Rustic Vegetable Stew/*Cianfotta*, 98–99

    Chicken Stew with Mushrooms and Onions/*Stufato di pollo con funghi e cipolle*, 134–135

    Citrus and Herb–Infused Scallop Stew/*Capesante in umido con erbe ed agrumi*, 130–131

    Fish Stew over Polenta/*Pesce in umido con la polenta*, 128–129

    meal planning, 91

    Roman Chicken, Pepper, and Tomato Stew/*Pollo in umido alla Romana*, 94–95

    Spiced Chickpea Stew/*Stufato di ceci alle spezie*, 100–101

    Tuscan Seafood Stew/*Cacciucco Livornese*, 34–35

    Veal, Potato, and Pepper Stew/*Spezzatino di vitello*, 150–151

Strawberries in Balsamic Vinegar/*Fragole in aceto balsamico*, 240

strawberry, 237, 240–241, 247

Stuffed Eggplant/*Melanzane ripiene*, 22–23

Stuffed Peppers/*Peperoni ripieni*, 24–25

stuzzichini, 299

sugar, 297

summer menu, x, 159–160, 184

Sunday dinner, ix, xi, 71, 196

Sweet-and-Sour Cabbage/*Cavoli acidi*, 163

sweet potato, 82–83, 124–125

swiss chard, 168–169

Swordfish with Olives, Capers, Herbs, and Tomatoes/*Pesce spade alla ghiotta*, 120–121

T

tax, 32

thyme, 299

tomato

    Braised, Stuffed Calamari with Tomato Sauce/*Calamari ripieni in salsa di pomodoro*, 112–113

    Cannellini Bean, Tomato, and Orzo Soup/*Zuppa di cannellini e pomodoro con pasta di riso*, 56–57

    diced, 140–141

    Fresh Tomato Sauce/*Salsa fresca di pomodoro*, 228–229

    grape, 108–109

    Mussels in Saffron-Tomato Broth/*Cozze in brodo di zafferano*, 110–111

    plum, 40–41, 104–105, 122–123, 228–229

    Red Pepper, Yellow Tomato, and Artichoke Salad/*Insalata di peperoni rossi, pomodori gialli, e carciofi*, 187

    Roman Chicken, Pepper, and Tomato Stew/*Pollo in umido alla Romana*, 94–95

    Roman-Style Rice and Herb–Stuffed Tomatoes/*Pomodori ripieni di riso alla Romana*, 20–21

    sauce, 22–23, 46–47, 78–79, 102–103, 154–155, 228–229

Spaghetti Squash "Pasta" with Shrimp, Tomatoes, and Basil/*"Pasta" di zucca con gamberi, pomodori, e basilico*, 62–63

sun-dried, 52–53, 118–119, 230

Swordfish with Olives, Capers, Herbs, and Tomatoes/*Pesce spade alla ghiotta*, 120–121

Tomatoes with Balsamic Vinegar/*Insalata di pomodori all'aceto balsamico*, 190

Trout Fillets with Sun-Dried Tomato and Cured-Olive Crust/*Filetti di trota impanati con pomodori secchi ed olive curate*, 118–119

Whole-Wheat Fusilli with Pesto and Cherry Tomatoes/*Fusilli con pesto e pomodori*, 66–67

tonnara, 73

Trapani-Style Almond Couscous/*Cuscus alla mandorla Trapanese*, 86–87

trisodium phosphate (TSP), 106

Trout Fillets with Sun-Dried Tomato and Cured-Olive Crust/*Filetti di trota impanati con pomodori secchi ed olive curate*, 118–119

tuna, 72–73, 116–117, 186

turkey, 146–149

Turnip Gnocchi with Herb Sauce/*Gnocchi di rapa con salsa d'erbe*, 84–85

Tuscan Buckwheat Pasta with Cheese, potatoes, and Greens/*Pizzoccheri della Valtellina*, 80–81

Tuscan Crudités with Olive Oil Dip/*Pinzimonio*, 5

Tuscan Farro Salad/*Insalata di farro alla Toscana*, 204–205

Tuscan Fig, Walnut, and Fennel Seed Torte/*Torta di ficchi, noci, e semi di finocchio*, 270–271

Tuscan Seafood Stew/*Cacciucco Livornese*, 34–35

Tyrolean Rye Bread with Fennel and Cumin/*Ur-Paarl della Val Venosta*, 212–213

U

Umbrian Frittata Skewers with Chickpea Dipping Sauce/*Spiedini di frittata con crema di ceci d'Umbria*, 14–15

unfiltered extra virgin olive oil, 299

United Nations Educational, Scientific and Cultural Organization (UNESCO), 6

unrefined sea salt, 299

V

Val d'Aosta–Style Dandelion Salad/*Insalata di dente di leone Valdostana*, 193

vanilla, 242–243

Vanilla-Scented Roasted Figs/*Ficchi vanigliati al forno*, 242

veal, 150–151, 299

Veal, Potato, and Pepper Stew/*Spezzatino di vitello*, 150–151

vegetable. *See also under specific type*

    Campania-Style Rustic Vegetable Stew/*Cianfotta*, 98–99

    Farmhouse Vegetable and Farro Soup/*Zuppa di verdure e farro*, 58–59

    Homemade Vegetable Stock/*Brodo di verdura*, 287

    Mixed Grilled Vegetables/*Verdure miste alla griglia*, 166–167

nutrition, 183

sagre, 31

Sicilian-Style Fish with Vegetables/*Dentice alla Siciliana con verdure al forno*, 122–123

Sicilian Sweet-and-Sour Vegetable Medley/*Caponata*, 6–7

side dishes (*contorni*), 159–160

Vegetable and Parmesan Carpaccio/*Carpaccio di verdure e parmigiano*, 12–13

Vegetable-Stuffed Turkey Breast/*Petto di tacchino ripieno di verdure*, 146–147

Vegetarian Feast menu, xi

Venetian-Style Beans with Swiss Chard/*Fagioli alla Veneziana con bietole*, 168–169

Venetian-Style Sole in a Sweet-and-Sour Sauce/*Sfogi in saor*, 126–127

Venetian-Style Whole-Wheat Spaghetti with Sauce/*Bigoli in salsa*, 76–77

Venice, 4

vinegar, 173, 294

vitamin, 183

viticulture, vii

W

walnut, 64–65, 193, 242, 270–271

wedding, 50–51

wheat, 32

white sesame, 299

Whole-Wheat and Honey Cookies/*Biscotti integrale al miele*, 251

Whole-Wheat Country Loaves/*Pane casareccio integrale*, 220–221

Whole-Wheat Cracker Rings with Black Pepper and Fennel Seeds/*Taralli integrali con pepe e finocchio*, 222–223

whole-wheat flour, 218–219, 222–223, 251

Whole-Wheat Fusilli with Pesto and Cherry Tomatoes/*Fusilli con pesto e pomodori*), 66–67

Whole-Wheat Orecchiette Pasta with Broccoli and Garlic/*Orecchiette integrale con broccoli*, 68–69

Whole-Wheat Rolls/*Panini di San Giovanni*, 218–219

Whole-Wheat Ziti with Goat Ragu/*Ziti integrale con ragu di capra*, 70–71

wine, vii–viii, 70–71, 294

winter menu, x, 159, 184

Y

yeast, 209–210, 216–217

yogurt, 235–236, 238–239, 243–246, 248–249, 259

Yogurt Gelato/*Gelato allo yogurt*, 259

Z

zucchini, 28, 44–45, 104–105, 161, 166–167, 173

Zucchini and Herb Croquettes/*Polpette di zucchine*, 104–105

Zucchini Carpaccio with Green Peppercorns/*Carpaccio di zucchine al pepe verde*, 28

Zucchini Soup with Crostini/*Zuppa di zucchini con crostini*, 44–45

zuppe, 33

Metric Equivalents

Liquid Measurement	Metric equivalent
1 teaspoon	5 mL
1 tablespoon *or* 1/2 fluid ounce	15 mL
1 fluid ounce *or* 1/8 cup	30 mL
1/4 cup *or* 2 fluid ounces	60 mL
1/3 cup	80 mL
1/2 cup *or* 4 fluid ounces	120 mL
2/3 cup	160 mL
3/4 cup *or* 6 fluid ounces	180 mL
1 cup *or* 8 fluid ounces *or* 1/2 pint	240 mL
1 1/2 cups *or* 12 fluid ounces	350 mL
2 cups *or* 1 pint *or* 16 fluid ounces	475 mL
3 cups *or* 1 1/2 pints	700 mL
4 cups *or* 2 pints *or* 1 quart	950 mL
4 quarts *or* 1 gallon	3.8 L

Weight Measurement	Metric equivalent
1 ounce	28 g
4 ounces *or* 1/4 pound	113 g
1/3 pound	150 g
8 ounces *or* 1/2 pound	230 g
2/3 pound	300 g
12 ounces *or* 3/4 pound	340 g
1 pound *or* 16 ounces	450 g
2 pounds	900 g

Dry Measurements	Metric equivalent
1 teaspoon	5 g
1 tablespoon	14 g
1/4 cup	57 g
1/2 cup	113 g
3/4 cup	168 g
1 cup	224 g

Length	Metric equivalent
1/8 inch	3 mm
1/4 inch	6 mm
1/2 inch	13 mm
3/4 inch	19 mm
1 inch	2.5 cm
2 inches	5 cm

Fahrenheit	Celsius	Fahrenheit	Celsius
275ºF	140ºC	400ºF	200ºC
300ºF	150ºC	425ºF	220ºC
325ºF	165ºC	450ºF	230ºC
350ºF	180ºC	475ºF	240ºC
375ºF	190ºC	500ºF	260ºC

Weights of common ingredients in grams							
Ingredient	1 cup	3/4 cup	2/3 cup	1/2 cup	1/3 cup	1/4 cup	2 Tbsp
Flour, all-purpose (wheat)	120 g	90 g	80 g	60 g	40 g	30 g	15 g
Flour, well-sifted, all-purpose (wheat)	110 g	80 g	70 g	55 g	35 g	27 g	13 g
Sugar, granulated cane	200 g	150 g	130 g	100 g	65 g	50 g	25 g
Confectioner's sugar (cane)	100 g	75 g	70 g	50 g	35 g	25 g	13 g
Brown sugar, packed firmly	180 g	135 g	120 g	90 g	60 g	45 g	23 g
Cornmeal	160 g	120 g	100 g	80 g	50 g	40 g	20 g
Cornstarch	120 g	90 g	80 g	60 g	40 g	30 g	15 g
Rice, uncooked	190 g	140 g	125 g	95 g	65 g	48 g	24 g
Macaroni, uncooked	140 g	100 g	90 g	70 g	45 g	35 g	17 g
Couscous, uncooked	180 g	135 g	120 g	90 g	60 g	45 g	22 g
Oats, uncooked, quick	90 g	65 g	60 g	45 g	30 g	22 g	11 g
Table salt	300 g	230 g	200 g	150 g	100 g	75 g	40 g
Butter	240 g	180 g	160 g	120 g	80 g	60 g	30 g
Vegetable shortening	190 g	140 g	125 g	95 g	65 g	48 g	24 g
Chopped fruits and vegetables	150 g	110 g	100 g	75 g	50 g	40 g	20 g
Nuts, chopped	150 g	110 g	100 g	75 g	50 g	40 g	20 g
Nuts, ground	120 g	90 g	80 g	60 g	40 g	30 g	15 g
Bread crumbs, fresh, loosely packed	60 g	45 g	40 g	30 g	20 g	15 g	8 g
Bread crumbs, dry	150 g	110 g	100 g	75 g	50 g	40 g	20 g
Parmesan cheese, grated	90 g	65 g	60 g	45 g	30 g	22 g	11 g